Dear Dr. Olson,

Thank you so much for training me, inspiring me and constantly pushing me to do and be better surgically.

Though I may do all my surgery robotically the techniques, appreciation for anatomy and principals are all the same from the Columbia days.

All the best

Techniques of Robotic Urinary Tract Reconstruction

Michael D. Stifelman · Lee C. Zhao
Daniel D. Eun · Chester J. Koh
Editors

Techniques of Robotic Urinary Tract Reconstruction

A Complete Approach

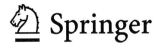 Springer

Editors
Michael D. Stifelman
Department of Urology
Hackensack Meridian Health School of
Medicine
Nutley, NJ
USA

Daniel D. Eun
Department of Urology
Lewis Katz School of Medicine at Temple
University
Philadelphia, PA
USA

Lee C. Zhao
Department of Urology
New York University Langone Medical Cent
Department of Urology
New York, NY
USA

Chester J. Koh
Division of Pediatric Urology
Texas Children's Hospital -
Baylor College of Medicine
Houston, TX
USA

ISBN 978-3-030-50195-2   ISBN 978-3-030-50196-9   (eBook)
https://doi.org/10.1007/978-3-030-50196-9

This Springer imprint is published by the registered company Springer Nature Switzerland AG
The registered company address is: Gewerbestrasse 11, 6330 Cham, Switzerland

Contents

Contents

List of Videos

Contributors

Ronney Abaza, MD, FACS OhioHealth Dublin Methodist Hospital, Dublin, OH, USA

Joseph Acquaye, MD Department of Urology, University of Minnesota, Minneapolis, MN, USA

Mutahar Ahmed, MD Hackensack Meridian Health, Hackensack University Medical Center, Hackensack, NJ, USA

Hackensack Meridian School of Medicine, Nutley, NJ, USA

Naif A. Aldhaam, MD Department of Urology, Roswell Park Comprehensive Cancer Center, Buffalo, NY, USA

Laith M. Alzweri, MD, MRCS, FECSM Urology, Tulane University School of Medicine, New Orleans, LA, USA

Division of Urology, Department of Surgery, University of Texas Medical Branch, Galveston, TX, USA

Ciro Andolfi, MD Department of Surgery, Chicago Medicine, Chicago, IL, USA

Monish Aron, MD USC Institute of Urology, Norris Comprehensive Cancer Center, Keck School of Medicine, University of Southern California, Los Angeles, CA, USA

Akbar N. Ashrafi, BHB, MD, FRACS (Urol) USC Institute of Urology, Norris Comprehensive Cancer Center, Keck School of Medicine, University of Southern California, Los Angeles, CA, USA

Olivier Belas Department of Urology, Polyclinique Le Mans Sud, Le Mans, France

Aylin N. Bilgutay, MD Pediatric Urology, Children's Healthcare of Atlanta and Emory University, Atlanta, GA, USA

Jill C. Buckley, MD Department of Urology, University of California, San Diego, San Diego, CA, USA

Grégoire Capon, MD Department of Urology, University of Bordeaux, Bordeaux, France

Vincent Cardot Department of Urology, Clinique Bizet, Paris, France

Nathan Cheng, MD Hackensack Meridian Health, Hackensack University Medical Center, Hackensack, NJ, USA

Hackensack Meridian School of Medicine, Nutley, NJ, USA

Gregory Chesnut, MD Urology Service, Department of Surgery, Memorial Sloan Kettering Cancer Center, New York, NY, USA

Michael Daugherty, MD Division of Pediatric Urology, Cincinnati Children's Hospital Medical Center, Cincinnati, OH, USA

Paolo Dell'Oglio, MD ORSI, Academy, Melle, Belgium

Department of Urology, OnzeLieve Vrouw Hospital, Aalst, Belgium

Unit of Urology, Division of Oncology, Urological Research Institute, IRCCS Ospedale San Raffaele, Milan, Italy

Frank Van Der Aa, MD Department of Urology, University of Leuven, Leuven, Belgium

Aurélien Descazeaud Department of Urology, University of Limoges, Limoges, France

Bethany Desroches, MD, MS Department of Urology, Hackensack University Medical Center, Hackensack, NJ, USA

Angelena B. Edwards, MD Department of Urology, Division of Pediatric Urology, Children's Health System Texas, University of Texas Southwestern, Dallas, TX, USA

Department of Urology, Division of Pediatric Urology, University of Iowa, Iowa City, IA, USA

Sean P. Elliott, MD, MS Department of Urology, University of Minnesota, Minneapolis, MN, USA

Jonathan S. Ellison, MD Children's Hospital of Wisconsin and Medical College of Wisconsin, Milwaukee, WI, USA

Ahmed S. Elsayed, MD Department of Urology, Roswell Park Comprehensive Cancer Center, Buffalo, NY, USA

Daniel D. Eun, MD Department of Urology, Lewis Katz School of Medicine at Temple University, Philadelphia, PA, USA

Georges Fournier Department of Urology, University of Brest, Brest, France

Thomas W. Fuller, MD Department of Urology, University of California, San Diego, San Diego, CA, USA

Xavier Gamé Department of Urology, University of Toulouse, Toulouse, France

Jonathan A. Gerber, MD Division of Pediatric Urology, Department of Surgery, Texas Children's Hospital, Houston, TX, USA

Scott Department of Urology, Baylor College of Medicine, Houston, TX, USA

Robert Steven Gerhard, MD OhioHealth Dublin Methodist Hospital, Dublin, OH, USA

Alvin C. Goh, MD Urology Service, Department of Surgery, Memorial Sloan Kettering Cancer Center, New York, NY, USA

Mohan S. Gundeti, MD Department of Surgery, Chicago Medicine, Chicago, IL, USA

Khurshid A. Guru, MD Department of Urology, Roswell Park Comprehensive Cancer Center, Buffalo, NY, USA

Jullet Han, MD USC Institute of Urology, Norris Comprehensive Cancer Center, Keck School of Medicine, University of Southern California, Los Angeles, CA, USA

Ashok K. Hemal, MD Department of Urology, Wake Forest University Baptist Medical Center, Winston-Salem, NC, USA

Sij Hemal, MD Department of Urology, Glickman Urological and Kidney Institute Cleveland Clinic, Cleveland, OH, USA

Jan Lukas Hohenhorst, MD Department of Urology and Urologic Oncology, Alfried-Krupp Krankenhaus, Essen, NRW, Germany

Ahmed A. Hussein, MD Department of Urology, Roswell Park Comprehensive Cancer Center, Buffalo, NY, USA

Micah Jacobs, MD Department of Urology, Division of Pediatric Urology, Children's Health System Texas, University of Texas Southwestern, Dallas, TX, USA

Min Suk Jan, DO, MS Crane Center for Transgender Surgery, Greenbae California, New York, NY, USA

Christina Kim, MD, FAAP Department of Urology, University of Wisconsin-Madison, Madison, WI, USA

Andrew J. Kirsch, MD Pediatric Urology, Children's Healthcare of Atlanta and Emory University, Atlanta, GA, USA

Joan Ko, MD Division of Urology, Children's Hospital of Philadelphia, Philadelphia, PA, USA

Chester J. Koh, MD Division of Pediatric Urology, Texas Children's Hospital - Baylor College of Medicine, Houston, TX, USA

Darko Kröpfl Department of Urology, Urologic Oncology and Pediatric Urology, Kliniken Essen-Mitte, Essen, Germany

Rana Kumar, MD Department of Urology, University of Chicago, Chicago, IL, USA

Alessandro Larcher, MD ORSI Academy, Melle, Belgium

Department of Urology, OnzeLieve Vrouw Hospital, Aalst, Belgium

Unit of Urology, Division of Oncology, Urological Research Institute, IRCCS Ospedale San Raffaele, Milan, Italy

Ziho Lee, MD Department of Urology, Temple University School of Medicine, Philadelphia, PA, USA

Heinrich Löwen, MD Department of Urology, Urologic Oncology and Pediatric Urology, Kliniken Essen-Mitte, Essen, Germany

Luis G. Medina, MD USC Institute of Urology, Norris Comprehensive Cancer Center, Keck School of Medicine, University of Southern California, Los Angeles, CA, USA

Michael J. Metro, MD, FACS Department of Urology, Temple University School of Medicine, Philadelphia, PA, USA

Kirtishri Mishra, MD Urology Institute, University Hospitals of Cleveland and Case Western Reserve University School of Medicine, Cleveland, OH, USA

Marcio Covas Moschovas, MD ORSI Academy, Melle, Belgium

Department of Urology, OnzeLieve Vrouw Hospital, Aalst, Belgium

Alexandre Mottrie ORSI Academy, Melle, Belgium

Department of Urology, OnzeLieve Vrouw Hospital, Aalst, Belgium

Ravi Munver, MD, FACS Department of Urology, Hackensack University Medical Center, Hackensack, NJ, USA

Hackensack Meridian School of Medicine at Seton Hall University, Nutley, NJ, USA

Michael Musch, MD Department of Urology, Urologic Oncology and Pediatric Urology, Kliniken Essen-Mitte, Essen, Germany

Paul H. Noh, MD University Urology, University of South Alabama, Mobile, Alabama, USA

Uzoamaka Nwoye, MD Division of Urology, Beth Israel Deaconess Medical Center, Boston, MA, USA

Joseph J. Pariser, MD Department of Urology, University of Minnesota, Minneapolis, MN, USA

Egor Parkhomenko, MD Department of Urology, Boston University School of Medicine/Boston Medical Center, Boston, MA, USA

Sunil H. Patel, MD Department of Urology, University of California, San Diego, San Diego, CA, USA

Ram A. Pathak, MD Department of Urology, Wake Forest University Baptist Medical Center, Winston-Salem, NC, USA

Benoit Peyronnet, MD Department of Urology, University of Rennes, Rennes, France

Anna Quian, BS Case Western Reserve School of Medicine, Cleveland, OH, USA

Courtney Rowe, MD Pediatric Urology, Connecticut Children's Medical Center, Hartford, CT, USA

Richard Sarle, MD Michigan State University, Lansing, MI, USA

Sparrow Hospital, Lansing, MI, USA

Ravindra Sahadev, MD Division of Urology, Children's Hospital of Philadelphia, Philadelphia, PA, USA

Nabeel Shakir, MD The University of Texas Southwestern Medical Center, Dallas, TX, USA

Aseem Shukla, MD Division of Urology, Children's Hospital of Philadelphia, Philadelphia, PA, USA

Rene Sotelo, MD USC Institute of Urology, Norris Comprehensive Cancer Center, Keck School of Medicine, University of Southern California, Los Angeles, CA, USA

Arun Srinivasan, MD Division of Urology, Children's Hospital of Philadelphia, Philadelphia, PA, USA

Robert J. Stein, MD Department of Urology, Glickman Urological and Kidney Institute Cleveland Clinic, Cleveland, OH, USA

Matthew E. Sterling, MD Department of Urology, Temple University School of Medicine, Philadelphia, PA, USA

Michael D. Stifelman, MD Department of Urology, Hackensack Meridian Health School of Medicine, Nutley, NJ, USA

Raju Thomas, MD, FACS, FRCS, MHA Urology, Tulane University School of Medicine, New Orleans, LA, USA

Johnson Tsui, MD Department of Urology, Hackensack University Medical Center, Hackensack, NJ, USA

Adrien Vidart Department of Urology, Foch Hospital, Suresnes, France

Anne Vogel, BSc Department of Urology, Urologic Oncology and Pediatric Urology, Kliniken Essen-Mitte, Essen, Germany

Mayya Volodarskaya, MD Department of Surgery, Rush University Medical Center, Chicago, IL, USA

Andrew A. Wagner, MD Division of Urology, Beth Israel Deaconess Medical Center, Boston, MA, USA

Aaron Wallace, MD Department of Surgery, Rush University Medical Center, Chicago, IL, USA

Shaun E. L. Wason, MD, FACS Department of Urology, Boston University School of Medicine/Boston Medical Center, Boston, MA, USA

Kevin K. Yang, MD Department of Urology, Lewis Katz School of Medicine at Temple University, Philadelphia, PA, USA

Lee C. Zhao, MD, MS NYU Langone Health, New York, NY, USA

If you have picked up this book, you too have had your robotic "aha" moment. Mine happened in 2003, when introduced to a three-arm, first generation intuitive system while struggling to learn laparoscopic suturing as a junior attending. It was clear this would become the great equalizer; one could maintain a steady camera with complete autonomy. Beyond that, the 3D imaging and endowrist technology made delicate dissection and complex suturing within grasp, coupled with a much shorter learning curve. Since the introduction of robotic surgery almost 2 decades ago, there have been innovators, early adopters, and pioneers all focused on robotic upper urinary tract reconstruction. Those that focused on urinary reconstruction surgery had diverse backgrounds including endourology, urologic oncology and urinary reconstruction. This varied and eclectic group of urologic surgeons provided a melting pot of ideas, and their willingness to share their techniques, successes, and failures allowed us to literally "build the plane as we were flying it." The progress made since the first publication on a robotic urinary tract reconstruction case has been remarkable. Leveraging the latest in robotic technology, incorporating perfusion imaging intraoperatively, and challenging the paradigm of managing proximal and mid ureteral strictures are just some of the accomplishments that have changed our patients' outcomes for the better. It has been the work of many and the relationships made while "building the plane" that allowed us to realize this book. The major catalyst, and the event that set the wheels in motion came in May 2018, while the 4 editors were sharing a beer, in San Francisco, after completing our third annual AUA course entitled "Robotic Urinary Tract Reconstruction: A Top to Bottom Approach." Despite three hours of content, it was just the tip of the iceberg. We all felt as if there was so much more to say and so many people to connect with that we were only scratching the surface. In addition, we wanted to spare the next generation of urologists from having to build their own plane from scratch. As we gathered collaborators for this book, we specifically looked for surgeons that were skilled at articulating their techniques in public. The authors chosen by the editors were those we operated with, moderated during live surgery, or personally observed teaching. This was to be a how-to book, focused on illustrating reproducible techniques. For each chapter there were specific objectives created by the editors and shared with the authors. Multiple edits were made to make sure these objectives were met. Finally, all images and videos were reviewed to ensure the best learning experience possible. We recognize that we stand on the shoulders of giants. It is the hope of the editors and authors that we may help the next generation of urologists build their foundation for greatness and advancement in urologic upper urinary tract reconstruction. Finally, we must acknowledge all of our spouses and those that support us. For it is their unwavering and unconditional love that has allowed us to dedicate the time and effort to create this textbook.

Why Robotic Surgery?

1

Sunil H. Patel, Thomas W. Fuller, and Jill C. Buckley

History of Robotics in Urinary Reconstruction

The first application of a robotic platform for surgery was the PUMA 200 robotic arm in a neurological procedure in 1985 [1]. Robotics in urology began in earnest 15 years later with the approval of the da Vinci® robotic system by the Food and Drug Administration (FDA) in 2000 (Fig. 1.1). The same year the first robotic-assisted radical prostatectomy (RALP) was performed followed closely by a radical nephrectomy in 2001 [2].

Robotics was applied quickly thereafter to upper urinary tract (UUT) urologic pathologies. The first series reported robotic pyeloplasty was published in 2002 [3]. From 2002 to 2006, a wider variety of reconstructive robotic surgeries were described. A retrospective review over this period describes the expanded use of robotics to ureteroureterostomy and ureteral reimplantation [4]. After only a decade of robotics in urology, a large proportion of common urologic cases were being done robotically. In 2009, 10.2% of pyeloplasties were performed laparoscopically, 44.7% were performed open, and 45.1% were robotic assisted [5]. In 2012, a large retrospective series of 759 patients compared outcomes of laparoscopic or robotic pyeloplasty. Results showed improved success rates and decreased need for the secondary procedure with the robotic platform over laparoscopic surgery [6].

Lower urinary tract reconstruction closely followed robotic pyeloplasty. An initial small comparison of open (n = 41) versus robotic (n = 25) ureteroneocystostomy showed comparable success rates between modalities. The robotic approach had decreased hospital stays, narcotic pain requirements, and estimated blood loss [7]. In a series of 14 patients, the feasibility, safety, and efficacy of robotic-assisted bladder neck reconstruction were also established. There was a 75% patency rate and

S. H. Patel · T. W. Fuller · J. C. Buckley (✉)
Department of Urology, University of California, San Diego, San Diego, CA, USA
e-mail: jcbuckley@ucsd.edu

© Springer Nature Switzerland AG 2022
M. D. Stifelman et al. (eds.), *Techniques of Robotic Urinary Tract Reconstruction*, https://doi.org/10.1007/978-3-030-50196-9_1

Fig. 1.1 The da Vinci®
robotic system – fourth
generation [23]

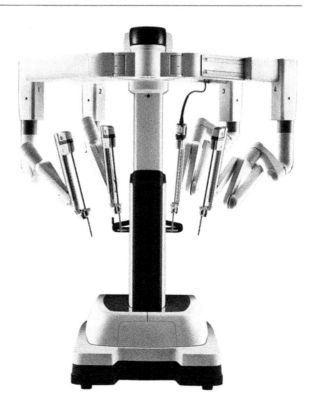

an 82% maintenance of continence at the 1-year follow-up. In addition, there were decreased blood loss and hospital stay compared to open perineal series [8].

Most recently, reconstructive surgeons have addressed ureteral strictures and rectourethral fistulas using the robotic platform. In a small case series, Zhao et al. described four patients undergoing ureteral reconstruction with buccal grafts. There were no intraoperative complications nor stricture recurrence at 15-month follow-up [9]. Chen et al. studied the management of rectourethral fistulas (RUF). They compared approaches including transperineal, transsphincteric, transanal, and transabdominal. The transabdominal approach was associated with greater morbidity and poor visualization [10]. The introduction of a minimally invasive surgical approach decreased patient morbidity and allowed for better visualization and suture placement deep in the pelvis [11].

Urinary Tract Reconstruction: Improved Visualization, Access to Narrow Anatomic Spaces, and Ergonomics

Robotic surgery improves both surgeon visualization and ergonomics. Muscle activation during robotic procedures is reduced compared to laparoscopic cases which decreases surgeon strain and fatigue. In a comparative assessment of ergonomics in robotic versus laparoscopic tasks by measuring upper arm EMG activity, it was demonstrated that robotic surgery was ergonomically favorable compared to laparoscopy [12]. This has translated to a decrease in musculoskeletal pain in urologists based on a survey of physician members of the Endourological Society and Society of Urologic Oncology [13].

Robotic surgery optics also provide a clear, magnified, three-dimensional image. Areas such as the deep pelvis where RUF and vesicourethral anastomotic stricture repairs are performed have visual limitations in open procedures. The system provides digital magnification (10–15×), 3D high-definition (HD) images, and motion scaling allowing for visualization superior to that of open or laparoscopic procedures.

The seven degrees of motion, which imitates the dexterity of the human wrist in small spaces, allows for accurate and precise dissection and suturing in narrow and challenging spaces [14]. This precision and enhanced visualization in a comfortable sitting position are major advantages over open surgery and make robotic-assisted complex genitourinary reconstruction ideal.

Technological Advances

Near-Infrared Fluorescence

Near-infrared fluorescence (NIRF) with indocyanine green (ICG) allows the identification of vascular structures or urinary luminal structures. Selective renal artery clamping with NIRF has been shown to improve short-term renal functional outcomes compared to a partial nephrectomy without selective arterial clamping [15, 16].

NIRF in urinary reconstruction can be helpful for identifying urinary tract structures such as the ureter or renal pelvis in the initial reconstruction, but its true value is in the ability to identify these structures in redo cases with severe scarring. Additionally, it can be helpful to identify both viable and nonviable tissue in the ureter or with bowel by demarcating perfused versus devascularized tissue (Fig. 1.2) [17, 18].

Single-Port Robotic Surgery

Single-port procedures, also known as laparoendoscopic single-site (LESS) surgery, was first described in urology in 2007. Raman et al. performed three LESS nephrectomies using a single transumbilical incision [19]. Shortly after in 2009, the first robot-assisted LESS (R-LESS) surgeries were reported by Kaouk et al. who performed a pyeloplasty, radical nephrectomy, and radical prostatectomy [20]. The Cleveland Clinic recently corroborated this experience in 2018 publishing a report of two single-port robot-assisted radical prostatectomies (Fig. 1.3). The surgeries were successful with no complications or deviations from standard postoperative care [21].

Fig. 1.2 Intraoperative images of a redo robotic-assisted pyeloplasty highlighting the identification of the ureter after luminal injection of ICG (**b**) in a field of dense scar tissue (**a**)

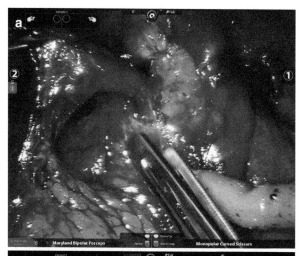

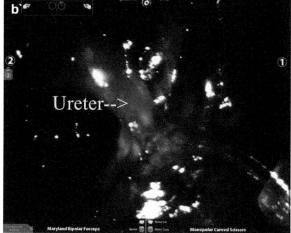

TilePro™

TilePro™ is a multi-image display mode of the da Vinci® surgical system that allows for a picture in picture display on the surgeon console. In genitourinary reconstruction, it is indispensable in rendezvous procedures such as when a cystoscope or ureteroscope is used to demarcate fistulous tracts, to identify obliterated lumens, or to help identify the optimal location for ureteral reimplantation in continent urinary diversions. Figure 1.4 shows the utility of TilePro™ by identifying the location of an obliterated bladder neck with the use of the cystoscopy using the screen in screen TilePro™ technology.

Fig. 1.3 The da Vinci®
robotic single-port
platform [23]

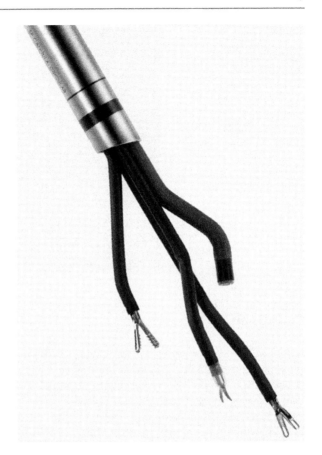

Simulation

The da Vinci® robotic platform provides new adopters of robotic technology and
trainees with a simulation package. Simulation has been shown to have a positive
correlation with intraoperative performance. Fundamental inanimate robotic skills
task (FIRST) and da Vinci® skills simulator (dVSS) virtual reality task performance has been shown to correlate with intraoperative prostatectomy performance
[22]. The authors of this study advocated for standardizing robotic simulation in
training curriculums.

Fig. 1.4 Intraoperative image of the use of TilePro™ during an obliterated bladder neck reconstruction using cystoscopy to identify the site of the true lumen

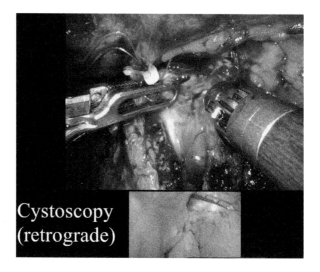

Conclusion

Robotic operative technology is advancing steadily and will continue to play an important and expanding role in urologic surgery and genitourinary reconstruction in particular. Data is rapidly emerging for its utility and benefit in a wide variety of complex urinary tract reconstruction procedures. Shorter hospital stays, decreased narcotic requirements, and earlier return to work are all patient benefits that have been shown with the robotic platform. Improved visualization, ergonomic comfort while operating, and access to deep narrow spaces improve the surgeon experience. As a combined result, the penetrance of robotics in reconstruction will likely increase in the years to come.

References

1. Kwoh YS, Hou J, Jonckheere EA, Hayati S. A robot with improved absolute positioning accuracy for CT guided stereotactic brain surgery. IEEE Trans Biomed Eng. 1988;35:153–60.
2. Binder J, Jones J, Bentas W, et al. Robot-assisted laparoscopy in urology. Radical prostatectomy and reconstructive retroperitoneal interventions. Der Urologe Ausg. 2002;41(2):144–9.
3. Gettman MT, Neururer R, Bartsch G, Reinhard P. Anderson-Hynes. Dismembered pyeloplasty performed using the da Vinci robotic system. Urology. 2002;60:509–13.
4. Mufarrij PW, Shah OD, Berger AD, et al. Robotic reconstruction of the upper urinary tract. J Urol. 2007;178:2002–5.
5. Monn MF, Bahler CD, Schneider EB, Sundaram CP. Emerging trends in robotic pyeloplasty for the management of ureteropelvic junction obstruction in adults. J Urol. 2013;189:1352–7.
6. Lucas SM, Sundaram CP, Wolf JS, Leveillee RJ, Bird VG, Aziz M, et al. Factors that impact the outcome of minimally invasive pyeloplasty: results of the multi-institutional laparoscopic and robotic pyeloplasty collaborative group. J Urol. 2012;187:522–7.

7. Isac W, Kaouk J, Altunrende F, Rizkala E, Autorino R, Hillyer SP, et al. Robot-assisted uretero-neocystostomy: technique and comparative outcomes. J Endourol. 2013;27:318–23.
8. Kirshenbaum EJ, Zhao LC, Myers JB, Elliott SP, Vanni AJ, Baradaran N, Alsikafi NF. Patency and incontinence rates after robotic bladder neck reconstruction for vesicourethral anastomotic stenosis and recalcitrant bladder neck contractures: the trauma and urologic reconstructive network of surgeons experience. Urology. 2018;118:227–33.
9. Zhao LC, Yamaguchi Y, Bryk DJ, Adelstein SA, Stifelman MD. Robot-assisted ureteral reconstruction using Buccal mucosa. Urology. 2015;86(3):634–8.
10. Chen S, Gao R, Li H, Wang K. Management of acquired rectourethral fistulas in adults. Asian J Urol. 2018;5(3):149–54.
11. Linder B, Frank I, Dozois E, Elliott D. V405 robotic transvesical rectourethral fistula repair following a robotic radical prostatectomy. J Urol. 2013;189(4):e164–5.
12. Lee GI, Lee MR, Clanton T, et al. Comparative assessment of physical and cognitive ergonomics associated with robotic and traditional laparoscopic surgeries. Surg Endosc. 2014;28(2):456–65.
13. Bagrodia A, Raman JD. Ergonomic considerations of radical prostatectomy: physician perspective of open, laparoscopic, and robot-assisted techniques. J Endourol Endourolog Soc. 2009;23:627–33.
14. Zárate Rodriguez JG, Zihni AM, Ohu I, Cavallo JA, Ray S, Cho S, Awad MM. Ergonomic analysis of laparoscopic and robotic surgical task performance at various experience levels. Surg Endosc. 2018; https://doi.org/10.1007/s00464-018-6478-4.
15. Mattevi D, Luciani LG, Mantovani W, Cai T, Chiodini S, Vattovani V, Malossini G. Fluorescence-guided selective arterial clamping during RAPN provides better early functional outcomes based on renal scan compared to standard clamping. J Robot Surg. 2018; https://doi.org/10.1007/s11701-018-0862-x.
16. Borofsky MS, Gill IS, Hemal AK, et al. Near-infrared fluorescence imaging to facilitate superselective arterial clamping during zero-ischaemia robotic partial nephrectomy. BJU Int. 2013;111:604–10.
17. Lee Z, Moore B, Giusto L, Eun DD. Use of Indocyanine green during robot-assisted ureteral reconstructions. Eur Urol. 2015;67(2):291–8.
18. Bjurlin MA, Gan M, McClintock TR, Volpe A, Borofsky MS, Mottrie A, Stifelman MD. Near-infrared fluorescence imaging: emerging applications in robotic upper urinary tract surgery. Eur Urol. 2014;65(4):793–801.
19. Raman JD, Bensalah K, Bagrodia A, et al. Laboratory and clinical development of single keyhole umbilical nephrectomy. Urology. 2007;70:1039–42.
20. Kaouk JH, Goel RK, Haber GP, et al. Robotic single-port transumbilical surgery in humans: initial report. BJU Int. 2009;103:366–9.
21. Kaouk J, Bertolo R, Eltemamy M, Garisto J. Single-port robot-assisted radical prostatectomy: first clinical experience using the SP surgical system. Urology. 2018; https://doi.org/10.1016/j.urology.2018.10.025.
22. Aghazadeh MA, Mercado MA, Pan MM, Miles BJ, Goh AC. Performance of robotic simulated skills tasks is positively associated with clinical robotic surgical performance. BJU Int. 2016;118:475–81.
23. https://www.intuitivesurgical.com/

Part II

Keys for Intraoperative Success: Principles of Urinary Tract Reconstruction

Michael D. Stifelman

In these three introductory chapters we tackle the use of stents vs. nephrostomy tubes in managing patients with upper urinary tract obstruction. We review the principals of reconstruction with a focus on assuring adequate blood supply, improving wound healing and techniques of appropriate spatulation. In addition we dedicate an entire chapter to tissue substitution, an ever evolving field. These chapters will lay the foundation for all following techniques represented in this book and provide the nuances required to perform successful robotic urinary tract reconstruction.

Ureteral Stenting and Percutaneous Nephrostomy Drainage for Urinary Tract Reconstruction

2

Shaun E. L. Wason and Egor Parkhomenko

Ureteral stents relieve obstruction, promote healing, and provide a diversion for urinary drainage [1, 2]. In our practice, we place a double-J stent for all reconstructive upper and lower urinary tract procedures with a ureteral anastomosis. In the pediatric literature, ureteral stents have been shown to decrease hospital stay and reduce postoperative complications following a pyeloplasty [3–5]. Recent literature, however, has challenged the benefit of ureteral stents in pediatrics for reconstructive procedures, and stentless/tubeless procedures have been described [6, 7]. In this population, ureteral stent placement tends to be based on surgeon preference. Although the advent of the da Vinci surgical system (Intuitive Surgical, Sunnyvale, CA) has greatly facilitated intracorporeal suturing, obviating the need for stenting in certain patients, in our opinion; however, the risks of stent placement is less than the risk of a urine leak or disruption of the anastomosis.

There is no clear consensus regarding the optimal timing of ureteral stent placement during pyeloplasty. Preoperative retrograde ureteral stent placement has the advantage of ensuring that a stent of ideal length has been correctly placed; however, it requires an additional procedure and may obscure the obstructing segment intraoperatively, and a decompressed redundant pelvis can occasionally lead to a challenging dissection. Furthermore, excision of the strictured segment and reconstruction may be more difficult in the presence of a pre-placed stent. For these reasons, we routinely place ureteral stents in an antegrade fashion intraoperatively.

Supplementary Information The online version of this chapter (https://doi.org/10.1007/978-3-030-50196-9_2) contains supplementary material, which is available to authorized users.

S. E. L. Wason (✉) · E. Parkhomenko
Department of Urology, Boston University School of Medicine/Boston Medical Center, Boston, MA, USA
e-mail: swason@bu.edu; egorpark@bu.edu

© Springer Nature Switzerland AG 2022
M. D. Stifelman et al. (eds.), *Techniques of Robotic Urinary Tract Reconstruction*, https://doi.org/10.1007/978-3-030-50196-9_2

The primary purpose of placing a percutaneous nephrostomy tube or ureteral stent is to relieve ongoing obstruction and alleviate symptoms. If a patient is obstructed but remains asymptomatic, we will typically proceed directly to the operating room for elective repair without a pre-placed nephrostomy tube or stent. In cases where the patient is obstructed and symptomatic, our preference is to place a percutaneous nephrostomy tube preoperatively, rather than a ureteral stent, in order to minimize periureteral inflammation, which can make the ureteral dissection more challenging. If a patient already has an indwelling ureteral stent in place, our practice is to exchange it for a nephrostomy tube 10–14 days prior to surgery.

The most common stent that we use in our practice is the Percuflex double-J stent (Boston Scientific, Boston, MA) with a hydrophilic coating, which facilitates placement intraoperatively. The short duration of stenting and the flexibility of silicone stents and a tapered tip make this ideally suited for reconstructive procedures. Other less common stent materials are biodegradable and metallic. Biodegradable stents have encountered difficulty with varying degradation rates, the need for a follow-up removal procedure and fragments entering the ureteral wall causing an inflammatory reaction [8–10]. New materials such as Uriprene® are actively being pursued to tackle these challenges [11]. Metallic stents have been employed for select cases of high-grade compressive ureteral obstruction due to malignancy [12]. Recent studies have utilized metallic stents for both malignant and benign causes of ureteral obstruction but with varying success for benign pathology [13, 14]. Urologists have yet to adapt the use of metallic stents to common practice, and further data is needed to outline the benefit of metallic stents over the commonly used silicone stents. The rigidity of the metallic stent, in addition to the need for a sheath and fluoroscopy for placement, makes this stent less ideal for benign reconstructive procedures.

The choice of a larger or smaller diameter stent remains controversial. The former may compress and compromise the vasculature of the ureter and promote fibrosis, while the latter may not provide adequate drainage through the lumen of the stent. Moon et al. investigated the use of 7F and 14F stents in pigs and concluded that there were no differences in outcomes such as stricture formation [15]. Given this, the selection of ureteral stent diameter is surgeon dependent, and in our practice, we have adopted the use of either 6F or 7F stents exclusively.

We typically use a fixed-length double-J stent chosen based on the length of the ureter from CT urography or retrograde pyelography or estimated based on a patients height [16]. We will also typically err on the side of choosing a longer stent in order to minimize the risk of stent migration often found with short ureteral stents. For instance, if the ureteral length measures 26 cm; then, we will often place a 28 cm stent. This also ensures that the proximal curl rests in the upper pole of the kidney away from the neoureteropelvic junction anastomosis. In select situations, such as ureteral reconstruction in a transplant or pelvic kidney, we will employ a 4.7F double-J stent as these are more commonly available in shorter lengths at our institution.

Placing a double-J stent across the anastomosis is either done in an antegrade or retrograde fashion. The antegrade approach has been shown to yield lower operative times and is the preferred technique in a recent multicenter review as well as in our practice [17, 18]. The timing of stent placement is at the discretion of the surgeon; however, the authors typically place the stent after half the anastomosis is complete. For antegrade stent placement during pyeloplasty, once the posterior anastomosis is complete, a stent pusher is placed through any sized port and directed down the ureter with the robotic needle drivers. Gentle manipulation is necessary to avoid excessive compression of the stent pusher. An angled 0.038in glide wire is passed through the stent pusher and directed down the ureter. An angled glide wire is used so that the floppy end curls within the bladder, and there is less risk of extrusion from the urethra. The pusher is held a few centimeters from the ureter to visualize the passage of the wire, ensuring resistance is not encountered early. At the point of resistance, the glide wire is grasped with the robotic needle drivers, and the stent pusher is removed. The double-J stent is passed with the tapered end over the glidewire. A hemostat forceps may be applied extracorporeally to hold the glidewire taut. Once the end of the stent reaches the robotic needle drivers, the console surgeon advances the stent antegrade down the ureter toward the bladder using a hand-over-hand technique. The stent is advanced until the proximal end is visualized, at which time the stent is stabilized, the glidewire is removed, and the proximal end of the stent is allowed to curl. The proximal curl can then be placed into the renal pelvis or an upper pole calyx, and the reconstruction can be completed. In the cases where there is no assistant port, a 14F intravenous cannula (angiocatheter) can be placed transcutaneously to allow passage of the glidewire and stent. To confirm stent placement, some centers have advocated filling the bladder with saline or methylene blue and clamping the foley so that the bladder is distended at the time of stent placement [19]. Reflux of fluid through the stent holes helps confirm appropriate placement. Other techniques to distend the bladder include clamping the foley 1 hour prior to stent placement and administering intravenous furosemide. We have found that this step is not always necessary unless there is a concern for a malpositioned stent.

For retrograde intracorporeal stent placement, as needed during a ureteroneocystostomy, stent placement can proceed in a similar fashion to that as previously described (Fig. 2.1) [20]. The console surgeon advances the stent toward the kidney

Fig. 2.1 0.038in Glidewire is advanced through the stent pusher into the distal ureter at the time of ureteroneocystostomy

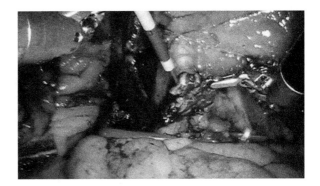

until the distal curl is visualized (Fig. 2.2), the glidewire is removed, and the distal curl is placed into the bladder, and reconstruction can be completed (Fig. 2.3). Our technique is outlined in Video 2.1.

The less common, retrograde technique for ureteral stent placement requires pre-placement of either a 5F or 6F ureteral catheter into the proximal ureter with a flexible cystoscope. The ureteral catheter is prepped into the sterile field so that it can be manipulated by the bedside assistant at the time of stent placement. The glide-wire can be passed through the ureteral catheter and is visualized intracorporeally entering the renal pelvis. The ureteral catheter can then be exchanged for an appropriate length stent over the glidewire. The stent pusher is subsequently passed over the wire, and the stent is advanced under direct vision by the console surgeon. Once the proximal curl is visualized, the stent is stabilized, and the wire is removed. A flexible cystoscope can be passed into the bladder to ensure an appropriate distal coil in the bladder.

Occasionally, intracorporeal stent placement will require manipulation of the stent both proximally and distally during ureteroureterostomy for mid-ureteral repair. In this scenario, the glidewire is passed through the stent directly to straighten one end of the stent. We usually pass the stent in a retrograde fashion toward the kidney first. The stent is stabilized, and the wire is removed. The entire stent is left intracorporeally, and the glidewire can be inserted through a side hole of the stent

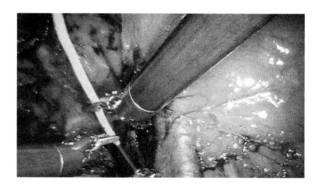

Fig. 2.2 The double-J stent is advanced by the console surgeon over the glidewire into the kidney

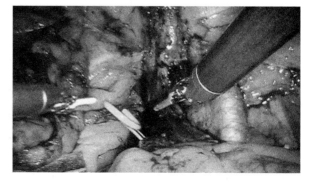

Fig. 2.3 The glidewire is removed, and the distal end of the stent is curled. A video of our technique for robotic intracorporeal double-J stent placement for urinary tract reconstruction is included

by the console surgeon until the distal curl is straightened. The distal end can be passed antegrade down the ureter into the bladder, and the glidewire is removed. We confirm stent placement with flexible cystoscopy at the end of the case as it is easy to do and the most reliable; however, a plain abdominal radiograph on the operating room table or a bedside ultrasound is also acceptable.

We typically remove ureteral stents 3 weeks after any reconstructive procedure involving the collecting system. However, in the literature, the ideal stent duration remains controversial. Kerbl *et al.* compared the effects of stent duration at 1, 3, and 6 weeks after an endoureterotomy in pigs and found favorable results in ureters stented for only 1 week [21]. A stent is thought to allow for regeneration of the ureter through a diversion of the urine while providing a platform upon which the ureter can heal [1, 2]. Yet, as a foreign body, ureteral stents can cause inflammation of the native tissue and predispose to infection [22]. Recently, Danuser *et al.* evaluated the efficacy of 1-week vs 4-week stent duration after a laparoscopic or robotic-assisted pyeloplasty. They found no significant differences between the two groups with respect to obstruction and concluded that 1-week stent duration is comparable to 4 weeks [23]. Nevertheless, there is a paucity of evidence for the optimal stent duration in humans, and thus, the final decision remains in the hands of the surgeon.

Ureteral stents have served as excellent tools for assisting in urinary diversion and ureteral healing for an assortment of urological procedures, but their use is not without morbidity. As temporary indwelling foreign bodies, they have been associated with urinary frequency, incontinence, hematuria, pain from daily activities, sexual dysfunction, infection, and encrustation [24]. Several treatment modalities have been explored to mitigate stent-related symptoms. Both alpha-blockers and anti-muscarinics alone or in combination have been used to successfully improve stent-related symptoms as assessed by the Ureteral Stent Symptom Questionnaire (USSQ) [25–27]. In the literature, nonsteroidal anti-inflammatory drugs (NSAIDs) have also been documented to improve renal colic [28]. Of note, a single dose of an NSAID prior to stent removal has been shown to reduce pain associated with stent removal and reduce the need for opioid analgesia [29]. Another commonly used analgesic that concentrates in the urine, phenazopyridine, can be used for dysuria, but recent studies have questioned its efficacy in improving USSQ scores [30]. Finally, a newer medication, pregabalin, in a recent randomized prospective study has shown an improvement in USSQ scores, particularly quality-of-life measures, as a stand-alone medication for patients with indwelling ureteral stents [31]. In our practice, intraoperative ketorolac (15 mg or 30 mg IV) is routinely employed following ureteral reconstructive procedures, barring any medical contraindication or renal insufficiency. Postoperatively, pain is managed using a combination of alpha-blockers, NSAIDs, acetaminophen and phenazopyridine with judicious oral narcotics (oxycodone 5 mg) for severe breakthrough pain, with a trend toward eliminating narcotics altogether.

Another common complication of ureteral stent utilization is the predisposition to infection. Farsi *et al.* have shown that indwelling ureteral stents are colonized within a few weeks [32]. A publication by Nevo *et al.* indicates that sepsis rates increase dramatically beyond the first month of ureteral stent placement [33]. Thus, stents should ideally be removed within 4 weeks to minimize infectious complications. For uncomplicated ureteral reconstructive procedures, stents can often be removed without sequelae within 2 weeks [20]. To minimize the risk of infection and stent-related morbidity, it is our current practice to obtain a urine culture 10–14 days postoperatively and to remove ureteral stents by the 21st day. If the urine culture is negative, a single dose of peri-procedural antibiotics is administered in accordance with the AUA Best Practice Policy on antimicrobial prophylaxis [34].

Substantial effort is currently being placed to delineate the ideal ureteral stent by way of design (grooved, spiral, self-expanding, etc.), coating (anti-microbial, encrustation resistance, etc.), and material (metallic, alternative plastics, biodegradable) in order to reduce the morbidity of stents [11, 35]. Interestingly, in an era of personalized medicine and technological advancement, researchers have begun to experiment with 3D printed stents. These can be customized and printed to the unique characteristics of each individual ureter. Del Junco *et al.* have studied 3D printed stents in an *ex vivo* porcine model and have shown comparable flow rates to commonly used stents [36]. Although no 3D printed stent is ready for use at this time, future development is promising.

Drains have an important role in any intra-abdominal surgery. In urology, drains are typically placed to identify a urine leak, lymphatic leak, and/or postoperative hemorrhage. For upper/lower urinary tract reconstructive procedures, we typically leave a closed-suction drain overnight, particularly if the patient underwent a bilateral staging pelvic lymph node dissection (BPLND). Drains after uncomplicated robotic-assisted radical prostatectomy (RARP) are not always necessary if a watertight anastomosis is confirmed. Some centers have eliminated their routine use without noting an increase in perioperative complications [37, 38]. These results however may not be generalizable to all surgeons, especially early in the learning curve or in all situations (i.e., difficult anastomosis, bladder neck reconstruction, prior TURP, increased blood loss, salvage RARP, and/or immunosuppression). At our institution, we typically leave an 18F Foley catheter and a 15F Blake drain at the end of a reconstructive procedure. For radical prostatectomy, drain output is measured at 8 hr. intervals and removed if drainage is less than 50 mL/8 hrs. If high drain output is observed, fluid is sent for creatinine to differentiate between lymphatic (equal to serum creatinine) or urine leak (higher than serum creatinine). If high volume output persists, the drain is taken off suction and left to gravity. For ease of care at discharge, the drain is cut 10–15 cm from the skin and secured within an ostomy appliance placed over the port site. The patient is then asked to return to the office to remove the drain once daily drain output is less than 150 mL. After ureteroneocystostomy, a uniform pathway has evolved as follows; the 15F Blake drain is removed on postoperative Day 1 once drain output is less than 50 mL/8 hrs. An office cystogram is performed on postoperative Day 5, and the Foley catheter is removed if there is no leak. The ureteral stent is removed 2 weeks post-operatively. For upper tract reconstruction, the Foley catheter is removed on the morning after discharge. If the drain output is less than 5–10 mL/hr, then the drain is removed.

The described technique of intracorporeal antegrade and retrograde double-J stent placement during robotic-assisted ureteral reconstruction is efficient, reproducible, and straightforward. It avoids the need for patient re-positioning, cystoscopy, and fluoroscopy, thereby avoiding increased operative time, expense, and radiation exposure.

References

1. Clayman RV, Basler JW, Kavoussi L, Picus DD. Ureteronephroscopic endopyelotomy. J Urol. 1990;144(2 Pt 1):246–51; discussion 251-242.
2. Denstedt JD. The endosurgical alternative for upper-tract obstruction. Contemp Urol. 1991;3(1):19–26. 31
3. McMullin N, Khor T, King P. Internal ureteric stenting following pyeloplasty reduces length of hospital stay in children. Br J Urol. 1993;72(3):370–2.
4. Sibley GN, Graham MD, Smith ML, Doyle PT. Improving splintage techniques in pyeloplasty. Br J Urol. 1987;60(6):489–91.
5. Woo HH, Farnsworth RH. Dismembered pyeloplasty in infants under the age of 12 months. Br J Urol. 1996;77(3):449–51.
6. Braga LH, Lorenzo AJ, Farhat WA, Bagli DJ, Khoury AE, Pippi Salle JL. Outcome analysis and cost comparison between externalized pyeloureteral and standard stents in 470 consecutive open pyeloplasties. J Urol. 2008;180(4 Suppl):1693–8; discussion1698–1699.
7. Kim J, Park S, Hwang H, et al. Comparison of surgical outcomes between dismembered pyeloplasty with or without ureteral stenting in children with Ureteropelvic junction obstruction. Korean J Urol. 2012;53(8):564–8.
8. Lingeman JE, Preminger GM, Berger Y, et al. Use of a temporary ureteral drainage stent after uncomplicated ureteroscopy: results from a phase II clinical trial. J Urol. 2003;169(5):1682–8.
9. Lingeman JE, Schulsinger DA, Kuo RL. Phase I trial of a temporary ureteral drainage stent. J Endourol. 2003;17(3):169–71.
10. Olweny EO, Landman J, Andreoni C, et al. Evaluation of the use of a biodegradable ureteral stent after retrograde endopyelotomy in a porcine model. J Urol. 2002;167(5):2198–202.
11. Brotherhood H, Lange D, Chew BH. Advances in ureteral stents. Transl Androl Urol. 2014;3(3):314–9.
12. Sountoulides P, Kaplan A, Kaufmann OG, Sofikitis N. Current status of metal stents for managing malignant ureteric obstruction. BJU Int. 2010;105(8):1066–72.
13. Liatsikos E, Kallidonis P, Kyriazis I, et al. Ureteral obstruction: is the full metallic double-pigtail stent the way to go? Eur Urol. 2010;57(3):480–6.
14. Patel C, Loughran D, Jones R, Abdulmajed M, Shergill I. The resonance(R) metallic ureteric stent in the treatment of chronic ureteric obstruction: a safety and efficacy analysis from a contemporary clinical series. BMC Urol. 2017;17(1):16.
15. Moon YT, Kerbl K, Pearle MS, et al. Evaluation of optimal stent size after endourologic incision of ureteral strictures. J Endourol. 1995;9(1):15–22.
16. Paick SH, Park HK, Byun SS, Oh SJ, Kim HH. Direct ureteric length measurement from intravenous pyelography: does height represent ureteric length? Urol Res. 2005;33(3):199–202.
17. Mufarrij PW, Woods M, Shah OD, et al. Robotic dismembered pyeloplasty: a 6-year, multi-institutional experience. J Urol. 2008;180(4):1391–6.
18. Arumainayagam N, Minervini A, Davenport K, et al. Antegrade versus retrograde stenting in laparoscopic pyeloplasty. J Endourol. 2008;22(4):671–4.
19. Mufarrij PW, Rajamahanty S, Krane LS, Hemal AK. Intracorporeal double-J stent placement during robot-assisted urinary tract reconstruction: technical considerations. J Endourol. 2012;26(9):1121–4.
20. Wason SE, Lance RS, Given RW, Malcolm JB. Robotic-assisted ureteral re-implantation: a case series. J Laparoendosc Adv Surg Tech A. 2015;25(6):503–7.

21. Kerbl K, Chandhoke PS, Figenshau RS, Stone AM, Clayman RV. Effect of stent duration on ureteral healing following endoureterotomy in an animal model. J Urol. 1993;150(4):1302–5.
22. Selmy GI, Hassouna MM, Begin LR, Khalaf IM, Elhilali MM. Long-term effects of ureteric stent after ureteric dilation. J Urol. 1993;150(6):1984–9.
23. Danuser H, Germann C, Pelzer N, Ruhle A, Stucki P, Mattei A. One- vs 4-week stent placement after laparoscopic and robot-assisted pyeloplasty: results of a prospective randomised single-centre study. BJU Int. 2014;113(6):931–5.
24. Joshi HB, Stainthorpe A, MacDonagh RP, Keeley FX, Jr., Timoney AG, Barry MJ. Indwelling ureteral stents: evaluation of symptoms, quality of life and utility. J Urol. 2003;169(3):1065–69.
25. Kwon JK, Cho KS, Oh CK, et al. The beneficial effect of alpha-blockers for ureteral stent-related discomfort: systematic review and network meta-analysis for alfuzosin versus tamsulosin versus placebo. BMC Urol. 2015;15:55.
26. Lamb AD, Vowler SL, Johnston R, Dunn N, Wiseman OJ. Meta-analysis showing the beneficial effect of alpha-blockers on ureteral stent discomfort. BJU Int. 2011;108(11):1894–902.
27. Zhou L, Cai X, Li H, Wang KJ. Effects of alpha-blockers, Antimuscarinics, or combination therapy in relieving ureteral stent-related symptoms: a meta-analysis. J Endourol. 2015;29(6):650–6.
28. Koprowski C, Kim C, Modi PK, Elsamra SE. Ureteral stent-associated pain: a review. J Endourol. 2016;30(7):744–53.
29. Tadros NN, Bland L, Legg E, Olyaei A, Conlin MJ. A single dose of a non-steroidal anti-inflammatory drug (NSAID) prevents severe pain after ureteric stent removal: a prospective, randomised, double-blind, placebo-controlled trial. BJU Int. 2013;111(1):101–5.
30. Norris RD, Sur RL, Springhart WP, et al. A prospective, randomized, double-blinded placebo-controlled comparison of extended release oxybutynin versus phenazopyridine for the management of postoperative ureteral stent discomfort. Urology. 2008;71(5):792–95.
31. Ragab M, Soliman MG, Tawfik A, et al. The role of pregabalin in relieving ureteral stent-related symptoms: a randomized controlled clinical trial. Int Urol Nephrol. 2017;49(6):961–6.
32. Farsi HM, Mosli HA, Al-Zemaity MF, Bahnassy AA, Alvarez M. Bacteriuria and colonization of double-pigtail ureteral stents: long-term experience with 237 patients. J Endourol. 1995;9(6):469–72.
33. Nevo A, Mano R, Baniel J, Lifshitz DA. Ureteric stent dwelling time: a risk factor for post-ureteroscopy sepsis. BJU Int. 2017;120(1):117–22.
34. Wolf JS Jr, Bennett CJ, Dmochowski RR, Hollenbeck BK, Pearle MS, Schaeffer AJ. Best practice policy statement on urologic surgery antimicrobial prophylaxis. J Urol. 2008;179(4):1379–90.
35. Mosayyebi A, Manes C, Carugo D, Somani BK. Advances in ureteral stent design and materials. Curr Urol Rep. 2018;19(5):35.
36. Del Junco M, Yoon R, Okhunov Z, et al. Comparison of flow characteristics of novel three-dimensional printed ureteral stents versus standard ureteral stents in a porcine model. J Endourol. 2015;29(9):1065–9.
37. Chenam A, Yuh B, Zhumkhawala A, et al. Prospective randomised non-inferiority trial of pelvic drain placement vs no pelvic drain placement after robot-assisted radical prostatectomy. BJU Int. 2018;121(3):357–64.
38. Musser JE, Assel M, Guglielmetti GB, et al. Impact of routine use of surgical drains on incidence of complications with robot-assisted radical prostatectomy. J Endourol. 2014;28(11):1333–7.

Principles of Reconstruction: Spatulation, Blood Supply, and Wound Healing

Ziho Lee, Matthew E. Sterling, and Michael J. Metro

Watertight Anastomosis

Creating a watertight anastomosis is essential during urinary tract reconstruction, and its importance cannot be overemphasized [1–3]. Urinary tract anastomoses, which may be performed in an interrupted or running fashion based on the surgeon's preference, must ensure a circumferential mucosa-to-mucosa approximation to minimize the risk of a urinary leak. At the same time, care must be taken to not place sutures with excessive force or too close together, as this may result in ischemia at the site of the anastomosis which may result in fistula or stricture formation [3]. Furthermore, a urethral catheter or ureteral stent may be used to facilitate the alignment and formation of a watertight anastomosis [4–6]. A discussion of the use of catheters and stents in urinary tract reconstruction may be found elsewhere in this book.

On the other hand, failure to create a watertight anastomosis can lead to a multitude of problems. Urinary leakage before epithelialization is complete can lead to abnormal reconstitution of the urinary tract. Although it does not change the pattern of urothelial regeneration, it does prolong regeneration and delay primary epithelialization [1, 7]. Also, urinary leakage through an anastomosis can cause considerable local disturbance, which can impair urinary tract healing. For example, it can lead to the formation of urinoma, abscess, fistula, and obstruction [6].

Z. Lee (✉) · M. E. Sterling · M. J. Metro
Department of Urology, Temple University School of Medicine, Philadelphia, PA, USA
e-mail: Ziho.Lee@tuhs.temple.edu; Michael.Metro@tuhs.temple.edu

© Springer Nature Switzerland AG 2022
M. D. Stifelman et al. (eds.), *Techniques of Robotic Urinary Tract Reconstruction*, https://doi.org/10.1007/978-3-030-50196-9_3

Graft Take: Imbibition and Inosculation

Understanding the principles surrounding graft take is critical for the reconstructive urologist, as grafting may be particularly useful during urinary tract reconstruction. Grafting refers to removing tissue from a donor site and transferring it to a recipient site without its native blood supply. As such, for adequate graft take, blood supply must be reestablished by imbibition and inosculation. Imbibition, which occurs in the first 48 h after tissue transfer, refers to the passive diffusion of nutrients and metabolic wastes between the graft tissue and host site. Inosculation, which occurs 48 h to 1 week after tissue transfer, refers to the formation of new vascular connections and capillary in-growth of host vasculature [8, 9].

Several different factors may play a role in survival and failure of the graft. Imbibition and inosculation may be optimized by a well-vascularized recipient bed and appropriate apposition and immobilization of the graft. However, fluid accumulation between the graft and recipient site inhibits the ability for inosculation and imbibition to occur. It is for this reason that an omental flap is an important adjunct during buccal mucosal graft ureteroplasty. The omental flap not only provides nutritional support to the graft and assists with neovascularization but also is porous enough to prevent hematoma, seroma, or urinoma formation between the host site and graft.

Gillies' Principles of Reconstructive Surgery

Sir Harold Delf Gillies (1882–1960) is widely considered to be the father of modern plastic surgery [10]. He was instrumental in pioneering many reconstructive surgical techniques, such as skin and tubed pedicle flaps and cartilage grafts, during World War I. In what was arguably his most valuable and enduring contribution to the specialty, he laid out the foundational principles pertaining to the practice of reconstructive surgery. Millard, who originally published these principles as the "Ten Commandments" in 1950 [11], described them as the "result of personal lessons learned from both successes and failures, retained in memory and crystallized into proverbs of short sentences spawned from long experience [12]." In 1957, Gillies and Millard modified and expanded upon these doctrines as "Gillies' Principles of Reconstructive Surgery [13]." Despite the continued refinement and development of surgical techniques, these principles are, to a large extent, valid today and can provide a strong framework for approaching any urinary tract reconstructive surgery:

- Principle 1: Observation is the basis of surgical diagnosis. Developing a keen sense of observation is invaluable in making an accurate diagnosis.
- Principle 2: Diagnose before you treat. A problem should be accurately determined before proceeding with an operation.

- Principle 3: Make a plan and a pattern for this plan. Although the nature of reconstructive surgery often requires intraoperative improvisation, it is important to preoperatively establish a goal and develop a method to reach that goal.
- Principle 4: Make a record. Rather than relying on memory, keeping accurate records of patient encounters may assist with coordinating patient care and provide legal protection.
- Principle 5: The lifeboat. Possible difficulties associated with a surgery should be anticipated, and a secondary plan should be devised in case the primary plan fails.
- Principle 6: A good style will get you through. Gillies and Millard defined surgical style as "the expression of personality and training exhibited by the movements of the fingers [13]." It is important that when developing one's own style, one is able to modify the style when required.
- Principle 7: Replace what is normal in a normal position and retain it there. Surgical reconstruction requires the ability to recognize what is normal in order to restore displaced parts to their correct place.
- Principle 8: Treat the primary defect first. Concern with secondary defects should not get in the way of treating the primary defect.
- Principle 9: Losses must be replaced in kind. When attempting reconstruction of damaged or lost body parts, like should be replaced with like (i.e., hairless skin with hairless skin). If an exact replacement is not available, a similar substitute should be made (i.e., urothelium with buccal mucosa).
- Principle 10: Do something positive. When faced with a particularly complex and difficult intraoperative problem, taking steps toward the final solution, regardless of how small or trivial the move may seem, is vital.
- Principle 11: Never throw anything away. In reconstructive surgery, never throw anything away unless one is sure that it is not needed.
- Principle 12: Never let routine methods become your master. While it is critical to master routine methods, one should be open to the advancement and innovation of surgical techniques.
- Principle 13: Consult other specialists. Obtaining assistance from the appropriate regional expert may not only allow for the dissemination of various solutions to problems in other specialties, but also allow for better patient care.
- Principle 14: Speed in surgery consists of not doing the same thing twice. It is more efficient to take the time to do things right the first time, than having to go back and fix it.
- Principle 15: The aftercare is as important as the planning. Making sure that a patient receives appropriate postoperative monitoring and care is crucial to maximize the chances for a successful surgery and, in some cases, may be more important than the surgery itself!
- Principle 16: Never do today what can honorably be put off till tomorrow. If there is danger or doubt associated with a particular surgical maneuver, consideration should be given to whether the decision may be delayed for another and safer day.

References

1. Hinman F Jr, Oppenheimer RO. The effect of urinary flow upon ureteral regeneration in the absence of splint. Surg Gynecol Obstet. 1956;103(4):416–22.
2. Brandes SB, McAninch JW. Reconstructive surgery for trauma of the upper urinary tract. Urol Clin North Am. 1999;26(1):183–99, x
3. Png JC, Chapple CR. Principles of ureteric reconstruction. Curr Opin Urol. 2000;10(3):207–12.
4. Franco I, Eshghi M, Schutte H, Park T, Fernandez R, Choudhury M, Addonizio JC. Value of proximal diversion and ureteral stenting in management of penetrating ureteral trauma. Urology. 1988;32(2):99–102.
5. Sieben DM, Howerton L, Amin M, Holt H, Lich R Jr. The role of ureteral stenting in the management of surgical injury of the ureter. J Urol. 1978;119(3):330–1.
6. Brandes S, Coburn M, Armenakas N, McAninch J. Diagnosis and management of ureteric injury: an evidence-based analysis. BJU Int. 2004;94(3):277–89. https://doi.org/10.1111/j.1464-410X.2004.04978.x.
7. Hinman F Jr, Oppenheimer R. Ureteral regeneration. VI. Delayed urinary flow in the healing of unsplinted ureteral defects. J Urol. 1957;78(2):138–44.
8. Greenwood J, Amjadi M, Dearman B, Mackie I. Real-time demonstration of split skin graft inosculation and integra dermal matrix neovascularization using confocal laser scanning microscopy. Eplasty. 2009;9:e33.
9. Bryk DJ, Yamaguchi Y, Zhao LC. Tissue transfer techniques in reconstructive urology. Korean J Urol. 2015;56(7):478–86. https://doi.org/10.4111/kju.2015.56.7.478.
10. Spencer CR. Sir Harold Delf Gillies, the otolaryngologist and father of modern facial plastic surgery: review of his rhinoplasty case notes. J Laryngol Otol. 2015;129(6):520–8. https://doi.org/10.1017/S0022215115000754.
11. Millard DR Jr. (1950) Plastic peregrinations. Plast Reconstr Surg. (1946) 5(1):26–53, illust.
12. Millard DR. Principlization of plastic surgery. 1st ed: Little Brown and Company; Boston, MA, USA 1986.
13. Sir Harold Gillies DRMJ. The principles and art of plastic surgery. 1st ed: Little Brown and Company; Boston, MA, USA 1957.

Tissue Substitution in Reconstruction

Joseph Acquaye, Joseph J. Pariser, and Sean P. Elliott

Oral Mucosa Graft

The use of buccal grafts for the purpose of genitourinary reconstruction was pioneered by Sapezkho in 1894 for the purpose of urethral reconstruction [1]. Buccal mucosa remains the primary preferred tissue used for substitution during urethroplasty due to its ease of harvest and low donor site morbidity. Additionally, it possesses excellent graft characteristics owing to a thin lamina propria while being hairless and compatible with a moist environment [2].

Additional uses of buccal grafts in genitourinary reconstruction have more recently been developed, including ureteral reconstruction. Classically, short strictures at the ureteropelvic junction have primarily been managed with pyeloplasty while strictures involving the majority of the ureter have been managed with ileal ureter or autotransplantation. However, there are some strictures, especially of the proximal ureter, which are too long for a pyeloplasty but not long enough to necessitate complete ureteral substitution. Buccal ureteroplasty, which can be performed using robotic techniques to minimize morbidity, is a viable option for these patients [3, 4].

The procedure involves reflection of the white line of Toldt to expose the retroperitoneum. The ureter is generally found coursing along the psoas muscle. Intraluminal indocyanine green or simultaneous ureteroscopy can assist the robotic surgeon in the identification of the ureter and strictured segment. It is anticipated that intravenous indocyanine green concentrated in the urine will become available to help ureteral identification. The stricture is incised longitudinally, and an appropriately long buccal graft is harvested.

J. Acquaye · J. J. Pariser (✉) · S. P. Elliott
Department of Urology, University of Minnesota, Minneapolis, MN, USA
e-mail: jpariser@umn.edu; selliott@umn.edu

© Springer Nature Switzerland AG 2022
M. D. Stifelman et al. (eds.), *Techniques of Robotic Urinary Tract Reconstruction*, https://doi.org/10.1007/978-3-030-50196-9_4

Buccal graft harvest is a standard technique for reconstructive urologists who perform urethroplasty. A retractor is used for the mouth, which can be minimalist using just sutures or include a Steinhauser, Denhardt, or Sluder-Jansen retractor. Stenson's duct, which is located just inferior to the upper second molar, is identified and avoided. Local anesthesia with epinephrine is infiltrated to facilitate hydrodissection, thus allowing a less painful and bloody field. The site is demarcated, and the borders are incised using a no. 15 blade. The graft is then harvested by dissecting in the plane superficial to the buccinator muscle (see Fig. 4.1 for an illustration). An overly deep dissection is bloodier, harms the muscle, and can lead to damage of the facial nerve. Focal bipolar electrocautery is used to stop bleeding after the harvest is complete. Closure or non-closure of the harvest site is surgeon preference as it remains unclear which approach is optimal. Several randomized trials have been published with disparate conclusions. Generally, we feel that there is no clear benefit to one approach or the other, but that wide grafts (2.5 cm or greater) should not

Fig. 4.1 Harvest of buccal graft (**a**), and closure with alloderm (**b**)

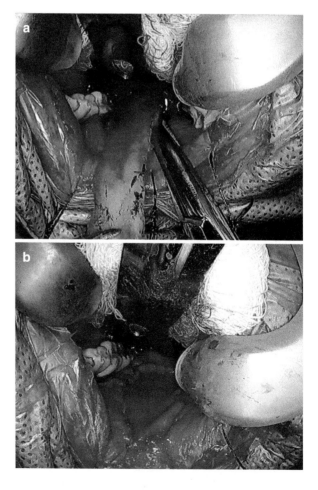

be closed given the risk of contracture. Generally, grafts do not need to be very wide (1.5–2 cm) for ureteral reconstruction. The graft is defatted prior to passing it intracorporeally through a port. The graft is sewn into place ensuring a watertight closure using fine absorbable suture. A double-J ureteral stent is positioned prior to completion of the anastomosis.

The graft relies on local blood supply for adequate take. Multiple methods have been trialed with good success. Options include quilting onto the psoas muscle belly or wrapping with omentum or mesenteric fat. We generally advocate for omental wrapping as it is readily available and provides adequate blood supply. Favorable outcomes of robotic buccal ureteroplasty have been reported [4–6]. For instance, a multi-institutional study published by Zhao et al. which examined 19 patients undergoing this procedure for median stricture lengths of 4.0 cm demonstrated an overall success rate of 90% at a 26-month median follow-up.

An alternative to oral mucosa is lingual mucosa from the underside of the tongue. As a positive, a unilateral lingual graft can yield a long area for harvest. When harvesting, there is less fat present on the underside of the mucosa. Care should be taken to avoid Wharton's duct and the lateral taste buds. Closure is generally recommended. Lingual mucosa can be used with similar indications as buccal mucosa, but we only recommend it only when oral mucosa is needed and bilateral buccal grafts have previously been harvested. This is primarily due to inferior outcomes associated with lingual mucosa and some increased donor site morbidity (such as dysgeusia) associated with its use. Another option is lower lip oral mucosa; however, we similarly recommend against using this tissue for primary harvest given its increased morbidity [7].

Rectus Flap

The rectus flap is another technique that can be utilized for the purpose of genitourinary reconstruction [8]. This flap has the advantage of a dual blood supply (derived from the superior and inferior epigastric arteries). Usually, the superior blood supply is sacrificed to allow mobility to the pelvis. In the urologic literature, it has been primarily utilized for pelvic reconstruction. The traditional "open" method of harvesting a rectus flap is associated with complications including abdominal wall hernia, infection, and seroma. Consequently, attempts have been made to harvest this flap using less invasive methods.

Laparoscopic rectus harvest has several technical challenges. Robotic surgery, however, has gained traction for this purpose owing to the easier learning curve, enhanced precision, and increased degrees of freedom. In urology, inferiorly based flaps can be utilized to reconstruct abdominopelvic defects where space obliteration or visceral protection is needed (e.g., abdominoperineal resection, radical cystoprostatectomy, pelvic exenteration, fistula repair, filling in a pubectomy site, and coverage of major vessels or visceral repairs) [9].

Positioning for this procedure involves placing the patient in either a supine or low lithotomy position; arms are tucked and the patient is secured in place. Port placement is marked along a line connecting the anterior axillary line and the anterior superior iliac spine. The midpoint between these two landmarks and 2 cm lateral to it is the desired location of the 12-mm camera port. On either side of the camera port, approximately four finger breadths away, or 1–2 cm from the costal margin and iliac crest, is the proposed location of the two 8-mm instrument ports. Of note, both this flap and the omental flap involve a high cephalad dissection. Thus, the da Vinci Xi (Intuitive Surgical, Sunnyvale, CA) is an improvement compared to prior models for such approaches, where there is the need to move between the upper abdomen and pelvis (see Fig. 4.2 for the illustration of robotic harvest).

Intraperitoneal access is obtained, and the abdomen is insufflated. The posterior rectus sheath is opened from the arcuate line to the upper abdomen, exposing the posterior surface of the rectus belly. When an inferiorly based rectus flap is being harvested robotically, the inferior epigastric vessels are gently dissected down to the external iliac vessels and freed. The muscle is then divided cephalad at the costal

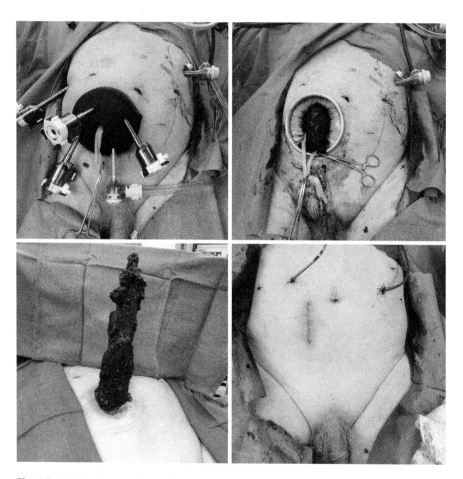

Fig. 4.2 Robotic harvest of rectus flap

margin and caudad between the symphysis pubis and the entrance of the pedicle into the muscle, thus isolating the muscle on the pedicle. The muscle is then dissected from the anterior abdominal fascia and directed into the pelvis for insetting. The abdominal wall relies on the anterior rectus fascia in this area. By avoiding a midline laparotomy, the surgeon does not further weaken this anterior sheath. However, inferior to the arcuate line, no fascial defect will be created as all of the layers of the rectus fascia run anterior to the rectus muscle.

Early studies by Ibrahim et al. have demonstrated the promise of this technique compared to the traditional technique of rectus flap harvest [9]. The rectus is a bulky muscle flap, ideal for pelvic reconstruction.

Omental Flap

In urology, the omental flap can be utilized for numerous indications including repair of various fistulas (including those involving the pubis, bladder, ureter, rectum, and vagina). These fistulas can have varied etiologies including iatrogenic causes, malignancy, trauma, or radiation. Principles of repair include exposure, gentle tissue handling, adequate dissection for separate closure, and interposition of healthy flap or graft. During laparotomy, the omentum is readily available. However, using older models of the da Vinci (Intuitive Surgical, Sunnyvale, CA), harvest of the omentum was more difficult as it often remained in the upper abdomen, especially in the Trendelenburg position. However, with the advent of the Xi, access to the omentum is more achievable, often without the need to re-dock or perform laparoscopic harvest. The indications for omental flap are very similar to those for rectus flap. In general, we prefer the omentum when it is available because the morbidity is much lower. Pelvic floor reconstruction after abdominoperineal resection remains one indication for which we still prefer a rectus flap.

The greater omentum is based off the greater curvature of the stomach. It derives its blood supply from the right and left gastroepiploic arteries. In general, one of these arteries is sacrificed to allow for an omental flap that can reach into the pelvis. While some authors describe a necessity to base the flap preferentially on the right or the left, we generally find that either grants adequate blood supply and sufficient length to reach the pelvis. When harvesting this flap, it is important to note that there is considerable blood supply in the omentum, so we generally utilize a LigaSure (Medtronic, Minneapolis, MN) device (or similar) to ensure hemostasis during dissection. Another note about the technique is that the bulkiest flap is achieved by dividing the short gastric arteries as they connect from the gastroepiploic artery to the omentum high against the greater curvature of the stomach. The omentum is then released from its reflection on the transverse colon. However, we rarely need such a bulky flap and find it to be much faster and easier to harvest the omentum by dividing it at the transverse colon reflection rather than the greater curvature of the stomach.

Alternative uses for omental flaps in urologic reconstruction include omental wrapping during ureterolysis, buccal ureteroplasty, or buccal fistula repair [10].

When performing omental wrapping for ureterolysis in the setting of retroperitoneal fibrosis, the goal is to maintain an intraperitoneal ureter. Often, the process is bilateral, and two omental flaps can be created by incising vertically through the omentum leaving left and right sided omental flaps based on their respective gastroepiploic arteries.

Peritoneal Flap

Peritoneal flaps are a less morbid and easier to harvest tissue interposition during fistula repair [11]. Although the omentum, gracilis, or rectus are still preferred for high-risk cases, peritoneum remains an option in low-risk situations or when the others are not available. Additionally, more novel uses for this flap including peritoneal vaginoplasty or ureteral reconstruction have been proposed. A peritoneal flap is best reserved for repair of relatively healthy, non-radiated tissue. When tissue integrity is in question, an omental or rectus flap is better.

Peritoneal vaginoplasty was first proposed by Davydov [12]. Indications include androgen insensitivity syndrome and gender affirmation surgery for transgender females. This can also be performed as a revision for neovaginal stenosis. Peritoneal vaginoplasty can be facilitated using a robotic approach to decrease morbidity [13]. For either indication, the procedure starts by incising the peritoneum over the rectovesical pouch. Dissection continues along Denonvilliers' fascia with great care taken to avoid injuring the rectum (see Fig. 4.3 for the illustration of robotic dissection of peritoneal flap). Simultaneous perineal dissection is performed for the distal aspect of the neovaginal space. Ultimately, these two dissections meet. Peritoneal based flaps are made (often one anterior and one posterior) and passed distally to line the neovaginal canal. Sutures lines are closed, and the peritoneum is closed from the neovaginal canal. The apex of the neovagina can be pexed to the peritoneal

Fig. 4.3 Robotic dissection of peritoneal flap

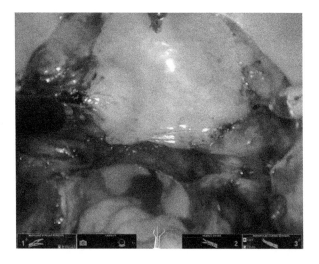

incision to decrease the risk of prolapse. The peritoneal incision is then closed robotically. When comparing peritoneal flap vaginoplasty to conventional skin grafting methods, peritoneal flaps have distinct advantages including their hairless nature and increased lubrication [13, 14].

A study by Bradao et al. used a porcine model do assess ureteral reconstruction with peritoneum in a tubularized fashion [15]. Outcome analysis demonstrated sub-optimal results with respect to patency of the repaired segment, endoscopic appearance, and functional outcomes (i.e., renal function). These suboptimal outcomes underscore the limitations of using a tubularized graft.

Gracilis Flap

The gracilis is the most superficial muscle of the medial thigh, which can be harvested for use in urologic reconstruction. Its uses include urethroplasty, rectourethral fistula repair, penoscrotal reconstruction, and for providing additional tissue for perineal wound closure [16–18]. Although the gracilis flap is ideal for transperineal urethral reconstruction and this book is focused on robotic intra-abdominal surgery, we present the gracilis flap here because recent advancements in urethral reconstruction techniques have included a combined transperineal and robotically assisted laparoscopic approach. In these situations, a rectourethral fistula, for example, can be exposed robotically, and a gracilis flap can be rotated in through a perineal incision.

Harvesting the gracilis flap is traditionally done in an open fashion though morbidity can be decreased by limiting the incision size [19]. An incision is initially made just distal to where the pedicle is expected at the origin at the profunda femoris artery. This is inferior to the adductor longus. This pedicle is located 8–10 cm from the pubic symphysis. After opening its connective tissue sheath, blunt dissection can be performed to isolate the muscle belly from the surrounding structures. The distal aspect of the muscle is tendinous in nature and is attached to the medial aspect of the femur above the condyle. This can be transected using a small counter incision (thus avoiding a long incision along the entire medial thigh). One advantage of a single long incision is that it is easy to follow the muscle along its entire length and ensure that the correct tendinous insertion is divided distally. If two smaller incisions are used, then the surgeon should take extra precaution when dividing distally. Great care is taken proximally where the pedicle is expected to ensure the blood supply is not sacrificed. There is some controversy regarding denervation. Benefits of denervation include the lack of flexing in the area where the muscle will eventually lie; however, one of the risks of denervation is the resultant muscle atrophy that can occur. The muscle is then tunnelled underneath a skin bridge medially to pass it through to the perineum for use (see Fig. 4.4 for an example of traditional open harvest of this graft). The thigh incisions are then closed in layers, and a drain is generally left in place.

Similar to other muscle flaps, there can be some morbidity associated with this procedure including neuropathic pain, reduced function, and scarring [19]. In light

Fig. 4.4 Traditional
harvest of gracilis flap

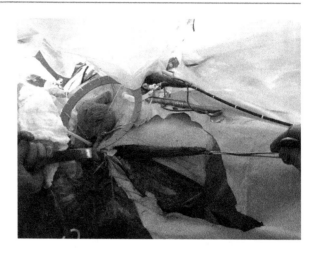

of this, endoscopic techniques have been postulated for gracilis flap harvest and
modeled in one cadaveric study by Mohammed et al [20]. While this study did demonstrate feasibility, drawbacks included technical difficulty, increasing bleeding
risk and increased costs compared to the traditional approach. Further refinement of
technique is warranted before application in live patients.

When utilizing the gracilis for urethroplasty, it can be used to wrap an entire
anastomosis or buttress an oral mucosal graft, especially when local tissue has poor
blood supply. Newer indications involving the gracilis include buttressing urethroplasty during primary neophallus creation or revision urethroplasty in the neophallus. When using the gracilis to optimize buccal graft take, some authors utilize a
prelaminated approach where the buccal graft is laid on the gracilis as a first-stage
procedure to later be harvested and transposed into the perineum [17]. Of note,
because its mobility is limited by its pedicle on the upper medial thigh, it does not
reach the abdomen easily and is primarily used in the perineal reconstruction.

Overall, the gracilis represents a viable option for well-vascularized, space-
filling tissue amenable for perineal use with relatively low morbidity and ease of
harvest.

Conclusion

When undertaking urologic reconstruction, surgeons should be familiar with the
commonly utilized grafts and flaps. At times, this may involve other specialties, and
we encourage liberal consultation with specialists (e.g., plastic surgeons) especially
if the surgeon is less experienced with a particular flap or graft harvest. Choosing
the optimal graft or flap is critical to the surgical outcomes of reconstructive procedures. We review common flaps and grafts used during robotic urologic reconstruction. However, this list is certainly not exhaustive. Other flaps used in urologic
reconstruction include anterolateral thigh (ALT), vastus lateralis, superficial

circumflex iliac artery perforator (SCIP), and radial forearm. Many of these options are more commonly used for external genitalia reconstruction. Robotic technology has been increasingly utilized for more complex reconstruction, and it behooves the surgeon to ensure that a sound operative plan is generated including optimal and backup options for tissue substitution when needed.

References

1. Korneyev I, Ilyin D, Schultheiss D, Chapple C. The first oral mucosal graft urethroplasty was carried out in the 19th century: the pioneering experience of Kirill Sapezhko (1857–1928). Eur Urol [Internet]. 2012 Oct 1 [cited 2018 Nov 19];62(4):624–7. Available from: http://www.ncbi.nlm.nih.gov/pubmed/22749735.
2. Rourke K, McKinny S, St. Martin B. Effect of wound closure on buccal mucosal graft harvest site morbidity: results of a randomized prospective trial. Urology [Internet]. 2012 Feb 1 [cited 2018 Nov 19];79(2):443–7. Available from: https://www.sciencedirect.com/science/article/pii/S0090429511024411.
3. Vasudevan VP, Johnson EU, Wong K, Iskander M, Javed S, Gupta N, et al. Contemporary management of ureteral strictures. J Clin Urol [Internet]. 2018 Jun 8 [cited 2018 Nov 19];205141581877221. Available from: http://journals.sagepub.com/doi/10.1177/2051415818772218
4. Kroepfl D, Loewen H, Klevecka V, Musch M. Treatment of long ureteric strictures with buccal mucosal grafts. BJU Int [Internet]. 2009 Oct 28 [cited 2018 Nov 19];105(10):1452–5. Available from: http://www.ncbi.nlm.nih.gov/pubmed/19874302.
5. Zhao LC, Weinberg AC, Lee Z, Ferretti MJ, Koo HP, Metro MJ, et al. Robotic ureteral reconstruction using buccal mucosa grafts: a multi-institutional experience. Eur Urol [Internet]. 2017 Nov 24 [cited 2018 Nov 19];73(3):419–26. Available from: http://www.ncbi.nlm.nih.gov/pubmed/29239749.
6. Badawy AA, Abolyosr A, Saleem MD, Abuzeid AM. Buccal Mucosa graft for ureteral stricture substitution: initial experience. Urology [Internet]. 2010 Oct [cited 2018 Nov 19];76(4):971–5. Available from: http://www.ncbi.nlm.nih.gov/pubmed/20932415.
7. Kamp S, Knoll T, Osman M, Häcker A, Michel MS, Alken P. Donor-site morbidity in buccal mucosa urethroplasty: lower lip or inner cheek? BJU Int [Internet]. 2005 Sep [cited 2018 Nov 19];96(4):619–23. Available from: http://doi.wiley.com/10.1111/j.1464-410X.2005.05695.x
8. Nigriny JF, Wu P, Butler CE. Perineal reconstruction with an extrapelvic vertical rectus abdominis myocutaneous flap. Int J Gynecol Cancer [Internet]. 2010 Dec [cited 2018 Nov 19];20(9):1609–12. Available from: http://www.ncbi.nlm.nih.gov/pubmed/21119371.
9. Ibrahim AE, Sarhane KA, Pederson JC, Selber JC. Robotic harvest of the rectus abdominis muscle: principles and clinical applications. Semin Plast Surg [Internet]. 2014 Feb [cited 2018 Nov 19];28(1):26–31. Available from: http://www.ncbi.nlm.nih.gov/pubmed/24872776.
10. Arora S, Campbell L, Tourojman M, Pucheril D, Jones LR, Rogers C. Robotic Buccal Mucosal graft ureteroplasty for complex ureteral stricture. Urology [Internet]. 2017 Dec [cited 2018 Nov 24];110:257–8. Available from: http://www.ncbi.nlm.nih.gov/pubmed/29153902.
11. Matei DV, Zanagnolo V, Vartolomei MD, Crisan N, Ferro M, Bocciolone L, et al. Robot-assisted vesico-vaginal fistula repair: our technique and review of the literature. Urol Int [Internet]. 2017 [cited 2018 Nov 19];99(2):137–42. Available from: http://www.ncbi.nlm.nih.gov/pubmed/28743109.
12. Davydov SN. [Colpopoeisis from the peritoneum of the uterorectal space]. Akush Ginekol (Sofiia) [Internet]. 1969 Dec [cited 2018 Nov 19];45(12):55–7. Available from: http://www.ncbi.nlm.nih.gov/pubmed/5381096.
13. Rangaswamy M, Machado NO, Kaur S, Machado L. Laparoscopic vaginoplasty: using a sliding peritoneal flap for correction of complete vaginal agenesis. Eur J Obstet Gynecol Reprod Biol

[Internet]. 2001 Oct 1 [cited 2018 Nov 19];98(2):244–8. Available from: https://www-science-direct-com.ezp3.lib.umn.edu/science/article/pii/S030121150100313X?via%3Dihub#BIB1

14. Kriplani A, Karthik SDS, Kriplani I, Kachhawa G. Laparoscopic peritoneal vaginoplasty for Mayer–Rokitansky–Küster–Hauser syndrome: an experience at a tertiary care center. J Gynecol Surg [Internet]. 2018 Apr 1 [cited 2018 Nov 19];34(2):63–7. Available from: http://www.liebertpub.com/doi/10.1089/gyn.2017.0076

15. Brandao LF, Laydner H, Akca O, Autorino R, Zargar H, De S, et al. Robot-assisted ureteral reconstruction using a tubularized peritoneal flap: a novel technique in a chronic porcine model. World J Urol [Internet]. 2017 Jan 5 [cited 2018 Nov 19];35(1):89–96. Available from: http://www.ncbi.nlm.nih.gov/pubmed/27151276.

16. Shibata D, Hyland W, Busse P, Kim HK, Sentovich SM, Steele G, et al. Immediate reconstruction of the perineal wound with gracilis muscle flaps following abdominoperineal resection and intraoperative radiation therapy for recurrent carcinoma of the rectum. Ann Surg Oncol [Internet]. 1999 Jan [cited 2018 Nov 24];6(1):33–7. Available from: http://link.springer.com/10.1007/s10434-999-0033-4

17. Palmer DA, Buckley JC, Zinman LN, Vanni AJ. Urethroplasty for high risk, long segment urethral strictures with ventral buccal mucosa graft and gracilis muscle flap. J Urol [Internet]. 2015 Mar 1 [cited 2018 Nov 24];193(3):902–5. Available from: https://www.sciencedirect.com/science/article/pii/S0022534714045467

18. Zinman L. The management of the complex recto-urethral fistula. BJU Int [Internet]. 2004 Dec 1 [cited 2018 Nov 24];94(9):1212–3. Available from: http://doi.wiley.com/10.1111/j.1464-410X.2004.05225.x

19. Deutinger M, Kuzbari R, Paternostro-Sluga T, Quittan M, Zauner-Dungl A, Worseg A, et al. Donor-site morbidity of the gracilis flap. Plast Reconstr Surg [Internet]. 1995 Jun [cited 2018 Nov 24];95(7):1240–4. Available from: http://www.ncbi.nlm.nih.gov/pubmed/7761511.

20. Mohammad JA, Shenaq SM. Minimally invasive endoscopic technique of harvesting free gracilis muscle flap to lower donor site morbidity: a feasibility study in cadavers. Can J Plast Surg [Internet]. 1999 Apr 1 [cited 2018 Nov 24];7(2):81–5. Available from: http://journals.sagepub.com/doi/10.1177/229255039900700204

Part III

Ureteropelvic Junction Obstruction

Chester J. Koh

In this section of the book, we encounter the most common robotic reconstructive procedure in children, robotic pyeloplasty for ureteropelvic junction obstruction (UPJO), which also occurs frequently in adults. Whether the source of the obstruction is intrinsic such as a thin caliber ureter or an aperistaltic segment of ureter at the level of the ureteropelvic junction, or is extrinsic such as crossing lower pole renal vessels, similar robotic techniques are utilized to address the obstruction. While dismembered pyeloplasty remains the gold standard for both open surgery and robotic surgery, other robotic techniques for robotic pyeloplasty have also been described.

Drs. Laith M. Alzweri and Raju Thomas describe the various surgical modalities of adult pyeloplasty for the treatment of UPJO from the gold standard of open pyeloplasty to more recent techniques using minimally invasive modalities including robotic surgery.

Drs. Michael Daughtery and Paul Noh note that robotic pyeloplasty has become increasingly utilized for UPJO in the pediatric population, and they describe their operative technique for this minimally invasive approach that avoids the use of a ureteral stent in some cases and can be done on an outpatient basis.

Since secondary pathologies or unusual anatomy can arise in patients undergoing pyeloplasty that necessitate additional surgical interventions, the chapter by Drs. Ram Pathak and Ashok Hemal delves into the management of UPJO with concomitant nephrolithiasis and for patients presenting with unusual urinary tract anatomy.

Drs. Ravindra Sahadev, Joan Ko, Arun Srinivasan, and Aseem Shukla noted that robotic repair of recurrent UPJO can be technically challenging. However, several studies have shown that, with adherence to sound surgical principles, success rates for this surgery are promising. Their chapter reviews various strategies used for robotic procedures that address recurrent UPJO that includes technical tips to improve the likelihood of success.

Adult Robotic Pyeloplasty

5

Laith M. Alzweri and Raju Thomas

Introduction

Ureteropelvic junction obstruction (UPJO) is the most common congenital anomaly of the ureter, affecting approximately 13,000 newborns with hydronephrosis in the United States every year [1]. UPJO presenting in adults could be congenital or acquired; majority of congenital cases are related to intrinsic or extrinsic causes, while acquired cases could be secondary to treatment of urolithiasis, inflammatory stricture, urothelial tumors, and iatrogenic [2]. Adult UPJO may present with intermittent flank pain, recurrent infections, and kidney stones with or without worsening renal function, evident biochemically and radiologically with various degrees of hydronephrosis (ultrasound, CT, and MRI) and obstruction reflected by evaluating T1/2 time on a diuretic nuclear medicine renogram. In addition, an increasing number of subclinical and asymptomatic UPJO are diagnosed incidentally on cross-sectional imaging studies [3].

Historically, open pyeloplasty was the gold standard for surgical management of UPJO, with published success rates consistently greater than 90% [1]. Open surgical pyeloplasty remains the international gold standard treatment option for UPJO with published intraoperative complications rate of 2%, and recurrent UPJO

Supplementary Information The online version of this chapter (https://doi.org/10.1007/978-3-030-50196-9_5) contains supplementary material, which is available to authorized users.

L. M. Alzweri
Urology, Tulane University School of Medicine, New Orleans, LA, USA

Division of Urology, Department of Surgery, University of Texas Medical Branch, Galveston, TX, USA

R. Thomas (✉)
Urology, Tulane University School of Medicine, New Orleans, LA, USA
e-mail: rthomas@tulane.edu

© Springer Nature Switzerland AG 2022
M. D. Stifelman et al. (eds.), *Techniques of Robotic Urinary Tract Reconstruction*, https://doi.org/10.1007/978-3-030-50196-9_5

requiring second intervention being 4% [3]. Pyeloplasty was described for the first time in 1886 by Trendelenburg [4]. Ureterotomy was introduced by Albarran as the first endosurgical repair in 1903, and then intubated ureterotomy was performed by Davis in 1943. Until the 1980s, the surgical treatment of UPJO was primarily open pyeloplasty and endopyelotomy. The era of minimally invasive approaches started in 1993 with Schuessler performing the first laparoscopic pyeloplasty [5]. The laparoscopic approach had overall comparable success rates and shorter postoperative recovery when compared with open pyeloplasty. Nevertheless, operative time was longer due to the technically demanding intracorporeal suturing; therefore, laparoscopic pyeloplasty was mainly relegated as a tertiary hospital procedure performed by experienced laparoscopic urological surgeons. The introduction of robotic laparoscopically assisted pyeloplasty in 2002 by Gettman [6] leveled the playing field and was a major advancement with improved quality of optics, acuity, and intracorporeal surgical abilities with robotic wrist movements. This led to significantly reduced operative time and learning curves for urological surgeons, including the laparoscopic naïve, and widespread adoption in both community and tertiary settings. In this chapter, we discuss our institution's experience and different techniques using the robotic approach for the management of adult pyeloplasty.

Indications

Ureteral obstruction is any impedance to normal antegrade urinary flow, which if left unaddressed will result in kidney injury and progressive loss of function.

Congenital causes are divided into intrinsic and extrinsic. UPJO from intrinsic causes includes ureteral smooth muscle maldevelopment resulting in the adynamic ureteral segment, which is the most common cause in the pediatric population. Insufficient recanalization during fetal development and persistent ureteral mucosal valvular folds are considered as being etiologic. Extrinsic causes include crossing aberrant/accessory vessel (lower pole, which is the most common cause in the adult population), high insertion of the ureter into the renal pelvis, and atypical renal anatomy which includes malrotated, ectopic, or horseshoe kidneys.

Acquired causes are severe vesicoureteral reflux, genitourinary trauma in general and instrumentation (iatrogenic), retroperitoneal fibrosis, and sequelae of urolithiasis management.

UPJO often presents with intermittent flank pain, usually post alcohol or diuretics (Dietl's crisis). Pyeloplasty indications also include progressive loss of renal function diagnosed classically with a diuretic nuclear medicine renogram showing prolonged drainage time as measured by T 1/2 time > 20 min and split function <40% for the obstructed kidney, associated with urolithiasis or upper tract infection. Nevertheless, in symptomatic cases with equivocal T1/2 (10–20 min) and worsening kidney function, pyeloplasty should be seriously considered. Open pyeloplasty is still performed in different parts of the world, where minimally invasive surgical training and equipment are not available or when extensive abdominal adhesions preclude a minimally invasive approach.

Contraindications

All approaches of pyeloplasty are contraindicated in the presence of active urine infection, uncorrected bleeding disorder, severe loss of renal function (<20% with recurrent kidney infections), or suspicious filling defect in the collecting system. In these cases, additional workup with ureteroscopy or extirpative surgery may be necessary. Additionally, it should be noted that minimally invasive pyeloplasty (laparoscopic or robotic) is the best option in cases of failed previous endopyelotomy, a very proximal ureteral stricture >1 cm, crossing vessel, severe hydronephrosis, and obstructed kidney with split function less than 25% [7].

Preoperative Care

Standard preoperative assessment includes routine laboratory tests: complete blood count, basic metabolic panel, PT/PTT if on anticoagulants, HbA1c for diabetics, EKG, and chest radiograph. Preoperative urine cultures should be obtained, and any urine infection should be adequately treated preoperatively.

Usually, patients should have some form of cross-sectional imaging, preferably a CT urogram showing the degree of hydronephrosis, related renal anatomy, stones, and crossing vessels. In addition, baseline diuretic renography is essential in assessing the degree of obstruction and split renal function of the two kidneys, and is used for follow-up.

Preoperative Cystoscopy

The patient would receive IV antibiotics at induction with second-generation cephalosporins with or without gentamicin, depending on allergies and previous urine culture results, and sequential pneumatic compression stockings are used for deep vein thrombosis (DVT) prophylaxis.

At our institution, cystoscopy with retrograde pyelogram is performed immediately prior to the definitive pyeloplasty. The cystoscopy would rule out any causes of urethral, prostatic, or bladder neck obstruction, and the retrograde pyelogram would assess for length and configuration of UPJO. In addition, it would rule out any unexpected ureteral strictures distal to the UPJO and any filling defects not consistent with stones. Leaving an in situ 5Fr ureteral catheter up to the UPJO would aid in identifying and transecting the ureter and facilitating retrograde placement of a guidewire and ureteral stent. The 5Fr ureteral catheter also facilitates direct intraluminal injection of indocyanine green (ICG) as an option to help identify the location of the ureter or renal pelvis should the need arise. Alternatively, surgeons can opt to use an antegrade technique to pass the ureteral stent through a port or percutaneously before completing the anastomosis.

Fig. 5.1 Port placement configuration for da Vinci Xi robot, all trocars are 8 mm, except for a trocar labeled 5 which is 14 mm

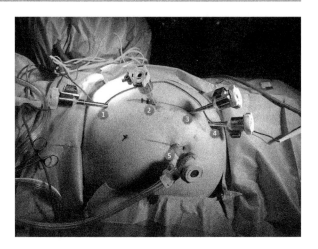

Positioning

Our preferred position is the modified lateral position. After initial cystoscopy and retrograde pyelography, the5Fr ureteral catheter and Foley catheter should be prepped into the sterile field to facilitate subsequent retrograde placement of the ureteral stent over a guidewire.

Our preference is to use a Veress needle to create pneumoperitoneum. Once pneumoperitoneum is established, robotic trocars are placed in the recommended straight-line configuration (da Vinci Xi) along a paramedian line with approximately 8 cm between each trocar. The second (camera) port is placed toward the renal hilum of the obstructed kidney. A 14-mm assistant port is also placed parallel and inferior to the straight line for suction and passage of needles (Fig. 5.1), a trocar labeled 5. A trocar labeled 4 is used for obese patients and those with retraction needs; it is not required in all patients.

Technique

1. The dissection starts along the white line of Toldt (Fig. 5.2) and the colon is reflected using the Maryland bipolar forceps and the monopolar scissors. This allows for access to the renal pelvis and ureter in the retroperitoneum. The ureter is then traced cephalad toward the renal pelvis.
2. The ureter can be identified by peristalsis and by the presence of the 5Fr ureteral catheter. Careful dissection in a manner so as to preserve the adventitial tissues and ureteral blood supply is performed. Then, the ureter is isolated in a vessel loop (Fig. 5.3). Injection of 5cc of ICG through the 5Fr ureteral catheter can help in early ureteral identification, especially in the obese, excessively fibrosed ureters, anomalous variants, and secondary UPJO repair. The renal

pelvis is dissected anteriorly and posteriorly (pelviolysis) to facilitate maximum mobilization for a tension-free anastomosis (Fig. 5.4).

3. The surgeon should assess for the presence of any crossing vessel, which might be present in approximately 40% of all cases of adult UPJO and even higher in patients undergoing secondary pyeloplasty [8]. Management of crossing vessels is discussed later in the chapter.

4. Stay sutures are placed in the renal pelvis and upper ureter, for assisting in dissection and minimizing tissue handling.

Fig. 5.2 Dissecting the colon (arrow) off the distended renal pelvis, along the white line of Toldt

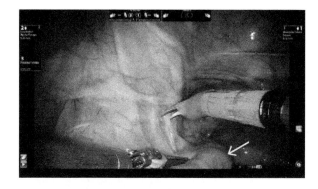

Fig. 5.3 The ureter is isolated with a vessel loop

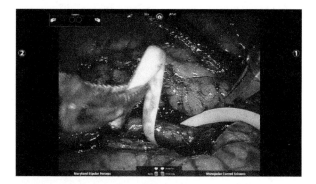

Fig. 5.4 The renal pelvis (yellow arrow) is dissected anteriorly and posteriorly (pelviolysis) to facilitate maximum mobilization for a tension-free anastomosis

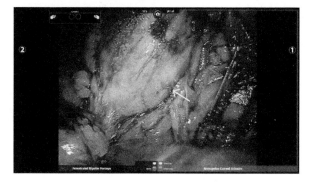

5. The UPJO is identified, and the ureter is transected just distal to the UPJ (Fig. 5.5). Prior to complete transection, while the ureter is stabilized, the ureteral end is spatulated (Fig. 5.6). The obstructed UPJO segment is then excised and sent for histopathology. Caution should be exercised so as to not transect the pre-placed 5Fr ureteral catheter or tamper with the integrity (bending and kinking) of the guidewire.

6. Careful evaluation of the renal pelvis and the ureter is then undertaken. Any additional scar tissue that may be visualized should be excised, and the two transected ends are mobilized to configure a tension-free anastomosis.

7. In case a crossing vessel has been identified, careful angiolysis is performed to ensure that the vessel descends posteriorly, so as to facilitate transposition of the collecting system superior to the crossing vessel, without any undue angulation or tension.

8. To optimize exposure to the UPJ area, we have often utilized a hitch stitch. This includes using a percutaneously placed Keith needle with 2-0 polyglactin suture

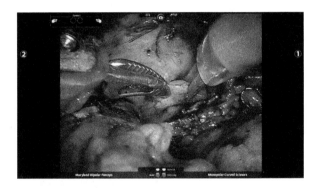

Fig. 5.5 UPJO is identified, and the ureter is transected just distal to the UPJ

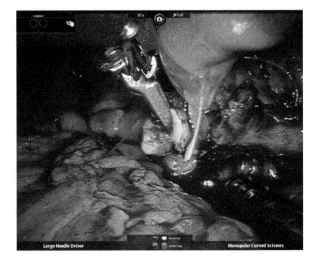

Fig. 5.6 The ureteral end is spatulated

that is passed through overlying abdominal wall and then utilizing this needle to apply traction on mobilized tissue, with the same needle, then exiting the abdominal wall. This exposes and provides traction on the operative area of interest without any impairment of vision from surrounding tissue. The hitch stitch can also be secured with surgical clips, securing any perinephric fat to the abdominal sidewall.

9. The posterior anastomosis is started by utilizing two 4-0 polyglactin sutures of different colors [dyed and undyed]. This anastomosis is performed similarly to the anastomosis technique van Velthoven described for the vesicourethral anastomosis for robotic radical prostatectomy (Fig. 5.7) [9]. The suturing is continuous, and each of these 4-0 sutures is circumferentially advanced in opposite directions until they meet anteriorly to complete the anastomosis. Use of interrupted sutures is another option and up to the surgeon's discretion.

10. Once the posterior portion of the anastomosis has been completed, the ureteral stent is placed. Our preference is to use the retrograde technique for placing the stent. For this, we use the pre-placed, 5Fr, open-ended ureteral catheter, and the bedside assistant passes the guidewire through the pre-placed, 5Fr open-ended catheter. The surgeon identifies and secures the guidewire with the robotic needle driver. Next, the Foley catheter is removed, as well as the 5Fr open-ended ureteral catheter, and the desired stent is then passed in a retrograde manner until it is visualized by the surgeon and determined to be secure and appropriately placed.

11. At the end of the procedure, flexible cystoscopy can be performed to ensure that the distal end of the ureteral stent is secured in the bladder.

12. The completed anastomosis of the UPJ is inspected, and the tied ends of the anastomotic sutures (yellow arrow) are confirmed to be securely knotted (Fig. 5.8).

13. An optional Jackson-Pratt drain or similar closed suction drain can be placed through one of the robotic trocars at the completion of the case.

Fig. 5.7 The ureteropelvic anastomosis is performed similar to the van Velthoven anastomosis for the vesicourethral anastomosis in robotic radical prostatectomy. The 5Fr ureteral catheter facilitates and protects the posterior ureteral wall

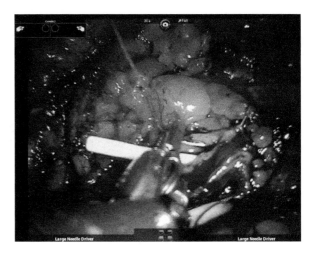

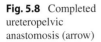**Fig. 5.8** Completed
ureteropelvic
anastomosis (arrow)

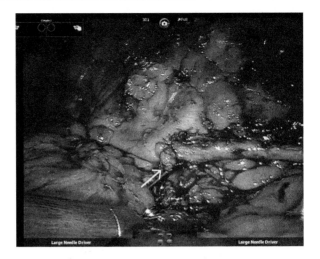

14. The kidney with its perinephric fat can be retroperitonealized by returning the colon back to its normal position. We believe this step is important in case one has to return to this area in the future.
15. The Foley catheter is reintroduced into the bladder, to promote low-pressure urinary drainage.

Transmesenteric Approach

This technique is utilized in pediatric patients or in very low-BMI adults who have a very thin mesocolon. In this instance, the colon does not have to be dissected from the sidewall, and the UPJO can be reached through the thin colonic mesentery. In such patients, one can observe the distended renal pelvis through the thin mesocolon. If a wide ureterolysis is required, it may be prudent to mobilize the colon rather than using this approach. The rest of the steps for the pyeloplasty are the same.

Retroperitoneal Approach

Though we have not utilized this technique, the retroperitoneal approach does provide direct access to the renal pelvis without accessing the peritoneal space. In a patient with a hostile abdomen, this approach could potentially lead to quicker recovery and less morbidity. However, the working space is significantly narrower, and one may not be able to readily evaluate the status of any crossing vessels. The technique for retroperitoneal access and dissection are similar for any retroperitoneal nephrectomy and partial nephrectomy. The pyeloplasty steps are otherwise similar to the previously described technique.

Dismembered Pyeloplasty

The dismembered pyeloplasty is the gold standard and most common technique for surgical management of UPJO. Using this versatile technique, the surgeon would be able to address the obstruction, excise the adynamic ureteral segment, preserve any crossing vessel, and optionally reduce redundant pelvic tissue (reduction pyeloplasty). After dissection of the upper ureter and renal pelvis, the ureter is isolated with a vessel loop, and angiolysis is performed for any crossing vessels. Traction sutures are placed on the medial and lateral aspects of the most dependent and redundant portion of the renal pelvis. Another two mirroring stay sutures are placed on the ureter, in a way that would preserve normal anatomical orientation for reconstruction (Fig. 5.9).

Reduction Pyeloplasty

Reduction of the renal pelvis is infrequently done. However, in patients who have a very capacious and redundant renal pelvis, it makes sense to taper the renal pelvis into a more efficient funnel, so as to decrease the transit time of the urine from the kidneys into the bladder. This option needs to be carefully considered because if the renal pelvis is massively dilated, it could slow down the urine transit time and postoperative imaging studies may show the persistence of hydronephrosis and/or delay of urinary transit time. In our practice, 6.4% of our patients [n = 248] have undergone a reduction pyeloplasty. Reduction of the renal pelvis is performed judiciously, because this maneuver should not compromise a tension-free anastomosis.

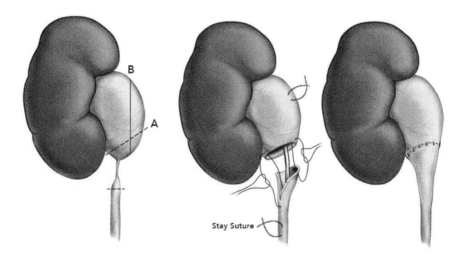

Fig. 5.9 Dismembered (line A) and reduction pyeloplasty (line B)

Foley Y-V Plasty

The Foley Y-V plasty is a non-dismembered technique that is best used in select UPJO cases with a high insertion of the ureter and no crossing vessel and in the absence of a dysplastic upper ureter. It requires more spatial visualization and surgical planning than classical dismembered technique. After exposing the renal pelvis and upper ureter, a long incision is made on the dependent aspect of the renal pelvis and continues along the lateral aspect of the upper ureter (Fig. 5.10(1)). The incision is carried inferiorly on the renal pelvis and anchoring sutures are taken (Fig. 5.10(2)). All limbs of the Y should be approximately equal in length. The apex of the V flap is advanced and sutured to the apex of the ureteral incision (Fig. 5.10(3)). A ureteral stent can be placed at this point before completing the anastomosis (Fig. 5.10(3)).

Vascular Hitch (Hellström Procedure)

This procedure was first described in 1949 by Hellström [11] to address UPJO associated with a crossing lower pole vessel without breaching the collecting system of the kidney. This technique first involves angiolysis, liberating the crossing vessel from the presumed underlying site of obstruction of the otherwise normal looking and peristalsing UPJ and ureter, with no obvious intrinsic obstruction. The crossing vessel is then mobilized cephalad from the UPJ site onto the renal pelvis and then fixed into position by imbricating the redundant wall of the pelvis around the crossing vessel using two or three absorbable sutures. This technique has mainly been applied to the pediatric population and to a lesser extent in adults. Interestingly, this technique has been reported to have comparable success rates to the classical dismembered pyeloplasty, in a small group of well-selected UPJO patients [12]. Given the paucity of data, this technique has not been widely adopted. We recommend adequate angiolysis to facilitate cephalad translocation of the crossing vessel whenever this anatomical configuration is encountered.

Spiral Flap

The spiral flap is best used for UPJO cases with a long ureteral stricture segment associated with dilated renal pelvis, where a dismembered pyeloplasty would result in excessive tension along with the anastomosis. Therefore, candidates for this option are those with the extrarenal pelvis, allowing for adequate tissue for the creation of a surgical flap. Careful planning with consideration of vascular blood supply to the flap is recommended to successfully implement this technique.

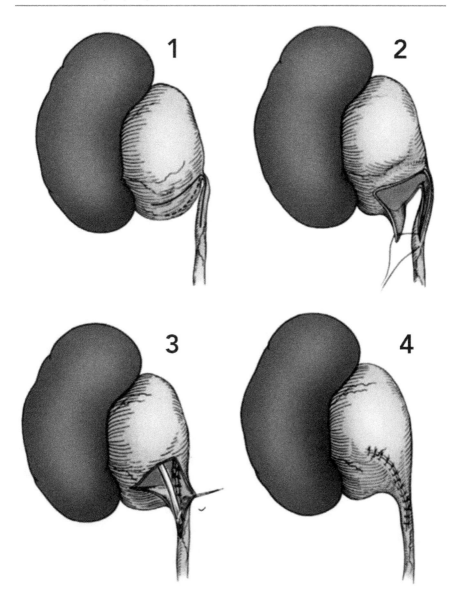

Fig. 5.10 The Foley Y-V plasty is, thus, a non-dismembered technique. (1)Incisions from the renal pelvis into the upper ureter. (2) Flap apex sutured to ureteral incision. (3) Stent in place. (4) Suture completed

H-M Repair

Heineke-Mikulicz repair is a non-dismembered technique to perform pyeloplasty in cases where the obstructed segment is short and in the absence of a dilated renal pelvis that may otherwise require reduction pyeloplasty. A longitudinal incision is extended through the obstructed UPJ segment and extended to expose normal caliber renal pelvis and ureter. The longitudinal incision is then closed transversely, thereby creating a wide-open lumen at the previously obstructed site.

Transposition of Crossing Vessels

We have carefully analyzed the rationale for and the techniques of transposition of crossing vessels. All patients with crossing vessels do not require transposition of the collecting vessels superior to the crossing vessels. Very often, adequate angiolysis and pelviolysis can free the renal pelvis and UPJ from the crossing vessels (Fig. 5.11). Once the UPJ area has been reevaluated following the pelviolysis and angiolysis, a decision can then be made regarding the need for transection and transposition of the urinary collecting system superior to any crossing vessel. Our preference is that the new UPJ anastomosis should be approximately 1 cm distal to the existing crossing vessel for optimum postoperative results [13].

Downward Nephropexy

For optimum success in any reconstructive procedure, lack of tension at the anastomotic site is crucial. If there is tension in a given case, the first option is usually to perform further pelviolysis and ureterolysis to gain further mobility. Another important option is to perform downward nephropexy when ureteral and renal pelvis

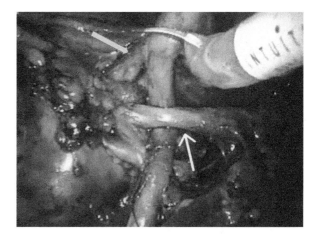

Fig. 5.11 Crossing vessel. The UPJO transection to transpose above the crossing vessel (yellow arrow) after ureterolysis. The renal pelvis is marked (green arrow)

mobilization has been maximized or ineffective. To execute a downward nephropexy, the entire kidney must be fully mobilized and perinephric fat dissected off the kidney and attached only at the renal hilum. The kidney is then transposed caudally toward the bladder and fixed to the lateral abdominal wall and to the psoas muscle. We prefer taking a total of three stitches an using absorbable 2-0 braided polyglactin suture with a CT-2 needle. This stitch is thrown with a wide, shallow capsular bite, including minimal renal parenchyma. We recommend placing all the sutures first and then sequentially tying them. The pyeloplasty is then continued as described above [7].

Calculi Associated with UPJO

Usually, in such patients, multiple calculi are encountered. These can be managed after transection of the UPJ and using a flexible nephroscope (flexible cystoscope), which is passed through one of the ports (Fig. 5.12). Details of this technique have been previously published [8].

Postoperative Care

In postoperative care, early patient mobilization is an important factor. Diet is given as tolerated, and we encourage minimizing the use of narcotics. If a JP drain has been placed, the output can be evaluated for a fluid creatinine level, and if

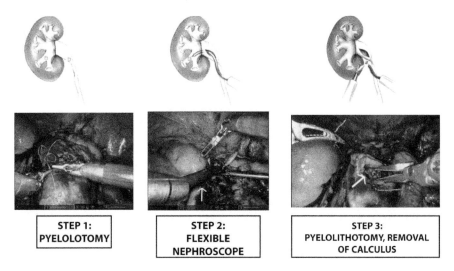

Fig. 5.12 Management of pelvic stone in patients with UPJO, performing pyelolithotomy. Step 1: pyelotomy: the renal pelvis is accessed after transection of the UPJ. Step 2: the flexible nephroscope (flexible cystoscope -arrow) is passed through the pyelotomy, and the stone is located, and continuous suction of the irrigation fluid is maintained. Step 3: pyelolithotomy: the stone (arrow) is removed either with robotic graspers or basketed with the flexible nephroscope

equal to the serum values, the closed suction drain is removed in 24–48 h. If there is continuing concern regarding the integrity of the anastomosis, the drain can be left in for a couple more days, and drain fluid creatinine level is remeasured. The Foley catheter is usually discontinued within 24 h, unless there are technical concerns of the anastomotic site or confirmed urinary drainage from the closed suction drain (JP).

Most patients can be discharged on postoperative day #1, and if needed, arrangements can be made for outpatient management of drains and catheters. Outpatient ureteral stent removal typically occurs at 6 weeks for the uncomplicated patient.

Follow-up imaging is variable among urologists. We prefer postoperative evaluation with a CT scan and a mercaptoacetyltriglycine-3 (MAG-3) diuretic renal scan in 6–12 weeks after stent removal. Even with our referred patients, we encourage postoperative imaging at the same hospital site, using the same equipment and personnel to optimize the comparison of pre- and postoperative follow-up studies. Patients are also assessed for the recurrence of flank pain and infections. Follow-up is maintained for at least 1 year, with the two major criteria for postoperative success being improvement in symptoms and improvement/stabilization of the functional status of the kidney.

Database

Our updated database includes 248 patients, with the age range of 9 months to 83 years and the median age of 42 years. In our cohort, we have 139 females vs 109 males and 107 left-sided vs 141 right-sided. Crossing vessels were found in 101 patients with only 47 requiring transposition (46.5%). Concomitant pyelolithotomy was performed in 24 cases (9.6%), and reduction pyeloplasty was only performed in 16 patients (6.4%). References (8, 10, 13–15) highlight our published techniques and results.

Conclusion

The management of UPJO has significantly advanced over the past three decades due to advances in endoscopic approaches, proliferation of laparoscopic techniques, and introduction of robotic surgery. Robotic surgery has changed the paradigm and leveled the playing field by enabling surgeons at the community level to offer robotic pyeloplasty to their patients. The results have been comparable to those reported with the so-called gold standard of open surgical "dismembered" pyeloplasty. This chapter has highlighted the robotic management of various pyeloplasty techniques. The foundations of gentle tissue handling, vascular preservation, precise mucosal realignment, and tension-free anastomosis continue to remain as keys to a successful pyeloplasty, regardless of approach.

References

1. Tripp BM, Homsy YL. Neonatal hydronephrosis–the controversy and the management. Pediatr Nephrol. 1995;9(4):503–9.
2. Lam JS, Breda A, Schulam PG. Ureteropelvic junction obstruction. J Urol. 2007;177(5): 1652–8.
3. Stephen Y, Nakada MD. FaSLBM. Management of Upper Urinary Tract Obstruction. In: Wein AJ, Kavoussi LR, Partin AW, Peters CA, editors. Campbell-Walsh urology. 11th ed. Philadelphia: Elsevier, Inc.; 2016. p. 1104–47.
4. Murphy LJT. History of urology. Springfield: C. Thomas; 1972.
5. Schuessler WW, Grune MT, Tecuanhuey LV, Preminger GM. Laparoscopic dismembered pyeloplasty. J Urol. 1993;150(6):1795–9.
6. Gettman MT, Peschel R, Neururer R, Bartsch G. A comparison of laparoscopic pyeloplasty performed with the daVinci robotic system versus standard laparoscopic techniques: initial clinical results. Eur Urol. 2002;42(5):453–7; discussion 7-8
7. Bergersen A, Thomas R, Lee BR. Robotic Pyeloplasty. J Endourol. 2018;32(S1):S68–s72.
8. Atug F, Castle EP, Burgess SV, Thomas R. Concomitant management of renal calculi and pelvi-ureteric junction obstruction with robotic laparoscopic surgery. BJU Int. 2005;96(9):1365–8. (1464-4096 (Print)
9. Van Velthoven RF, Ahlering TE, Peltier A, Skarecky DW, Clayman RV. Technique for laparoscopic running urethrovesicalanastomosis: the single knot method. Urology. 2003;61(4):699–702.
10. Atug F, Woods M, Burgess SV, Castle EP, Thomas R. Robotic assisted laparoscopic pyelo-plasty in children. J Urol. 2005;174(4 Pt 1):1440–2.
11. Hellström J Giertz G, Lindblom K. Pathogenesis and treatment of hydronephrosis. In: VIII Congreso de la Sociedad International de Urologia; Paris, 1949.
12. Gundeti MS, Reynolds WS, Duffy PG, Mushtaq I. Further experience with the vascular hitch (laparoscopic transposition of lower pole crossing vessels): an alternate treatment for pedi-atric ureterovascular ureteropelvic junction obstruction. J Urol. 2008;180(4 Suppl):1832–6. discussion 6
13. Boylu U, Oommen M, Lee BR, Thomas R. Ureteropelvic junction obstruction secondary to crossing vessels-to transpose or not? The robotic experience. J Urol. 2009;181(4):1751–5.
14. Mufarrij PW, Woods M, Shah OD, Palese MA, Berger AD, Thomas R, et al. Robotic dismem-bered pyeloplasty: a 6-year, multi-institutional experience. J Urol. 2008;180(4):1391–6.
15. Mendez-Torres F, Woods M, Thomas R. Technical modifications for robot-assisted laparo-scopic pyeloplasty. J Endourol. 2005;19(3):393–6.

Pediatric Robotic Pyeloplasty

6

Michael Daugherty and Paul H. Noh

Introduction

Pyeloplasty is considered the gold standard treatment for ureteropelvic junction obstruction. This may be performed using both open and minimally invasive approaches. The minimally invasive approach can be performed with conventional laparoscopy as well as with robotic assistance. With the widespread adoption of robot-assisted laparoscopic surgery by urology residency training programs along with the benefits of wristed instrumentation and optics with depth perception provided by robotic surgical systems, many pediatric urologists opt to perform a minimally invasive pyeloplasty using the robotic platform [1–3]. Although patient factors affect the feasibility of robotic pyeloplasty especially regarding patient size, it has been successfully performed with comparable outcomes in infants [4, 5].

Indications/Contraindications

The indications for patients undergoing robotic pyeloplasty are those diagnosed with ureteropelvic junction obstruction. This has been offered to families with

Supplementary Information The online version of this chapter (https://doi.org/10.1007/978-3-030-50196-9_6) contains supplementary material, which is available to authorized users.

M. Daugherty
Division of Pediatric Urology, Cincinnati Children's Hospital Medical Center,
Cincinnati, OH, USA
e-mail: michael.daugherty@cchmc.org

P. H. Noh (✉)
University Urology, University of South Alabama, Mobile,
Alabama, USA
e-mail: pnoh@health.southalabama.edu

© Springer Nature Switzerland AG 2022
M. D. Stifelman et al. (eds.), *Techniques of Robotic Urinary Tract Reconstruction*, https://doi.org/10.1007/978-3-030-50196-9_6

infants as young as 4 weeks of age, with the smallest size being performed at our institution of 4.5 kg. Contraindications are consistent with those of any transabdominal laparoscopic surgery, including multiple previous open abdominal surgeries or poor pulmonary function that would not allow for abdominal insufflation.

Preoperative Preparation and Evaluation

Routine preoperative evaluation often includes a serum blood urea nitrogen and creatinine level along with a urine culture. Imaging studies typically include a renal ultrasound and a nuclear diuretic renogram. A computerized tomography scan is occasionally utilized in emergency rooms for children presenting with symptoms consistent with renal colic. An intravenous pyelogram is rarely utilized currently. Patients often undergo a preoperative bowel preparation using polyethylene glycol prior to surgery. This is not mandatory, but we prefer using it to help facilitate colon reflection and to maintain good exposure of the retroperitoneum. Symptomatic children may have a ureteral stent or nephrostomy tube placement prior to a definitive repair; however, it is preferred to avoid these drains prior to surgery, since they can cause tissue inflammation prior to the repair.

Patient Position

For the robotic portion of the procedure, the patient is placed in a varying flank position based on surgeon preference, with completely secure support to the operating room table. Gel rolls and foam padding may be utilized (Fig. 6.1a). The patient is placed with the umbilicus at the level of table flexion. The table is flexed to create more working space. The kidney rest is not utilized. An axillary roll is typically not needed when not using a full flank position. A lateral arm board can be used for positioning the lower arm, with padding such as foam or pillows to support the upper arm. An alternative is to place the ipsilateral arm along the body in its natural position (Fig. 6.1b). For the very small infants, the arm board for the operating table is often too large, where an intravenous access securement board can be used to act as an appropriately sized arm board. The patient is secured to the table with safety straps and/or tape over the chest, hips, legs, and head, with padding placed under all pressure points, to keep the patient completely immobilized (Fig. 6.1c,d). Positioning is tested with the table tilted as much as possible in both directions to ensure the patient is properly secured (Fig. 6.1e). Some surgeons use a supine position, but this may not be reliable for optimizing the view for all cases.

Trocar Placement

For the da Vinci Xi robot, three robotic trocars (8 mm) are typically utilized. A trocar is placed via an open technique through the umbilicus. Two additional trocars are then placed under direct visualization. Typically, a trocar is placed in the midline above and below the umbilicus (Fig. 6.2a). In some cases, with very small infants,

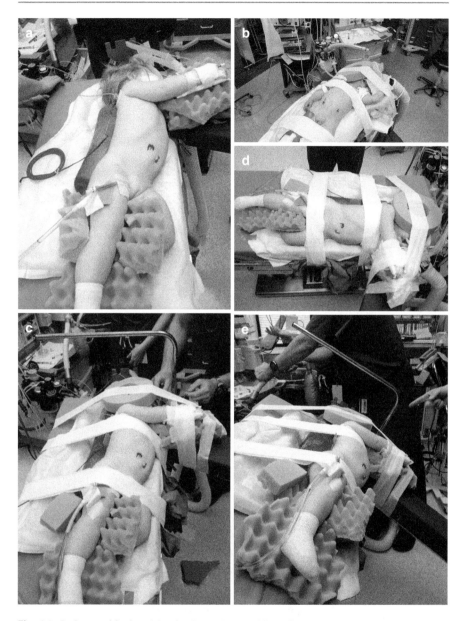

Fig. 6.1 Patient positioning: (**a**) gel roll and foam padding; (**b**) arm along the side of the body in natural position; (**c** and **d**) safety straps and tape across head, chest, and hips; (**e**) full tilt used to confirm secure immobilization

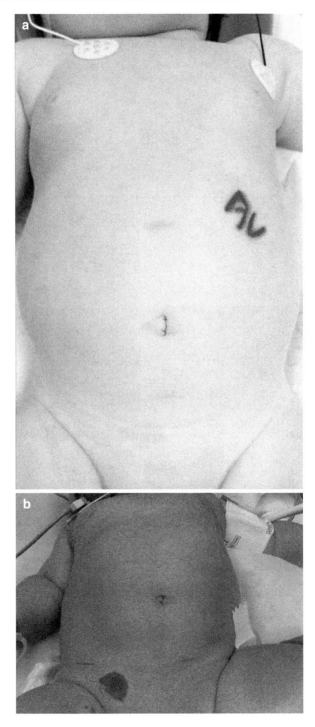

Fig. 6.2 Trocar positioning: (**a**) postoperative appearance after midline trocars; (**b**) postoperative appearance after umbilical and Pfannenstiel trocars

two trocars are placed in the midline above the umbilicus. When this occurs, the camera will be placed in the middle trocar. These working trocars are all placed under direct vision. Some surgeons prefer the lower trocar in the ipsilateral lower quadrant, similar to the placement for a conventional laparoscopic pyeloplasty. The minimal space that is felt to be necessary to adequately perform the operation is approximately 2.5 cm between the trocars. Another alternative for the trocar position is to utilize the umbilicus with the other trocars placed along the Pfannenstiel line (Fig. 6.2b) [6, 7]. The lower midline trocar would be used for the camera.

Step-by-Step Procedure

The procedure may begin with cystoscopy and a retrograde ureteropyelogram on the side of the intended repair. The retrograde ureteropyelogram allows for the identification and localization of ureteral pathology (Fig. 6.3a–d). The additional information obtained regarding the ureteral anatomy can help with surgical planning. Some surgeons prefer to place a retrograde ureteral stent at the beginning of the procedure, which may include leaving the dangler string in place exiting the urethra to facilitate future removal without the need for another general anesthetic session.

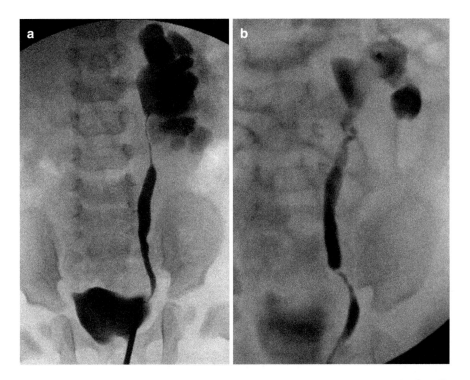

Fig. 6.3 Retrograde pyelograms: (**a**) demonstrating long gap proximal ureteral atresia; (**b**) solitary kidney with concomitant distal ureteral valve; (**c**) crossing vessels; (**d**) mid ureteral obstruction

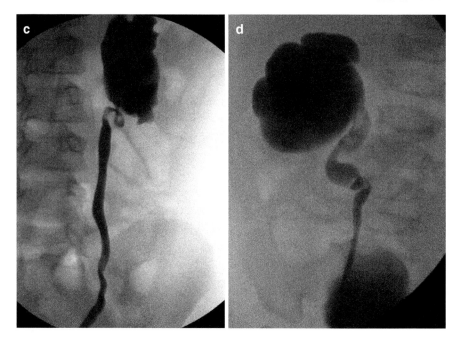

Fig. 6.3 (continued)

If an antegrade ureteral stent placement is planned in small infants, a wire or ureteral catheter left across the ureterovesical junction at the beginning of the procedure may be beneficial to help facilitate passing the stent through a tight ureterovesical junction antegrade later during the procedure. A Foley catheter is placed prior to the positioning for a pyeloplasty.

The patient is positioned to the appropriate flank position. Open access can be obtained through a vertical transumbilical incision after everting the umbilicus. Care is taken to avoid making the fascial opening larger than the robotic trocar, to prevent slippage of the trocar or gas leak after insufflation and docking. An 8 mm robotic port is placed, and the abdomen is insufflated after confirming intraperitoneal trocar placement with direct visualization. The abdomen is insufflated with a very slow flow rate, to help minimize the potential for postoperative pain from a rapid stretch of the abdominal wall. Two additional working trocars are placed under direct vision. The robot is then positioned appropriately over the patient, and the trocars are docked to the robot (Fig. 6.4). Our preferred instruments for pyeloplasty are the micro bipolar forceps, monopolar scissors, and a suture cut needle driver. Our preferred camera is the 30-degree lens in the down direction.

We prefer to reflect the colon to optimize exposure. Some surgeons prefer a transmesenteric approach, which is feasible for many left-sided procedures (Fig. 6.5). The colon is reflected medially with sharp and blunt dissection. The psoas muscle can be used as a landmark to maintain proper orientation. The ureter

Fig. 6.4 Robot docked with midline trocar placement

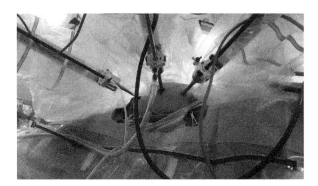

Fig. 6.5 Transmesenteric window with obstructing accessory lower pole renal vessels exposed

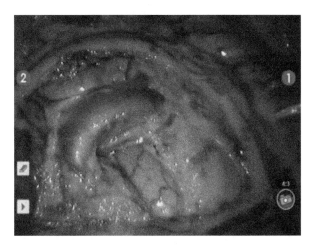

is identified and circumferentially dissected near the level of the lower pole of the kidney. This dissection is then continued proximally toward the renal hilum. It is imperative to identify any crossing vessels, as these may be a key factor leading to the obstruction (Fig. 6.5). Percutaneous traction sutures for the renal pelvis may facilitate performing the procedure without requiring additional trocars for the bedside assistant or the fourth robotic arm. If needed, the traction suture is placed as early as possible. Our preferred method is to use a small Prolene suture on a Keith needle (Fig. 6.6). Care must be taken to secure the tail of this suture outside of the abdomen. The needle is passed through the renal pelvis and then back out through the abdominal wall in a similar location. The location of the percutaneous traction suture should allow for optimal retraction to facilitate dissection and subsequent reconstruction. The traction suture can also be placed with a curved needle, with straightening of the needle if needed to allow for easier passage through the abdominal wall.

Dissection is completed to optimize exposure of the renal pelvis, the ureter, and the location of obstruction, in preparation for dismemberment and reconstruction. A rind of tissue encasing the renal pelvis and ureter may be found, often in

Fig. 6.6 Percutaneous traction suture using a Keith needle

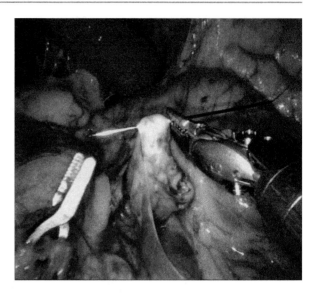

symptomatic patients. If bleeding is encountered, a small sponge, such as a neuro sponge pattie, can be introduced through a robotic trocar while holding pressure, to subsequently help achieve hemostasis. If brisk bleeding is encountered, additional access may be beneficial to safely control bleeding without requiring open conversion. If crossing vessels are a component of the obstruction, the UPJ is transected with cold scissors and then transposed anteriorly to the vessels for the anastomosis. If there are no crossing vessels present, the UPJ is transected with cold scissors on an angle that facilitates anastomosis after ureteral spatulation. Renal pelvis reduction is typically not performed. Our preference is to achieve a symmetric size lumen of the renal pelvis to the spatulated ureter, to obviate a need to close any residual opening of the renal pelvis after UPJ reconstruction. The ureter is spatulated in a direction to optimize the reconstruction, typically laterally. In some cases, such as a medial high insertion of the ureter into the renal pelvis or lateral ectopic insertion close to the parenchyma, repositioning the UPJ to a more dependent position on the renal pelvis may be preferable for reconstruction. Most procedures do not require complex reconstruction with a renal pelvis flap. For reoperative procedures after a failed previous pyeloplasty, an augmented reconstruction using buccal mucosa can be used if needed [8].

Depending on the patient size, we prefer 5-0 or 6-0 polyglactin absorbable suture for the anastomosis. Typically, a 6-0 suture is used with a BV-1 needle. Sutures are passed into the abdomen through one of the robotic trocars by the bedside assistant, or a bedside assistant accessory trocar per surgeon preference. We prefer using a micro bipolar forceps and the suture cut needle driver for suturing during the reconstruction. The suture cut needle driver allows for higher efficiency and the minimization of instrument exchanges when cutting sutures.

While it is more common to perform a running anastomosis, we prefer interrupted sutures for the anastomosis. In our experience, interrupted sutures, spaced about a half mm to 1 mm apart, allows for a watertight tubeless pyeloplasty (Fig. 6.7a,b) [9]. Typically, the distal apex is approximated first, with careful attention to prevent a twist in the alignment of the ureter to the renal pelvis. During the anastomosis, it may be necessary to adjust the tension on the traction suture during suture placement and knot tying. For interrupted suturing, the knots are typically extraluminal; however, this is not mandatory. At times, some of the sutures are placed with an intraluminal knot to facilitate suture placement, especially for the youngest patients with more delicate tissues. For very small infants undergoing robotic pyeloplasty, there may be a large amount of body wall motion during ventilation. It may be helpful to have the anesthesiologist hold respirations during these suture placements.

Prior to completing the reconstruction, a decision needs to be made regarding stenting across the anastomosis. With the interrupted suture technique, we routinely perform a tubeless pyeloplasty. If a decision is made to stent across the anastomosis,

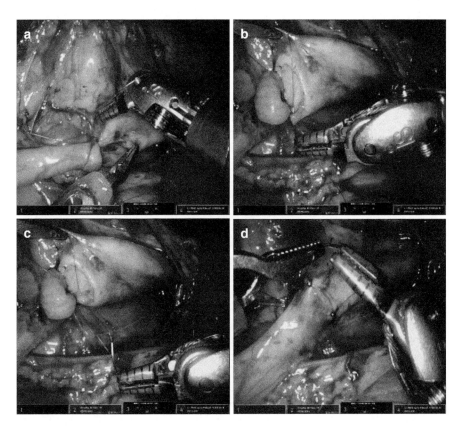

Fig. 6.7 Interrupted anastomosis: (**a**) apex approximation; (**b**) lateral posterior wall suture placement; (**c**) lateral posterior wall suture pulled through; (**d**) mid anterior wall suture; (**e**) medial anterior wall suture placement; (**f**) medial anterior wall suture being tied; (**g**) completed reconstruction anterior wall; (**h**) completed reconstruction posterior wall

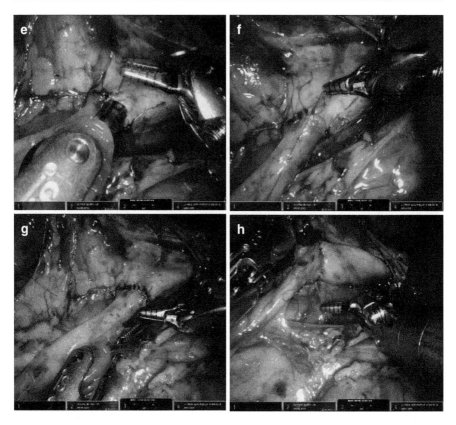

Fig. 6.7 (continued)

we prefer antegrade stent placement [10]. The stent can be passed through the abdominal wall using a percutaneous 14-gauge angiocatheter (Fig. 6.8). The stent can be passed over a wire or passed as a single unit with the wire in place. To help confirm the appropriate stent position in the bladder, the bladder can be filled with methylene blue-stained saline, to look for retrograde refluxing fluid (Fig. 6.9). Another option is to use intraoperative ultrasound of the bladder to identify the stent. A drain external to the anastomosis is generally not needed. We prefer to avoid leaving a stent with a retrieval string exiting the urethra. An alternative to an indwelling ureteral stent may include a nephrostomy tube, which may be placed through the renal pelvis or a calix or an externalized nephroureteral catheter to stent across the anastomosis.

Any residual fluid in the abdomen should be removed to help limit postoperative ileus. This can be performed with a suction irrigator or by using a sterile tube placed through one of the trocars, with passive drainage from gas insufflation pressure (Fig. 6.10a, b). A final inspection is performed to confirm hemostasis. Subsequently, the trocars are removed, and the fascia openings are closed. Local anesthesia is injected around the trocar sites for postoperative pain management.

Fig. 6.8 A percutaneous 14 gauge angiocatheter used for antegrade ureteral stent placement over a wire, which can also be used to vent smoke

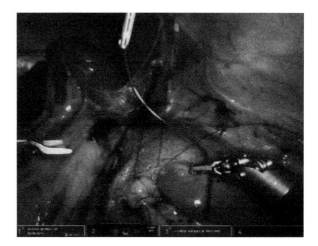

Fig. 6.9 Methylene blue-stained saline refluxing retrograde from bladder confirming stent position

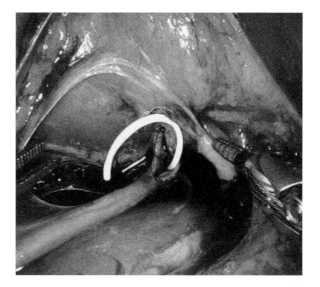

Postoperative Management

At our institution, these are outpatient procedures, where the Foley catheter is removed immediately at the end of the procedure. Patients are discharged as per recovery room protocol without an extended stay. Narcotic-free pain management strategies include alternating ibuprofen and acetaminophen on a scheduled regimen. Alpha blockers and diazepam are also used as adjuncts. Patients who stay for overnight observation receive scheduled intravenous acetaminophen and ketorolac, without requiring any narcotics. If an indwelling ureteral stent was utilized, it is

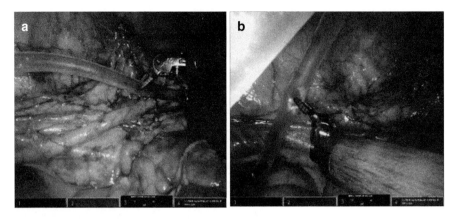

Fig. 6.10 Passive suctioning with a soft catheter passed through trocar: (**a**) catheter removal fluid near hilum; (**b**) catheter removing fluid in pelvis

typically removed 4–6 weeks after pyeloplasty, although many surgeons prefer sooner. Postoperative imaging usually includes a renal ultrasound at 3 months and subsequent renal ultrasounds 6 to 12 months later. Postoperative renography is not routinely utilized and only is performed if significant improvement of hydronephrosis is not observed by ultrasound assessment.

Complications

Rates of complications have been reported to be similar for both open and robotic/laparoscopic approaches, between 2.0 and 28.0% [11–24]. The majority tend to be Clavien grade 1 and grade 2 complications [12]. Complications that have been reported include anastomotic leakage, obstruction, urinary tract infection, trocar site hernia, stent dislodgement, and ileus [23]. The reoperation rate for robotic pyeloplasty is low and has been reported to be 0.7–3.0% [24].

References

1. Bowen DK, Lindgren BW, Cheng EY, Gong EM. Can proctoring affect the learning curve of robotic-assisted laparoscopic pyeloplasty? Experience at a high-volume pediatric robotic surgery center. J Robot Surg. 2017;11(1):63–7.
2. Reinhardt S, Ifaoui IB, Thorup J. Robotic surgery start-up with a fellow as the console surgeon. Scand J Urol. 2017;51(4):335–8.
3. Tasian GE, Wiebe DJ, Casale P. Learning curve of robotic assisted pyeloplasty for pediatric urology fellows. J Urol. 2013;190(4 Suppl):1622–6.
4. Bansal D, Cost NG, DeFoor WR Jr, et al. Infant robotic pyeloplasty: comparison with an open cohort. J Pediatr Urol. 2014;10(2):380–5.
5. Paradise HJ, Huang GO, Elizondo Saenz RA, Baek M, Koh CJ. Robot-assisted laparoscopic pyeloplasty in infants using 5-mm instruments. J Pediatr Urol. 2017;13(2):221–2.

6. Gargollo PC. Hidden incision endoscopic surgery: description of technique, parental satisfaction and applications. J Urol. 2011;185(4):1425–31.
7. Hong YH, DeFoor WR Jr, Reddy PP, Schulte M, Minevich EA, VanderBrink BA, Noh PH. Hidden incision endoscopic surgery (HIdES) trocar placement for pediatric robotic pyeloplasty: comparison to traditional port placement. J Robot Surg. 2018;12(1):43–7.
8. Ahn JJ, Shapiro ME, Ellison JS, Lendvay TS. Pediatric robot-assisted redo pyeloplasty with buccal mucosa graft: a novel technique. Urology. 2017;101:56–9.
9. Fichtenbaum EJ, Strine AC, Concodora CW, Schulte M, Noh PH. Tubeless outpatient robotic upper urinary tract reconstruction in the pediatric population: short-term assessment of safety. J Robot Surg. 2018;12(2):257–60.
10. Noh PH, DeFoor WR, Reddy PP. Percutaneous antegrade ureteral stent placement during pediatric robot-assisted laparoscopic pyeloplasty. J Endourol. 2011;25(12):1847–51.
11. Chan YY, Durbin-Johnson B, Sturm RM, Kurzrock EA. Outcomes after pediatric open, laparoscopic, and robotic pyeloplasty at academic institutions. J Pediatr Urol. 2017;13(1):49.e1–6.
12. Dangle PP, Akhavan A, Odeleye M, et al. Ninety-day perioperative complications of pediatric robotic urological surgery: a multi-institutional study. J Pediatr Urol. 2016;12(2):102.e1–6.
13. Dangle PP, Kearns J, Anderson B, Gundeti MS. Outcomes of infants undergoing robot-assisted laparoscopic pyeloplasty compared to open repair. J Urol. 2013;190(6):2221–6.
14. Franco I, Dyer LL, Zelkovic P. Laparoscopic pyeloplasty in the pediatric patient: hand sewn anastomosis versus robotic assisted anastomosis--is there a difference? J Urol. 2007;178(4) Pt 1:1483–6.
15. Lee RS, Retik AB, Borer JG, Peters CA. Pediatric robot assisted laparoscopic dismembered pyeloplasty: comparison with a cohort of open surgery. J Urol. 2006;175(2):683–7; discussion 7
16. Minnillo BJ, Cruz JA, Sayao RH, et al. Long-term experience and outcomes of robotic assisted laparoscopic pyeloplasty in children and young adults. J Urol. 2011;185(4):1455–60.
17. Olsen LH, Rawashdeh YF, Jorgensen TM. Pediatric robot assisted retroperitoneoscopic pyeloplasty: a 5-year experience. J Urol. 2007;178(5):2137–41; discussion 41
18. Riachy E, Cost NG, Defoor WR, Reddy PP, Minevich EA, Noh PH. Pediatric standard and robot-assisted laparoscopic pyeloplasty: a comparative single institution study. J Urol. 2013;189(1):283–7.
19. Singh P, Dogra PN, Kumar R, Gupta NP, Nayak B, Seth A. Outcomes of robot-assisted laparoscopic pyeloplasty in children: a single center experience. J Endourol Endourol Soc. 2012;26(3):249–53.
20. Sorensen MD, Delostrinos C, Johnson MH, Grady RW, Lendvay TS. Comparison of the learning curve and outcomes of robotic assisted pediatric pyeloplasty. J Urol. 2011;185(6 Suppl):2517–22.
21. Subotic U, Rohard I, Weber DM, Gobet R, Moehrlen U, Gonzalez R. A minimal invasive surgical approach for children of all ages with ureteropelvic junction obstruction. J Pediatr Urol. 2012;8(4):354–8.
22. Yee DS, Shanberg AM, Duel BP, Rodriguez E, Eichel L, Rajpoot D. Initial comparison of robotic-assisted laparoscopic versus open pyeloplasty in children. Urology. 2006;67(3):599–602.
23. Cundy TP, Harling L, Hughes-Hallett A, Mayer EK, Najmaldin AS, Athanasiou T, Yang GZ, Darzi A. Meta-analysis of robot-assisted vs conventional laparoscopic and open pyeloplasty in children. BJU Int. 2014;114(4):582–94.
24. Boysen WR, Gundeti MS. Robot-assisted laparoscopic pyeloplasty in the pediatric population: a review of technique, outcomes, complications, and special considerations in infants. Pediatr Surg Int. 2017;33(9):925–35.

Managing Stones: Unusual Anatomy in a Patient with UPJ Obstruction

7

Ram A. Pathak and Ashok K. Hemal

Introduction

The management of ureteropelvic junction obstruction in the adult and pediatric patients has been refined over the years with a greater emphasis on minimally invasive alternatives over traditional open surgery. Initially, the laparoscopic approach gave way to robotic assistance allowing for easier dissection and reconstruction [1]. Excellent perioperative and intermediate results have been achieved utilizing the robotic approach with a mean operative time of 194 minutes, estimated blood loss of 50 ml, and perioperative complication rate of 6% [2]. Although outcome analysis of robotic pyeloplasty has been overwhelmingly effective [3], on occasion, secondary pathologies or unusual anatomy in these patients arise prompting additional surgical interventions. This chapter delves into the management of UPJ obstruction with concomitant nephrolithiasis and patients presenting with unusual anatomy.

Management of Nephrolithiasis in Patients with Ureteropelvic Junction Obstruction

Up to 30% of patients with UPJ obstruction have concomitant nephrolithiasis [4] (Fig. 7.1). The management of both primary UPJ obstruction and extraction of renal lithiasis is key in caring for these patients. The pathophysiology of calculus formation in patients with UPJ obstruction is the resultant urinary stasis and delayed

Supplementary Information The online version of this chapter (https://doi. org/10.1007/978-3-030-50196-9_7) contains supplementary material, which is available to authorized users.

R. A. Pathak (✉) · A. K. Hemal
Department of Urology, Wake Forest University Baptist Medical Center, Winston-Salem, NC, USA
e-mail: rpathak@wakehealth.edu; ahemal@wakehealth.edu

© Springer Nature Switzerland AG 2022
M. D. Stifelman et al. (eds.), *Techniques of Robotic Urinary Tract Reconstruction*, https://doi.org/10.1007/978-3-030-50196-9_7

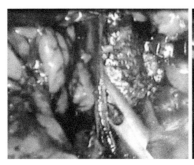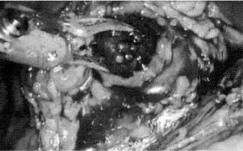

Fig. 7.1 Nephrolithiasis with concomitant UPJ obstruction. Left-sided image depicts left robot-assisted pyelolithotomy and extraction of staghorn calculus. Right-sided image depicts right pyelolithotomy and extraction of staghorn calculus

excretion of stone crystalline aggregates; in turn, calculus formation via the processes of nucleation, crystal growth, and aggregation is hastened. In fact, successful pyeloplasty repair yields to exceedingly low stone recurrence rates [5].

Preoperative Considerations

The technical aspects of the procedure are similar to both the adult and pediatric pyeloplasty operations with the exception of adjunctive procedures for stone removal.

Preoperative and Operative Room Setup

Preoperative planning is critical in guiding patient position, for example, semi-flank position for a horseshoe kidney and supine for a pelvic kidney. A CT angiogram can be obtained to review and assess spatial anatomy with a relationship to the vasculature. A KUB plain X-ray should also be reviewed to define relevant nephrolithiasis. As both endoscopic instrumentation and robotic instrumentation are utilized for these procedures, surgeons may face significant space constraints with additional light/video towers, laser machines, etc. The robotic light source, insufflator machine, and energy source towers are kept at the foot of the bed. Endoscopic towers for holmium laser lithotripsy and video equipment should flank the robotic tower in such a manner to avoid significant cord collusions.

Caveats to Port Placement

Robotic port placement can be reviewed elsewhere [6] and is identical to traditional robotic-assisted pyeloplasty (Fig. 7.2). A 5 mm or 12 mm assistant port can be useful for the introduction of various basket extractors or flexible ureteroscopy/nephroscopy (with corresponding increase in trocar diameter) for stone retrieval. In

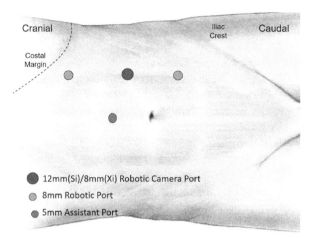

Fig. 7.2 Port placement for concomitant pyeloplasty and pyelolithotomy. The camera port is placed lateral and cranial to the umbilicus along the lateral border of the rectus sheath with flanking robotic trocars approximately 6–8 cm apart. A 5 mm assistant port is placed cranial to the umbilicus in the midline. Typically, a 3-arm approach is needed

patients with scoliosis or history of spinal fusion, we recommend midline placement of robotic trocars.

Tips and Tricks

The operative technique for initial kidney dissection and renal pelvis exposure has been described in the previous two chapters for both adult and pediatric patients. When dealing with calculi, certain caveats to traditional pyeloplasty must be mentioned. Many patients with UPJ obstruction and kidney stones have likely undergone prior stone procedures in the past including SWL or PCNL or even have a history of pyelonephritis. Therefore, the peripelvic and periureteral fat may be adherent to underlying inflammation. Dissection in this area is critical as the development of Gil-Vernet's plane allows appropriate exposure to the major calyces if needed for concomitant handling of large staghorn stones. The renal pelvis should be dissected away from the overlying renal vasculature without dissection of the renal moiety. If a calyceal diverticulum is suspected, then kidney dissection and diverticulectomy should be performed. Care is taken to preserve branches of the renal artery that may be intimately involved with the renal pelvis.

In cases without concomitant pyeloplasty, a V-shaped pyelotomy is performed with extension to the infundibulum as needed as dictated by the size and location of the stone. In cases with UPJ obstruction, excision of UPJ is undertaken if a prominent crossing vessel is present and transposition of the ureter is necessary. Simultaneous pyeloscopy can be performed if a multitude of stones are present. Usually, the stones are extracted via the same pyelotomy incision unless calyceal diverticular stone removal is planned (see below for techniques regarding stone extraction via pyelotomy). Using monopolar scissors (or Potts scissors for pediatric patients), the renal pelvic mucosa can be dissected off the adherent stone and manipulated in such a manner such that the smallest diameter is extracted first to enhance delivery.

We first implement the suction/irrigation system to dislodge any stones with sterile saline fluid. For stones deemed too large for simple extraction, utilization of holmium laser or ultrasonic lithotripter can be utilized [7]. Alternatively, an additional nephrotomy can be created along with the pyelotomy to manipulate large staghorn calculi [8]. If the calculi are unable to be extracted through a robotic trocar, the stones may be transferred to a specimen bag in situ and extracted after procedure completion. Persistent stones may require flexible nephroscopy which can be introduced into the abdomen via the assistant trocar (12 mm) or the cranial robotic trocar (8 mm). When accessing the different calyces, pressurized irrigation should be instituted. Various baskets or flexible grasper may be used for smaller stone extraction. Oftentimes, a specimen bag can be used to collect the stones for later retrieval.

Discussion

Several institutions have published their robotic series for concomitant pyeloplasty and pyelolithotomy [3, 9–13] (Table 7.1). The mean operative time of the studies examined is 169.8 minutes with averaged estimated blood loss and length of stay at 50.1 ml and 2.26 days. Stone-free rates are excellent (>80%) with minimal morbidity (<5%). Thus, robotic pyeloplasty with pyelolithotomy is not only safe and feasible but also efficacious.

Table 7.1 Perioperative outcomes of concomitant pyeloplasty and pyelolithotomy

Study (series with a minimum of 10 patients)	Operative time (min)	Estimated blood loss	Hospital stay	Stone-free rate (%)	Complication %
Atug	275.8 (180–345)	48.6 (10–100)	1.1 (1–2)	100	0
Mufarrij	235.9 (145–348)	60.8 (10–200)	2 (1–5)	100	0
Nayyar	130 (72–180)[a]	50[a]	2.7 (2–6)	80	0
Gupta	121 (63–278)[b]	45[b]	2.5 (2–5)	88	0
Hemal	105 (86–135)	77 (50–250)[c]	N/A	93.2	3.4[b]
Jensen	151 (128–185)	20 (0–50)	3 (2–4)	83	0

[a]Describes entire cohort of robotic pyeloplasty (n = 29), not specific to patients with stones (n = 10/29)
[b]Describes entire cohort of robotic pyeloplasty (n = 85), not specific to patients with stones (n = 16/85)
[c]Describes entire cohort of robotic lithotomy (n = 50), not specific to patients with secondary stones from UPJ obstruction (n = 29/50)
[d]1Patient had hematuria requiring selective angioembolization

Unusual Anatomy in Patients Undergoing Ureteropelvic Junction Obstruction Repair

Patients may present atypically with UPJ obstruction found in ectopic, malrotated, or horseshoe kidneys [14]. Patients with upper tract anomalies may complicate surgery secondary to difficult exposure, anomalous crossing vessels, nondependent nature of ureteropelvic junction, and potentially longer stricture length [15]. Patients with giant hydronephrosis [12] and mega-ureter [16] often require drainage of urine, excision of redundant ureter, and extensive repair [17]. Patients undergoing UPJ repair of a duplex pelvis may result in inadvertent harm to the ipsilateral unaffected pelvis by tissue manipulation and ischemic means [18]. These unique presentations are challenging even for those surgeons with considerable robotic experience. Regardless of location of the UPJ obstruction or upper tract anomaly encountered, similar robotic principles apply. The techniques of dismembered pyeloplasty are similar with the following caveats: (1) patient positioning, (2) port placement, and (3) use of adjunctive procedures (nephropexy/nephroplication).

Horseshoe Kidney

Horseshoe kidney, occurring in about 1 in 500 people, is the most common renal fusion anomaly [19]. There is an increased incidence of UPJ obstruction in this patient population secondary to high ureteral insertion, the potential for multiple aberrant vessels, and geometric functional anatomy of the renal unit [11]. Depending on the laterality of the affected renal unit, the patient is placed in a semi-lateral position with an affected/ipsilateral side up. An 8/12 mm camera port (Xi vs. S/Si) is placed 2 cm lateral to the umbilicus with 2 8 mm robotic trocars placed 2 cm below the subcostal line and 3 cm above the inguinal ligament in the mid-clavicular line (Fig. 7.3). Alternatively, the patient may be placed in supine/Trendelenburg with the camera port placed 3–4 cm inferior to the umbilicus with flanking robotic working trocars. The robot, in this instance, should be docked over the patient's head.

Technical challenges in repairing UPJ obstruction in horseshoe kidneys include frequent aberrant lower pole vessels, caudal position of the renal moiety, and the presence of the renal isthmus. Obtaining a CT angiogram in these cases can help the surgeon anticipate aberrant and accessory vasculature. Moreover, the renal pelvis is located at the level of the umbilicus and anterior. Use of retrograde catheter and injection of indocyanine green (ICG) can help delineate this structure [20] (Fig. 7.4). Robotic management by way of dismembered pyeloplasty in a horseshoe kidney is rare with less than 20 reported cases [11, 21]. Operative time can range from 90–210 minutes with average estimated blood loss ranging from 25 to 100 ml [21]. The procedure is deemed safe and efficacious with minimal reports of postoperative morbidity and complications.

A 39-year-old female presented as a referral for intermittent left-sided upper quadrant pain for 3 months and CT findings demonstrated a horseshoe kidney and left renal moiety hydronephrosis (Fig. 7.5). Lasix renal scan confirmed obstruction

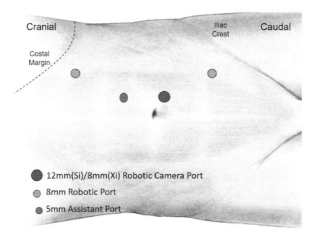

Fig. 7.3 Port placement for pyeloplasty in horseshoe kidney (left-sided). Camera port is placed lateral to the umbilicus by 2 cm, and 8 mm robotic trocars are placed in subcostal and iliac fossa, respectively. A 5 mm assistant trocar is placed cranial to the camera port

Fig. 7.4 Injection/ instillation of ICG can confirm the presence of crossing vessels and/or intrinsic lesions within the ureter

Ureteral / UPJ Obstruction

– Vascular Injection to confirm crossing vessels

– ICG pyelogram allows identification of intrinsic lesions

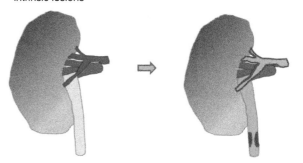

of the left renal moiety and intraoperative images of robotic pyeloplasty of horseshoe kidney are depicted in Fig. 7.6. The patient underwent successful robotic-assisted pyeloplasty of horseshoe kidney with total estimated blood loss of 25 ml and length of stay of 1 day. Follow-up imaging demonstrated an unobstructed system with resolution of pain.

Ectopic, Pelvic and Malrotated Kidney

Pelvic kidney occurs at an incidence rate of about 1 in 2200 to 1 in 3000 [22] with a majority of patients who have hydronephrosis exhibit concomitant UPJ

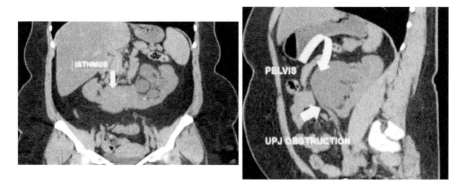

Fig. 7.5 A 39-year-old female presented with intermittent LUQ pain and findings of obstruction from a left renal moiety of a horseshoe kidney

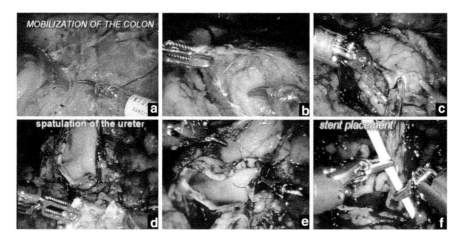

Fig. 7.6 Key operative steps in performing robotic dismembered pyeloplasty in a horseshoe kidney. (**a**) Mobilization of the colon along the white line of Toldt. (**b**) Dissection of the readily identifiable UPJ given its anterior location. (**c**) Incision and excision of redundant renal pelvis (**d**) excision of aperistaltic segment and subsequent spatulation of the proximal ureter. (**e**) Anastomosis of the proximal ureter in dependent fashion using running 5–0 monocryl. (**f**) Antegrade placement of a ureteral double-J stent

obstruction [23]. For ectopic pelvic kidneys, patients may be placed in low lithotomy and steep Trendelenburg, offering adequate exposure to the pathology [11]. Port placement should be amended based on the location of the target organ. In patients with pelvic kidney, the robotic camera port is placed in the supra-umbilical position with flanking robotic trocars (Fig. 7.7). Assistant ports can be placed as needed and lateral to the robotic trocars [23].

Pelvic kidneys often have aberrant vasculature making dissection difficult. The kidney is often visualized as a bulge underneath the lower mesentery of the bowel. Once the bowel is mobilized off the surface of the kidney, the renal pelvis is

Fig. 7.7 Port placement for pyeloplasty in the ectopic pelvic kidney (left-sided). Camera port is placed cranial to the umbilicus with flanking robotic trocars on the lateral border of the rectus sheath. A 5 mm assistant port can be placed laterally

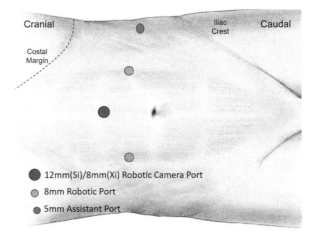

encountered anteriorly. Mobilization of the kidney is cumbersome and unnecessary. Again, retrograde catheter placement and instillation of saline of ICG can aid in visualization. Lastly, in patients with malrotated kidneys additional maneuvers such as nephropexy/nephroplication can enhance drainage of the affected kidney [11]. The application of robotic technology to this arena has greatly improved outcomes and lessened the learning curve by facilitating complex intracorporeal reconstruction, tissue dissection, and stone extraction.

History of Extensive Prior Surgery

Prior surgery can often distort internal anatomical structures greatly enhancing the difficulty of surgery. As a referral to our center, a 25-year-old female with significant past medical history of rhabdomyosarcoma of the retroperitoneum status post surgery and adjuvant radiation therapy at the age of 8 months presented after left-sided PCNL with hydronephrosis at the level of the UPJ/proximal ureter and recurrent urinary tract infections (Fig. 7.8). Positioning and port placement were challenging given the resultant scoliosis with posterior lumbar interbody fusion (PLIF) spanning T10-S1 (Fig. 7.9). The patient underwent successful repair of UPJ stricture with postoperative renal scan demonstrating t ½ < 10 minutes bilaterally. Keys to dissection include careful navigation of post-radiated tissue planes and the use of ICG to highlight important anatomical landmarks.

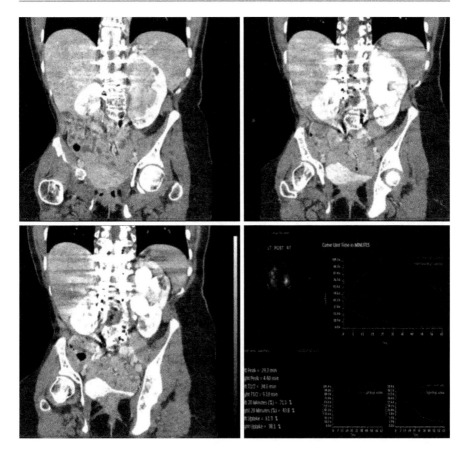

Fig. 7.8 A 25-year-old female s/p retroperitoneal rhabdomyosarcoma resection and adjuvant XRT with resultant severe scoliosis and PLIF demonstrates obstructed left kidney after Left-sided PCNL

Fig. 7.9 Midline port placement with three midline and one lateral ports. Careful dissection of post-radiated planes resulted in successful UPJ stricture repair

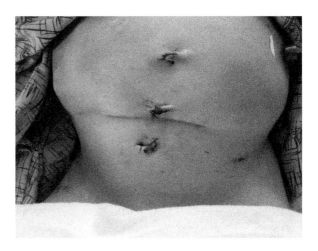

Conclusion

Robotic-assisted pyeloplasty in unique patient populations such as those with stones or unusual anatomy can be highly successful and completed in a safe and expeditious manner. Herein, we describe various techniques, tips, and tricks to complement the reconstructive robotic urologist in the management of UPJ obstruction in the pediatric and the adult patient.

References

1. Hemal A, Mukherjee S, Singh, K. Laparoscopic pyeloplasty versus robotic pyeloplasty for ureteropelvis junction obstruction: a series of 60 cases performed by a single surgeon.
2. Singh I, Hemal A. Robot-assisted pyeloplasty: review of the current.
3. Gupta N, Nayyar R, Hemal A. Outcome analysis of robotic pyeloplasty: a large single-centre experience.
4. Skolarikos A, Dellis A, Knoll T. Ureterpelvic obstruction and renal stones: Etiology and treatment.
5. Bernardo N, Liatsikos EDC, et al. Stone recurrence after endopyelotomy. Urology. 2000;56:378.
6. Pathak RP, Patel M, Hemal A. Comprehensive approach to port placement templates for robot-assisted laparoscopic urologic surgeries. J Endourol. 2017;31:1269–76.
7. Badalato G, Hemal A, Menon M, et al. Current role of robot-assisted Pyelolithotomy for the Management of Large Renal Calculi: a contemporary analysis. J Endourol. 2009;23:1719–22.
8. Badani K, Hemal A, Fumo M, et al. Robotic extended pyelolithotomy for treatment of renal calculi: a feasibility study. World J Urol. 2006;24:198–201.
9. Atug F, Castle E, Burgess S, et al. Concomitant management of renal calculi and pelvi-ureteric junction obstruction with robotic laparoscopic surgery. BJU Int. 2005;96:1365–8.
10. Mufarrij P, Woods M, Shah O, et al. Robotic dismembered pyeloplasty: a 6-year, multi-institutional experience. J Urol. 2008;180:1391–6.
11. Nayyar R, Gupta N, Hemal A. Robotic management of complicated ureteropelvic junction obstruction. World J Urol. 2010;28:599–602.
12. Hemal A, RIshi N, Narmada G, et al. Experience with robotic assisted laparoscopic surgery in upper tract urolithiasis. Can J Urol. 2010;17:5299–305.
13. Jensen P, Berg K, Azawi N. Robot-assisted pyeloplasty and pyelolithotomy with ureterpelvic junction stenosis. Scand J Urol. 2017;51:323–8.
14. Madi R, Hemal A. Robotic pyelolithotomy, extended pyelolithotomy, nephrolithotomy, and anatrophic nephrolithotomy. J Endourol. 2018;32:73–81.
15. Bove P, Ong A, Rha K, et al. Laparoscopic management of ureteropelvic junction obstruction in patients with upper urinary tract anamoalies. J Urol. 2004;171:77–9.
16. Hemal A, Nayyar R, Rao R. Robotic repair of primary symptomatic obstructive megaureter with intracorporeal or extracorporeal ureteric tapering and ureteroneocystostomy. J Endourol. 2009;23:2041–6.
17. Jindal L, Gupta A, Mumtaz F, et al. Laparoscopic nephroplication and nephropexy as an adjunct to pyeloplasty in UPJO with giant hydronephrosis. Int Urol Nephrol. 2006;38:443–6.
18. Metzelder M, Petersen C, Ure B. Laparoscopic pyeloplasty is feasible for lower pole pelv-ureteric obstruction in duplex systems. Pediatr Surg Int. 2007;23:907–9.
19. Natsis K, Piagkou M, Skotsimara A, et al. Horseshoe kidney: a review of anatomy and pathology. Surg Radiol Anat. 2014;36(6):517–26.
20. Pathak R, Hemal A. Intraoperative ICG-fluorescence imaging for robotic-assisted urologic surgery: current status and review of literature. Int Urol Nephrol. 2019;51:765–71.

21. Oderda MCG, Allasia M, et al. Robot-assisted laparoscopic pyeloplasty in a pediatric patient with horseshoe kidney: surgical technique and review of literature. Urologia. 2017;84:55–60.
22. Zafar F, Lingeman J. Value of laparoscopy in the management of calculi complicating renal malformations. J Endourol. 1996;10:379–83.
23. Nayyar R, Singh P, Gupta N. Robot-assisted laparoscopic Pyeloplasty with stone removal in an ectopic kidney. JSLS. 2010;14:130–2.

Recurrent Ureteropelvic Junction Obstruction

8

Ravindra Sahadev, Joan Ko, Arun Srinivasan, and Aseem Shukla

Introduction

Pyeloplasty is a commonly performed surgical procedure in pediatric urology with excellent outcomes. However, a small subset of patients may have suboptimal outcomes requiring additional procedures. The decision to reoperate on a failed pyeloplasty is often challenging due to discrepancies in clinical symptoms and radiological appearances. Proving a definitive anatomical obstruction can often be difficult. Finally, the secondary intervention can be complicated by inflammation, fibrosis, or infection from previous leak/stricture, leading to increased risk of morbidity and lower success rates than primary repair [1, 2].

This chapter highlights approaches to failed pyeloplasty: evaluation, surgical planning, and possible interventions, with particular emphasis on robot-assisted laparoscopic reoperative reconstructions and other salvage procedures based on recent literature and the authors' experience.

Failure of Pyeloplasty

A review of a national database yielded an estimate that 1 out of 9 children who undergo pyeloplasty require a secondary procedure for recurrent or persistent ureteropelvic junction obstruction (UPJO) regardless of the initial surgical approach [3]. The report found that despite attempts at stent placement or endoscopic

Supplementary Information The online version of this chapter (https://doi.org/10.1007/978-3-030-50196-9_8) contains supplementary material, which is available to authorized users.

R. Sahadev · J. Ko · A. Srinivasan · A. Shukla (✉)
Division of Urology, Children's Hospital of Philadelphia, Philadelphia, PA, USA
e-mail: srinivasana3@email.chop.edu; shuklaa@email.chop.edu

intervention to remedy the obstruction, a considerable number of patients require major reoperative procedures. Most secondary procedures were performed within 1 year of the index procedure.

There have been no modifiable predictors of pyeloplasty failure identified in any previous reviews. Although there are concerns regarding younger age (under 6 months), poor preoperative differential function, and crossing vessels as risk factors, they do not seem to be independent predictors of surgical failure [4–7].

Technical factors associated with failure include ischemia of the ureter or renal pelvis, nondependent anastomosis, tension on the anastomosis, twisting of the ureter, inadequate spatulation of the stenotic portion of the ureter, and rough handling of the tissue margins resulting in ischemia. Dismembered pyeloplasty with an unsuitable anatomy, such as small intrarenal pelvis, long ureteral stricture, or high ureteral insertion may increase the risk of complications and failure, as they often predispose to aggressive ureteral mobilization and difficult dissection around the hilum [8, 9].

Evaluation

Children with persistent or recurrent symptoms of flank pain, Dietl's crisis, urinary tract infection, or worsening or persistent severe hydronephrosis should be evaluated. The abovementioned features may themselves be sufficient to undertake an intervention, but it is prudent to investigate the drainage pattern, recent functional status, and the anatomy of the renal pelvis, renal vasculature and ureter.

In addition to a complete renal bladder ultrasound study, a MAG-3 Lasix renogram or, when available, a magnetic resonance urography (MRU) is advocated [5, 10]. Knowing the current renal functional status, renal pelvi-calyceal anatomy, and ureteral status assists in parental counseling and improved surgical planning. In addition, when nephrostomy tubes are placed, they can be used for antegrade contrast studies or Whitaker pressure studies.

Surgical Options

Possible options for secondary intervention include stenting, endopyelotomy (laser, cold knife), balloon dilatation, redo pyeloplasty, ureterocalicostomy, appendiceal/intestinal interposition, inferior nephropexy, autotransplantation, or nephrectomy. More recently, ureteric augmentation using buccal mucosa graft has shown promise for long strictures that occur after failed pyeloplasty.

Interim measures such as stenting/double stenting with subsequent routine exchanges may alleviate symptoms secondary to edema or inflammation of the ureter or ureteropelvic junction in the immediate postoperative period, but the majority of strictures (about 87%) require intervention within a year [3]. Additionally, nonfunctional kidneys or kidneys with negligible function that fail to improve after adequate drainage should undergo nephrectomy.

Although endopyelotomy has been shown to be effective in some series, the results are not uniform and do not compare favorably with pyeloplasty or ureterocalicostomy [11]. The outcomes of different techniques of endopyelotomy (cold knife, electrocautery, laser, Acucise, and balloon dilatation) appear to be similar [11]. Complications rates after endopyelotomy are higher, and the presence of a crossing vessel is a contraindication. The summary of outcomes of each of these procedures is summarized in Tables 8.1, 8.2, and 8.3.

Table 8.1 Outcomes of endourological interventions for recurrent UPJO

Intervention	Authors	Number of cases	Follow-up in months	Success rate[a]
Stenting/Stent exchange	Romao et al. [12]	16	56	6%
Endopyelotomy	Romao et al. [12]	18	56	50%
	Corbett et al. [11]	92	31	75% (25–100)
	Kim et al. [13]	31	31	94%
	Veenboer et al. [14]	11	20	70%
	Parente et al. [15]	9	39.3	100%
	Abdrabuh et al. [16]	27	17	81.5%

[a]The success rate is as defined by the respective authors in their publication

Table 8.2 Outcomes of reoperative pyeloplasty

Intervention	Authors	Number of cases	Follow-up in months (mean/median)	Success rate[a]
Redo pyeloplasty: open	Romao et al. [12]	13	56	92%
	Helmy et al. [24]	16	28	100%
	Abdrabuh et al. [16]	16	21	93.8%
Redo pyeloplasty: lap	Abdel-Karim et al. [25]	24	31.5	91.7%
	Moscardi et al. [26]	8	57.9	100%
	Basiri et al. [27]	15[b]	14.1	100%
Redo pyeloplasty: robot-assisted	Davis et al. [1]	23	26	83%
	Jacobson et al. [28]	31	40	100%
	Baek et al. [29]	10	13.6	100%
	Asensio et al. [30]	5	24.36	100%
	Hemal et al. [31]	9	7.4	100%
	Niver et al. [32]	20[b]	26	94.1%

[a]The success rate is as defined by the respective authors in their publication.
[b]Predominantly adult patients

Table 8.3 Outcomes of ureterocalicostomy for recurrent UPJO

Intervention	Authors	No of cases	Follow-up in months	Success rate[a]
Robotic ureterocalicostomy	Jacobson et al. [28]	5	40	100%
	Casale et al. [33]	9	12	100%
Laparoscopic uretero-calicostomy	Lobo at al. [34]	1	12	100%
	Moscardi at al. [26]	3	30.7	100%

[a]The success rate is as defined by the respective authors in their publication

Techniques

Since most children with recurrent obstruction require definitive reconstruction [3, 6, 17, 18], robot-assisted laparoscopic reconstruction offers a means of excellent visualization, meticulous dissection, and precise reconstruction and is preferred over the conventional laparoscopic approach whenever feasible due to the steep and challenging learning curve of laparoscopic pyeloplasty [19, 20].

Robot-Assisted Laparoscopic Reoperative Pyeloplasty

Redo pyeloplasty is considered the gold standard for secondary intervention. It is preceded by a retrograde pyelogram to assess overall anatomy as well as the location and extent of stricture. A ureteral stent or open-ended catheter is placed to aid in the identification and dissection of the ureter. Of note, some authors have reported difficult dissection owing to extensive inflammation in a long-term stented system and perform a stent removal a few weeks prior to the scheduled pyeloplasty [12].

Patient Positioning

In anticipation of intraoperative cystoscopy, stent placement, and/or ureteroscopy, the patient should be placed in a modified lithotomy position. After the endoscopic portion of the case is completed, the patient can be repositioned to the modified flank position for reconstruction. Alternatively, the patient can be kept in lithotomy with a bump placed under the ipsilateral flank if endoscopic access will be necessary during the reconstruction. The robot is typically docked from the ipsilateral side. The port placement is similar to that for a primary pyeloplasty (Fig. 8.1). A camera port is placed at the umbilicus, one working port is placed in the midline in a subxiphoid position, and one working port is placed either in the ipsilateral midclavicular line below the level of the umbilicus (taking care to avoid the inferior epigastric vessels) or in the lower midline above the pubis (in younger children). Assistant ports are typically only used when necessary. The authors pass sutures and tissue through the robotic ports and use a hitch stitch to retract redundant pelvic tissue, as well as pass stents and 4.7 French nephrostomy drainage tubes through a 14-gauge angiocath that traverses the abdominal wall to obviate the need for an assistant port.

Fig. 8.1 Patient position and proposed port positions for robotic pyeloplasty

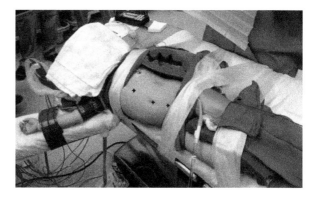

Steps

After confirming safe entry into the peritoneum, adequate exposure of the kidney, hilum, and ureter are achieved by incising the line of Toldt and reflecting the colon medially from the splenic/hepatic flexure.

The proximal ureter is dissected carefully toward the UPJ by blunt and sharp dissection, taking care not to overlook a missed crossing vessel. It is helpful to start the dissection in an area without scarring to better delineate the anatomical planes of dissection. The inflammatory rind on the pelvis is cleared. Care must be given to preserve the vascularity of the ureter/pelvis by staying outside the adventitial layer.

At this point, the dissection may be aided by the use of a hitch stitch on the renal pelvis to provide adequate traction to expose the entire UPJ and proximal ureter.

Before incising the pelvis, in the setting of a long stricture and a redundant extra-renal pelvis, it is important to consider the potential need for a renal pelvic flap pyeloplasty.

The UPJ is transected, and the ureter is transposed over the crossing vessel, if any. The fibrotic segment of the ureter is excised. Again, careful attention must be paid to ensuring healthy tissue edges, orienting the ureter properly, and minimizing the potential for tension on the anastomosis before spatulating the ureter. Once the ureter has been spatulated, we use three interrupted absorbable monofilament sutures at the corner of the anastomosis before running the suture between the pelvis and ureter toward the hitch stitch. Stenting is recommended as it keeps the anastomosis patent and facilitates functional healing while minimizing the risk of leak and subsequent fibrosis. Ensuring its correct placement can avoid unnecessary complications. Alternatively, an externalized pyelo-ureteral catheter can be used since it has comparable outcomes in primary pyeloplasty [21].

In the setting of previous leaks and extensive fibrosis, intraureteral injection of Indocyanine green (ICG) dye and subsequent visualization under near-infrared fluorescence (NIRF) (Fig. 8.4) can aid in safe, rapid, and accurate ureteral dissection and precise localization of the strictured segment, where excision is of paramount importance in redo pyeloplasties [2, 22, 23].

If a tension-free anastomosis can be achieved with ureteral mobilization alone, redo pyeloplasty is a feasible option. However, as noted above, in the setting of a long stricture and a redundant renal pelvis, a flap pyeloplasty may be necessary.

Fig. 8.2 Utilization of laparoscopic sonography to locate the calyx position

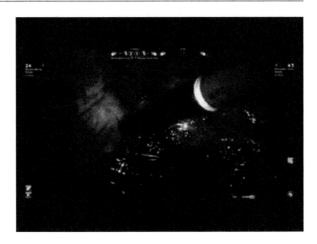

Vertical flap and spiral flaps both are options for performing a non-dismembered pyeloplasty in patients with a long strictured segment of the ureter at the UPJ. The vertical flap is typically performed in patients with an extrarenal pelvis that has a significant amount of redundancy lateral to the ureter as the flap is taken from that tissue. Spiral flaps are used when the ureter is already in a dependent position on the renal pelvis. The location of the apex is dependent on the length of the strictured ureter and can extend from anterior to posterior or posterior to anterior, depending on the approach. Both types of flaps can be performed robotically with the use of a well-placed hitch stitch.

Robot-Assisted Laparoscopic Ureterocalicostomy

A predominantly intrarenal pelvis or extensive scarring at the UPJ can preclude a satisfactory pyeloplasty. Therefore, one should be prepared for possible ureterocalicostomy even in patients who appear to be amenable to redo pyeloplasty on preoperative imaging.

Intraoperative laparoscopic ultrasound (Fig. 8.2) can aid in identifying the area of parenchyma that would need to be resected to access the inferior calyx. Ideally, this layer of parenchyma should be fairly thin in order to perform a technically feasible and safe ureterocalicostomy.

It may be prudent to isolate the vessels at the renal hilum for vascular control if needed in case significant uncontrolled bleeding from the nephrotomy edges occurs. Also, an additional port may be necessary for uninterrupted suction/irrigation.

A combination of electrocautery and vessel-sealing energy devices are then used to excise the renal parenchyma overlying the inferior calyx. An argon beam laser is then used to adequately achieve hemostasis.

The spatulated edge of the ureter is then sutured to the urothelium of the calyx without including the renal parenchyma (Fig. 8.3). Barbed running sutures (e.g., Covidien V-loc) can be used on either side to achieve a watertight anastomosis.

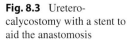

Fig. 8.3 Uretero-
calycostomy with a stent to
aid the anastomosis

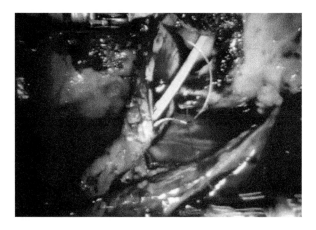

   As previously noted, a double-J stent with or without nephrostomy is recommended for postoperative drainage.

Robot-Assisted Ureteroplasty with Buccal Mucosa Graft (BMG)

Renal units complicated by long ureteral/UPJ strictures that are not amenable to the
above reconstructive techniques can still be salvaged without having to resort to
more morbid procedures such as bowel interposition or autotransplantation. Buccal
mucosal graft (BMG) augmentation of the deficient ureter has been reported in the
literature as a viable alternative with promising results [2, 22, 23].

Technique Port placement is similar to pyeloplasty. An assistant port can be
placed for the passage of the graft into the patient. After dissection of the ureter
(with or without the assistance of ICG), if the gap between the pelvis/lower pole
and the proximal healthy ureteral edge is too long for redo pyeloplasty or ureterocalicostomy (usually 2–8 cm), the decision can be made to perform BMG
reconstruction.

   Based on the length of the gap, an adequately sized graft can be harvested from
the mucosa of the lower lip or cheek after hydro dissection with lidocaine and
epinephrine.
   A pedicled flap of the omentum is used to provide vascularity to the graft.
Alternatively, a flap of perirenal fat or appendiceal mesentery can be used when
omentum is deficient. During the harvest of this flap, intravenous ICG can be used
to determine its viability (Fig. 8.4).

Onlay/Inlay Ureteroplasty In cases of ureteral narrowing with luminal continuity, the diameter can be increased by partially augmenting the ureter wall with
BMG by an onlay or inlay technique, depending on the situation. For dorsal

Fig. 8.4 Ureteral dissection-intraureteral ICG injection to aid the identification of healthy and strictured part of the ureter in white light and near-infrared light (fluorescent green color taken up by healthy ureter). (Image courtesy of Dr. Daniel D. Eun)

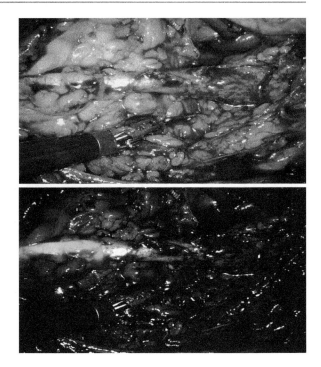

inlays, an omental flap is sutured in place dorsally, underlying the ureterotomy. In those with ventral onlay grafts, the omentum is sutured to the graft after the onlay is complete.

The BMG is introduced into the abdomen through an assistant port and sutured onto the ureterotomy edges in running fashion using absorbable monofilament sutures (Fig. 8.5). In addition, the graft also needs to be anchored to the omentum as described above. A flexible ureteroscope or stent may be placed in the ureter during the anastomosis to prevent the misplacement of the suture into the back wall of the ureter. Once the anastomosis is complete, ureteroscopy can be performed to confirm a patent and watertight anastomosis. A drain is kept near the anastomosis.

Augmented Anastomotic Ureteroplasty For patients in whom the ureter is transected due to a segment with complete obliteration of the lumen, the posterior wall of the ureter is re-anastomosed, and both ends of the ureter are spatulated on the anterior side. The BMG is then placed into the anterior defect to increase the luminal diameter. Again, the omentum is used to provide a vascular bed for the graft (Table 8.4).

Fig. 8.5 Incised stricture and measurement of the gap: Buccal graft onlay ureteroplasty completed. (Image courtesy of Dr. Daniel D. Eun)

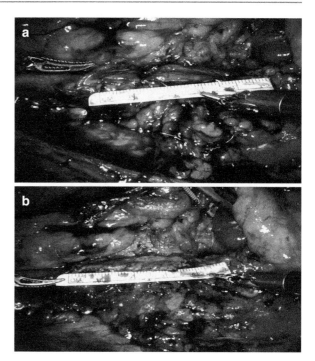

Table 8.4 Outcomes of robot-assisted buccal mucosal graft ureteroplasty

Intervention	Authors	No of cases	Follow-up in months (mean/median)	Success rate[a]
Buccal graft ureteroplasty	Ahn et al. [2]	3	10	100%
	Zhao et al. [22]	19[b]	26	90%

[a]The success rate is as defined by the respective authors in their publication
[b]Predominantly adult patients

Summary

Strategies

- Adequate assessment of the pathologic anatomy with preoperative MRU or intraoperative RGP and other novel techniques (ICG)
- Flexible surgical planning
- Transperitoneal approach with the reflection of the colon and mesentery for wider exposure

- Identification and careful dissection of ureter and UPJ
- Attention to rule out crossing vessel, twisted or kinked ureter, nondependent UPJ
- Adequate excision of scar tissue/fibrosis to obtain supple healthy margins
- Tension-free anastomosis of the healthy, vascularized ends
- Adoption of promising reconstructive techniques such as buccal ureteroplasty in select cases of long strictures
- Stenting, drain placement, and adequate bladder drainage
- Routine postoperative imaging and close follow-up

Annexures

Videos: Ureterocalicostomy (Video 8.1), Flap pyeloplasty (Video 8.2).

References

1. Davis T, Burns A, Corbett S, Peters C. Reoperative robotic pyeloplasty in children. J Pediatr Urol. 2016;12(6):394.e1–7.
2. Ahn J, Shapiro M, Ellison J, Lendvay T. Pediatric robot-assisted redo pyeloplasty with Buccal Mucosa Graft: a novel technique. Urology. 2017;101:56–9.
3. Dy G, Hsi R, Holt S, Lendvay T, Gore J, Harper J. National trends in secondary procedures following pediatric pyeloplasty. J Urol. 2016;195(4):1209–14.
4. Kawal T, Srinivasan AK, Shrivastava D, Chu DI, Van Batavia J, Weiss D, Long C, Shukla AR. Pediatric robotic-assisted laparoscopic pyeloplasty: does age matter? J Pediatr Urol. 2018. pii: S1477-5131(18)30215-8; https://doi.org/10.1016/j.jpurol.2018.04.023.
5. Weiss DA, Kadakia S, Kurzweil R, Srinivasan AK, Darge K, Shukla AR. Detection of crossing vessels in pediatric ureteropelvic junction obstruction: clinical patterns and imaging findings. J Pediatr Urol. 2015;11(4):173.e1–5. https://doi.org/10.1016/j.jpurol.2015.04.017.
6. Thomas JC, DeMarco RT, Donohoe JM, Adams MC, Pope JC IV, Brock JW III. Management of the failed pyeloplasty: a contemporary review. J Urol. 2005;174:2363e6.
7. Pettersson S, Brynger H, Henriksson C, Johansson S, Nilson AE, Ranch T. Autologous renal transplantation and pyelocystostomy after unsuccessful pyeloplasty. J Urol. 1983;130(2):234–9.
8. Tasian GE, Casale P. The robotic-assisted laparoscopic pyeloplasty: gateway to advanced reconstruction. Urol Clin North Am. 2015;42(1):89–97. https://doi.org/10.1016/j.ucl.2014.09.008.
9. Diamond DA, Nguyen HT. Dismembered V-flap pyeloplasty. J Urol. 2001;166(1):233–5.
10. Kirsch AJ, McMann LP, Jones RA, Smith EA, Scherz HC, Grattan-Smith JD. Magnetic resonance urography for evaluating outcomes after pediatric pyeloplasty. J Urol. 2006;176(4 Pt 2):1755–61.
11. Corbett H, Mullassery D. Outcomes of endopyelotomy for pelviureteric junction obstruction in the paediatric population: a systematic review. J Pediatr Urol. 2015;11(6):328–36.
12. Romao R, Koyle M, Pippi Salle J, Alotay A, Figueroa V, Lorenzo A, et al. Failed pyeloplasty in children: revisiting the unknown. Urology. 2013;82(5):1145–9.
13. Kim EH, Tanagho YS, Traxel EJ, Austin PF, Figenshau RS, Coplen DE. Endopyelotomy for pediatric ureteropelvic junction obstruction: a review of our 25-year experience. J Urol. 2012;188:1628e33.
14. Veenboer PW, Chrzan R, Dik P, Klijn AJ, de Jong TP. Secondary endoscopic pyelotomy in children with failed pyeloplasty. Urology. 2011;77:1450e4.
15. Parente A, Angulo J, Burgos L, Romero R, Rivas S, Ortiz R. Percutaneous endopyelotomy over high pressure balloon for recurrent ureteropelvic junction obstruction in children. J Urol. 2015;194(1):184–9.

16. Abdrabuh A, Salih E, Aboelnasr M, Galal H, El-Emam A, El-Zayat T. Endopyelotomy versus redo pyeloplasty for management of failed pyeloplasty in children: a single center experience. J Pediatr Surg. 2018;53(11):2250–5.
17. Braga LH, Lorenzo AJ, Bagli DJ, et al. Risk factors for recurrent ureteropelvic junction obstruction after open pyeloplasty in a large pediatric cohort. J Urol. 2008;180:1684.
18. Lindgren BW, Hagerty J, Meyer T, et al. Robot assisted laparoscopic reoperative repair for failed pyeloplasty in children: a safe and highly effective treatment option. J Urol. 2012;188:932.
19. Tasian GE, Wiebe DJ, Casale P. Learning curve of robotic assisted pyeloplasty for pediatric urology fellows. J Urol. 2013;190(4 Suppl):1622–6. https://doi.org/10.1016/j.juro.2013.02.009. Epub 2013 Feb 11.
20. O'Brien ST, Shukla AR. Transition from open to robotic-assisted pediatric pyeloplasty: a feasibility and outcome study. J Pediatr Urol. 2012;8(3):276–81. https://doi.org/10.1016/j.jpurol.2011.04.005.
21. Chu DI, Shrivastava D, Van Batavia JP, Bowen D, Tong CC, Long CJ, Weiss DA, Shukla AR, Srinivasan AK. Outcomes of externalized pyeloureteral versus internal ureteral stent in pediatric robotic-assisted laparoscopic pyeloplasty. J Pediatr Urol. 2018. pii: S1477-5131(18)30182–7; https://doi.org/10.1016/j.jpurol.2018.04.012.
22. Zhao LC, Weinberg AC, Lee Z, Ferretti MJ, Koo HP, Metro MJ, Eun DD, Stifelman MD. Robotic ureteral reconstruction using buccal mucosa grafts: a multi-institutional experience. Eur Urol. 2017. pii: S0302-2838(17)31000-X; https://doi.org/10.1016/j.eururo.2017.11.015.
23. Lee Z, Waldorf BT, Cho EY, Liu JC, Metro M, Eun DD. Robotic ureteroplasty with Buccal Mucosa Graft for the management of complex ureteral strictures. J Urol. 2017;198(6):1430–5. https://doi.org/10.1016/j.juro.2017.06.097.
24. Helmy T, Sarhan O, Hafez A, Elsherbiny M, Dawaba M, Ghali A. Surgical management of failed pyeloplasty in children: single-center experience. J Pediatr Urol. 2009;5(2):87–9.
25. Abdel-Karim A, Fahmy A, Moussa A, Rashad H, Elbadry M, Badawy H, et al. Laparoscopic pyeloplasty versus open pyeloplasty for recurrent ureteropelvic junction obstruction in children. J Pediatr Urol. 2016;12(6):401.e1–6.
26. Moscardi P, Barbosa J, Andrade H, Mello M, Cezarino B, Oliveira L, et al. Reoperative laparoscopic ureteropelvic junction obstruction repair in children: safety and efficacy of the technique. J Urol. 2017;197(3):798–804.
27. Basiri A, Behjati S, Zand S, Moghaddam SM. Laparoscopic pyeloplasty in secondary ureteropelvic junction obstruction after failed open surgery. J Endourol. 2007;21:1045–51; discussion 1051.
28. Jacobson DL, Shannon R, Johnson EK, Gong EM, Liu DB, Flink CC, Meyer T, Cheng EY, Lindgren BW. Robot-assisted laparoscopic reoperative repair for failed pyeloplasty in children: an updated series. J Urol. 2018; https://doi.org/10.1016/.juro.2018.10.021.
29. Baek M, Silay MS, Au JK, Huang GO, Elizondo RA, Puttmann K, Janzen NK, Seth A, Roth DR, Koh CJ. Quantifying the additional difficulty of pediatric robot-assisted laparoscopic Re-Do pyeloplasty: a comparison of primary and Re-Do procedures. J Laparoendosc Adv Surg Tech A. 2018;28(5):610–6. https://doi.org/10.1089/lap.2016.0691.
30. Asensio M, Gander R, Royo GF, Lloret J. Failed pyeloplasty in children: is robot-assisted laparoscopic reoperative repair feasible? J Pediatr Urol. 2015;11(2):69.e1–6. https://doi.org/10.1016/j.jpurol.2014.10.009. Epub 2015 Feb 24
31. Hemal AK, Mishra S, Mukharjee S, Suryavanshi M. Robot assisted laparoscopic pyeloplasty in patients of ureteropelvic junction obstruction with previously failed open surgical repair. Int J Urol. 2008;15:744e6.
32. Niver BE, Agalliu I, Bareket R, Mufarrij P, Shah O, Stifelman MD. Analysis of robotic-assisted laparoscopic pyeloplasty for primary versus secondary repair in 119 consecutive cases. Urology. 2012;79(3):689–94. https://doi.org/10.1016/j.urology.2011.10.072.
33. Casale P, Mucksavage P, Resnick M, Kim S. Robotic ureterocalicostomy in the pediatric population. J Urol. 2008;180(6):2643–8.
34. Lobo S, Mushtaq I. Laparoscopic ureterocalicostomy in children: the technique and feasibility. J Pediatr Urol. 2018;14(4):358–9. https://doi.org/10.1016/j.jpurol.2018.06.012.

Part IV

Proximal and Mid Ureteral Strictures

Michael D. Stifelman

In this section of the book, we encounter some of the most difficult ureteral reconstruction challenges of the upper urinary tract – proximal and mid-ureteral strictures. These procedures require a detailed preoperative evaluation with patient history and imaging to identify length of stricture and viability of tissue based on previous insults and mechanism of ureteral injury. The surgeon must plan for anything and be familiar with and consider all of the options outlined in this section. Meticulous dissection, respect of tissue, generous use of intraoperative vascular confirmation, and a flexible openminded approach to potential roadblocks are mandatory. These chapters prepare you for this challenge by identifying adjunct technology and intraoperative pearls that will help guide you in planning and executing the best and least invasive repair. The editors of this book will follow in the path of Sir Harold Gillies, the father of plastic surgery, for the theme of this section by modeling their initiatives around the core principles of "replace like with like," and "don't waste a living thing."

Proximal Ureteral Reconstruction: Ureteroureterostomy, Buccal Mucosa Graft, Retrocaval Ureter

9

Nabeel Shakir, Min Suk Jan, and Lee C. Zhao

Introduction

Mid- and proximal ureteral strictures, which are long or refractory to endoscopic management, have historically presented a treatment quandary. Surgical challenges for definitive repair are compounded when the disease etiology involves prior abdominopelvic radiation or ischemic insult or the patient has undergone multiple prior interventions, resulting in a poor periureteral blood supply, tenuous or obliterated ureteral plate, and abnormal tissue planes [1]. Salvage procedures for these scenarios, including renal autotransplantation or ileal interposition, may require significant technical expertise and increased perioperative risk.

To repair recalcitrant proximal strictures with well-vascularized, healthy tissue, surgeons have refined or repurposed techniques ranging from traditional ureteroureterostomy (UU) to oral mucosa grafts and appendiceal flaps. However, the success of any surgical approach also relies on adequate exposure and mobilization of the diseased ureteral segment; in the open setting, especially where long bladder flaps or downward nephropexy is also performed to achieve a tension-free anastomosis, this may result in considerable morbidity not only from the incision but also with each added step in a potentially hostile, reoperative field.

Supplementary Information The online version of this chapter (https://doi.org/10.1007/978-3-030-50196-9_9) contains supplementary material, which is available to authorized users.

N. Shakir
The University of Texas Southwestern Medical Center, Dallas, TX, USA

M. S. Jan
Crane Center for Transgender Surgery, Greenbae California, New York, NY, USA

L. C. Zhao (✉)
NYU Langone Health, New York, NY, USA
e-mail: Lee.zhao@nyulangone.org

© Springer Nature Switzerland AG 2022
M. D. Stifelman et al. (eds.), *Techniques of Robotic Urinary Tract Reconstruction*, https://doi.org/10.1007/978-3-030-50196-9_9

Laparoscopic ureteral reconstruction, first described in 1992 by Nezhat et al. for UU, may result in improved recovery and cosmesis as compared to open approaches, but has not been adopted widely owing to the challenges of precise visualization, dissection, and suturing with limited working space [2, 3]. In response to this dilemma, beginning in 2007, robotic-assisted management of ureteral obstruction became more widely reported [4]. The robotic platform may be particularly suited to this application due to its advantages of three-dimensional, magnified vision, improved articulation, and potential for concurrent use of adjuncts to aid in the identification of diseased tissues such as indocyanine green (ICG) [5]. We describe several valuable additions to the robotic reconstructive armamentarium, building on fundamental principles derived from open surgical approaches to proximal ureteral strictures.

Preoperative Planning

Patients with ureteral stricture commonly present with hydronephrosis and renal colic with or without pyelonephritis. The workup at this time often includes a CT scan, showing hydroureteronephrosis with a distinct ureteral transition point suggestive of a ureteral stricture. These patients will often have ureteral stents placed in the acute setting. The workup should include a renal scan to assess function, as nephrectomy may be appropriate for kidneys contributing less than 20% function.

Our first step in the diagnostic period is percutaneous nephrostomy placement, typically performed by interventional radiology. The existing stent can aid in percutaneous access as the stent is an echogenic target that may be identified with ultrasonography. Alternatively, the interventionist can place a Foley catheter and instill the bladder with irrigants. This will reflux and induce hydronephrosis, providing a larger target for the interventionist. The stent is then removed to allow for a period of "ureteral rest" during which the ureteral stricture is allowed to fully declare itself, a concept analogous to the well-accepted practice of "urethral rest" in anterior urethral strictures [6].

After 4–6 weeks of ureteral rest, we routinely study the ureter with antegrade/retrograde ureterography and ureteroscopy as necessary. Attention is given to the location, length, and grade of obstruction. Importantly, this provides an opportunity to definitively rule out malignancy as the cause of obstruction. At this point, the patient is counseled on the findings and prepared for definitive repair.

Operating Room Preparation, Positioning, and Instrumentation

Women are placed in modified dorsal lithotomy with the ipsilateral side bumped up. The genitalia are prepped and included in the field to facilitate lower urinary tract access. Lithotomy is not required in men as the genitalia can be prepped into the field in lateral decubitus position, and a flexible cystoscope is used to gain retrograde access to the ureter. The nephrostomy tube should be capped and prepped into the field. The endotracheal tube is taped to the side of the mouth laying downward to facilitate buccal mucosa harvest should it be needed.

Surgical Technique

Initial access is obtained at the midline above the umbilicus. The robotic ports are then placed vertically along the midclavicular line from two finger breadths below the costal margin to two finger breadths above the iliac crest. While this is the ideal setup, patients often have had prior abdominal surgery, and the presence of adhesions may dictate the location of these ports. We prefer to use Maryland bipolar forceps, monopolar scissors, and ProGrasp forceps.

Cystoscopy is performed at the beginning of each case, and a guidewire is placed, facilitating flexible ureteroscopy. The ureteroscope is advanced to the level of the stricture where it remains. The white light of the ureteroscope can aid in ureteral identification as the Firefly™ near-infrared camera can detect the light through tissue. Of note, digital flexible ureteroscopes do not emit the near-infrared spectrum and will not be detected by the Firefly™ system. Another method to enhance ureteral identification is to inject indocyanine green (ICG) intraluminally via nephrostomy or in a retrograde fashion (Fig. 9.1). Of note, once in contact with urothelium, it will be present for the duration of the case, compromising its utility in assessing ureteral vascularity. Intravenous ICG is another useful tool one should consider to assess the blood supply to the ureter. Once administered, well-perfused tissue will glow green under the near-infrared camera within seconds. If the proximal or distal extent of the ureterotomy is not well perfused, one should consider extending the ureterotomy until a well-perfused ureter is encountered. IV ICG can also be useful in delineating the blood supply to an appendiceal flap.

The final steps of ureteroplasty are the same regardless of technique. Ureteroscopy is used to confirm patency and a water-tight closure. A guidewire is placed, and a

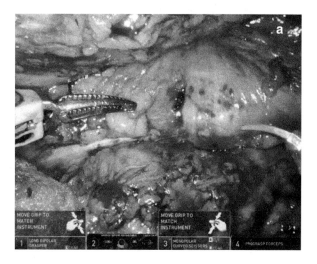

Fig. 9.1 The near-infrared camera can identify the white light of the ureteroscope through tissue to aid with ureteral identification. (**a**) Normal camera mode looking at the ureteroscope within the ureter. (**b**) Near-infrared camera mode detects the white light through tissue

Fig. 9.1 (continued)

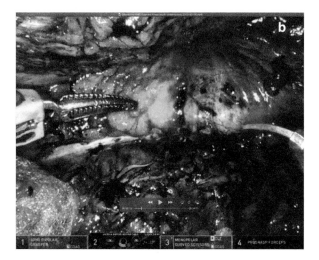

6 French ureteral stent is placed in the usual fashion cystoscopically. If the nephrostomy tube is no longer needed, it is removed while grasping the ureteral stent to
avoid accidental dislodging. A closed suction drain is then placed.

Ureteroureterostomy

For relatively short (<3 cm) strictures of the proximal ureter, UU is a viable and
potentially straightforward option. It is our preferred technique in cases of complete
luminal obliteration. Lee et al. reported the first robotic-assisted UU in 2010 in a
case series ultimately expanded to 12 patients in 2013, with only one recurrence at
midterm follow-up [3, 7]. The largest series in the literature reports similar outcomes
with a mean operative time of 2.5 h [8]. However, circumferential ureteral dissection can risk disruption of blood supply, especially with longer or radiation-induced
strictures, and therefore, this technique may be better suited to unifocal stenoses in
a nonirradiated field amenable to tension-free excision and anastomosis [4].

Ureteroureterostomy requires circumferential mobilization of the ureter. The
diseased ureter is excised, leaving flanking segments of healthy ureter both proximally and distally. In all cases of proximal ureteral stricture in the Lee et al. series,
concomitant downward nephropexy was performed to facilitate a tension-free anastomosis, which also required full dissection of the proximal ureteral segment. The
capsular adhesions that fix the kidney in situ are detached, and the kidney is relo-
cated to a more inferior location. 0 V-Loc™ (Covidien, Mansfield, MA) is then used
to fix the kidney to the psoas fascia. While this technique has proven efficacy, our
algorithm for longer, obliterative ureteral strictures obviates the need for downward
nephropexy. Instead, we prefer the augmented anastomotic buccal ureteroplasty as

described in the next section. The ends of the ureter are then spatulated 1–2 cm on opposing sides, and the anastomosis is completed using fine absorbable suture in a running fashion.

Oral Mucosa Graft Onlay

First described in an animal model by Somerville and Naude in 1984, and subsequently by Naude for open ureteral stricturoplasty in humans in 1999, buccal mucosa grafts (BMG) carry several advantages for the reconstruction of proximal ureteral defects, including in a radiated or multi-operative field [9, 10]. The graft has a well-vascularized yet thin lamina propria, an epithelium adapted to wet environments, and is associated with minimal donor site morbidity. These qualities have contributed to the success and increasing prominence of BMG in urethral reconstruction over the past two decades [11]. Robotic BMG ureteroplasty was reported initially by Zhao et al. in 2015, with this series subsequently expanded to a multicenter analysis of 19 patients with a median stricture length of 4 cm [12, 13]. In this report, the majority of repairs were with onlay graft and covered with omental wrap, and 90% were without recurrence at median follow up of 26 months.

As compared to UU, relatively minimal ureteral dissection is required, allowing for improved preservation of blood supply. Moreover, where there is severe periureteral fibrosis, only the ventral ureter may need to be dissected for an onlay BMG. For non-obliterative strictures, this approach can limit further devascularization. Furthermore, the ureter may be densely adherent to the underlying iliac vessels posteriorly, and circumferential dissection comes at the cost of significant risk of bleeding. It is for this reason that we now prefer anterior onlay ureteroplasty for all non-obliterative ureteral strictures. For short obliterative strictures (1.5-3 cm), an augmented anastomotic ureteroplasty can be performed, avoiding an end-to-end anastomosis to potentially unhealthy tissue [4]. Regardless of the location of the graft, it can be supported by any pedicled flap, including but not limited to omentum, perinephric fat, or psoas muscle. The use of BMG in these settings, particularly for patients with prior abdominopelvic radiation, renal insufficiency, short bowel syndrome, or inflammatory bowel disease, may avoid the need for more morbid interventions such as ileal interposition or autotransplant. Nevertheless, such options remain available in the event of graft failure. By analogy with urethral reconstruction, tubularized grafts should be eschewed in favor of onlay with well-vascularized tissue backing and avoided altogether where there is a long obliterative ureteral segment [11].

Once the ureter is exposed, a small anterior ureterotomy is made and extended the length of the ureteral stricture. IV ICG may be used to confirm adequate blood supply to the ureters beyond the apices. Once confirmed, the apices are marked with a stay suture. If the ureteral lumen is obliterated, the obliterated section is excised, and the ventral portion of the two ureteral ends are spatulated. The dorsal side of

Fig. 9.2 Anterior onlay of buccal mucosal graft onto the left ureter. The medial anastomosis is in progress. The lateral anastomosis has not begun. A ureteral stent lays in front of the ureteral plate with the buccal graft seen medially (below)

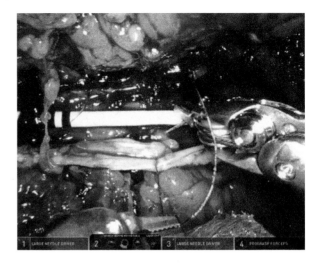

the transected ureter is then anastomosed with fine absorbable suture in a running fashion, establishing the posterior ureteral plate. This leaves a ventral ureteral defect onto which the buccal mucosa graft can be placed.

Once the length of the stricture is determined, BMG harvest is performed. A headlamp is useful since the robot may block the path of the overhead lamp. Holding sutures are placed on the lip for retraction and Stenson's duct is identified. The required graft size is then marked; the grafts are tailored to be the length of the ureteral stricture and 1 cm in width. Hydrodissection of the buccal mucosa is performed with lidocaine and epinephrine. The graft is then harvested sharply, leaving the buccinator muscle in situ. The BMG is defatted and placed in saline until needed. Electrocautery is used to control bleeding at the harvest site. The defect may be closed or left open at the surgeon's prerogative. Once the graft is delivered into the field, the edges are anastomosed with 3-0 Stratafix. (Fig. 9.2). The omentum is then sutured over the graft with 4-0 Vicryl sutures.

Appendiceal Flap

The use of the appendix for ureteral interposition was described first in 1912 by Melnikoff with an end-to-end anastomosis [14]. While this technique presented some apparent advantages, including relatively easy mobilization of the appendix together with its blood supply, small surface area with negligible absorption of urine, and potential use for total ureteral segmental loss, for nearly a century after its promulgation, the appendiceal interposition was rarely performed [15, 16]. Disadvantages, in addition to the possibility of prior appendectomy, include variable appendiceal length and caliber especially in the setting of vascular compromise, potential scarring due to inflammation, and possible anastomotic stricture with an end-to-end approach given the relatively narrow luminal diameter. Left-sided ureteral repair, while technically feasible, may be difficult and has hitherto been described in the pediatric population [17].

In recent years, interest has increased in minimally invasive iterations of this technique. In 2009, Reggio et al. described laparoscopic appendiceal onlay flap ureteroplasty for a right-sided non-obliterative proximal stricture, involving longitudinally incising of the diseased ureteral segment, thereby preserving posterior ureteric blood supply and anastomosing the detubularized appendix to the posterior ureteral wall [18]. The same group expanded on this technique in 2015 with a review of six patients with a mean stricture length of 2.5 cm, all right-sided; at mean follow-up of 16 months, all patients were without recurrence [19]. Subsequently, Yarlagadda et al. reported a 5 cm iatrogenic obliterative proximal and mid-right ureteric stricture managed with robotic-assisted tubularized appendiceal interposition in an isoperistaltic fashion [20]. The patient was without recurrence of symptoms 10 months postoperatively. Similarly, Gn et al. in 2018 described robotic-assisted complete appendiceal replacement of the right ureter for iatrogenic avulsion, albeit also necessitating right lower pole calycostomy, downward nephropexy, and psoas hitch [21].

We have used the appendiceal onlay flap preferentially when possible as outcomes are excellent without the donor site morbidity of BMG harvest. One might even consider this technique as prophylaxis against appendicitis. While port placement is similar to the previously described setup, a 12 mm port will need to be placed to accommodate a laparoscopic stapler, which will be used to segment the appendiceal flap from the cecum. Once harvested, the two ends of the appendix are opened, and the lumen is cleared with suction and irrigation. The appendix is opened longitudinally sharply along its antimesenteric border. The mesentery of the appendix is carefully mobilized to facilitate a tension-free anastomosis. IV ICG can be useful during this maneuver as it will highlight the main vascular pedicle of the mesoappendix, which is to be avoided (Fig. 9.3). Anastomosis is performed similarly to that previously described for buccal grafts (Fig. 9.4). If the appendix is not appropriate for ureteroplasty, the mesentery is divided, and appendectomy is completed.

Fig. 9.3 IV ICG shows adequate perfusion to the harvested appendiceal flap

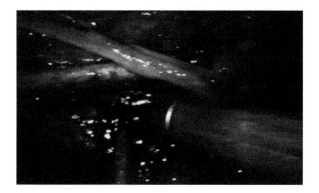

Fig. 9.4 A suture is being placed into the ureter. The appendix is visible in the foreground

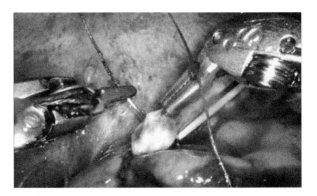

Retrocaval Ureter

For patients with symptomatic ureteral obstruction secondary to retrocaval ureter, traditional options have included UU or pyelopyelostomy to reroute the ureter. During laparoscopic transperitoneal approaches, the most time-consuming portion of the procedure can be the intracorporeal anastomosis [22]. Robotic-assisted UU for retrocaval ureter was first reported in 2006 in the pediatric population and elaborated on in 2011 by LeRoy et al [22, 23]. In the latter case, the retrocaval segment of the ureter was left in situ, and the normal ureter was transected and transposed anteriorly to the vena cava. Whether to dissect and preserve the retrocaval segment remains controversial; there is a theoretical risk of malignancy if it is retained. Simforoosh et al. reported six cases in which no resection of the retrocaval segment was performed and suggest that as long as this portion does not appear dysplastic or otherwise grossly abnormal, it can be left in place [24]. In order to minimize the likelihood of stricture recurrence, minimal dissection of the distal ureter is recommended [25].

Postoperative Care

The Foley catheter is removed on postoperative day (POD) 1. The drain is removed shortly thereafter, and the patient is discharged on the same day. Irrespective of technique, the stent is removed in the clinic 4 weeks later, and a renal ultrasound is performed 6 weeks after that. In the absence of any symptoms, a diuretic renal scan will be done 6 months postoperatively. This can be performed sooner if indicated based on ultrasound findings or symptoms consistent with ureteral obstruction.

Discussion

Many techniques exist in the ureteroplasty armamentarium. We take an algorithmic approach when faced with a proximal ureteral stricture. While ureteroureterostomy is a well-accepted technique, we avoid it if possible as it requires circumferential ureterolysis, stripping the ureter of its local blood supply. The ureter must then rely on its longitudinal blood supply, which is interrupted with transection. We feel that this concept is particularly important in the case of reoperation and in irradiated fields where vascular supply is compromised. It is our practice to make a ventral ureterotomy. Appendiceal ventral onlay flap is our first option. If the appendix is unavailable or if the mesentery is too short, then buccal mucosa graft ureteroplasty is performed. It is important to counsel the patient preoperatively on the possibility of an ileal ureter in case it becomes apparent intraoperatively that other techniques will not suffice. Autotransplantation can be performed as a salvage procedure.

Conclusion

We are frequently referred patients who have endured years of management of ureteral strictures with serial stent exchanges, who are told that there is no surgical cure for their condition. Using the algorithm outlined above, we have been able to offer a durable surgical cure to most of our patients, freeing them of their reliance on indwelling hardware.

References

1. Knight RB, Hudak SJ, Morey AF. Strategies for open reconstruction of upper ureteral strictures. Urol Clin North Am. 2013;40:351–61.
2. Nezhat C, Nezhat F, Green B. Laparoscopic treatment of obstructed ureter due to endometriosis by resection and Ureteroureterostomy: a case report. J Urol. 1992;148:865–8.
3. Lee Z, et al. Single surgeon experience with robot-assisted ureteroureterostomy for pathologies at the proximal, middle, and distal ureter in adults. J Endourol. 2013;27:994–9.
4. Tracey AT, et al. Robotic-assisted laparoscopic repair of ureteral injury: an evidence-based review of techniques and outcomes. Minerva Urol Nefrol. 2018; https://doi.org/10.23736/S0393-2249.18.03137-5.
5. Lee Z, Moore B, Giusto L, Eun DD. Use of Indocyanine Green during robot-assisted ureteral reconstructions. Eur Urol. 2015;67:291–8.
6. Terlecki RP, Steele MC, Valadez C, Morey AF. Urethral rest: role and rationale in preparation for anterior urethroplasty. Urology. 2011;77:1477–81.
7. Lee DI, Schwab CW, Harris A. Robot-assisted Ureteroureterostomy in the adult: initial clinical series. Urology. 2010;75:570–3.

8. Buffi NM, et al. Robot-assisted surgery for benign ureteral strictures: experience and outcomes from four tertiary care institutions. Eur Urol. 2017;71:945–51.
9. Somerville JJF, Naude JH. Segmental ureteric replacement: an animal study using a free non-pedicled graft. Urol Res. 1984;12
10. Naude JH. Buccal mucosal grafts in the treatment of ureteric lesions. BJU Int. 2001;83:751–4.
11. Wessells H, et al. Male urethral stricture: American urological association guideline. J Urol. 2017;197:182–90.
12. Zhao LC, Yamaguchi Y, Bryk DJ, Adelstein SA, Stifelman MD. Robot-assisted ureteral reconstruction using buccal mucosa. Urology. 2015;86:634–8.
13. Zhao LC, et al. Robotic ureteral reconstruction using buccal mucosa grafts: a multi-institutional experience. Eur Urol. 2018;73:419–26.
14. Melnikoff A. Sur le replacement de l'uretere par anse isolee de l'intestine grele. Rev Clin Urol. 1912;1:601–3.
15. Richter F, Stock JA, Hanna MK. The appendix as right ureteral substitute in children. J Urol. 2000;163:1908–12.
16. Juma S, Nickel JC. Appendix interposition of the ureter. J Urol. 1990;144:130–1.
17. Deyl RT, Averbeck MA, Almeida GL, Pioner GT, Souto CAV. Appendix interposition for total left ureteral reconstruction. J Pediatr Urol. 2009;5:237–9.
18. Reggio E, Richstone L, Okeke Z, Kavoussi LR. Laparoscopic ureteroplasty using on-lay appendix graft. Urology. 2009;73:928.e7–10.
19. Duty BD, Kreshover JE, Richstone L, Kavoussi LR. Review of appendiceal onlay flap in the management of complex ureteric strictures in six patients: Appendiceal onlay flap in management of ureteric strictures. BJU Int. 2015;115:282–7.
20. Yarlagadda VK, Nix JW, Benson DG, Selph JP. Feasibility of intracorporeal robotic-assisted laparoscopic appendiceal interposition for ureteral stricture disease: a case report. Urology. 2017;109:201–5.
21. Gn M, Lee Z, Strauss D, Eun D. Robotic Appendiceal interposition with right lower pole calycostomy, downward nephropexy, and psoas hitch for the management of an iatrogenic near-complete ureteral avulsion. Urology. 2018;113:e9–e10.
22. LeRoy TJ, Thiel DD, Igel TC. Robot-assisted laparoscopic reconstruction of Retrocaval ureter: description and video of technique. J Laparoendosc Adv Surg Tech A. 2011;21:349–51.
23. Gundeti MS, Duffy PG, Mushtaq I. Robotic-assisted laparoscopic correction of pediatric retrocaval ureter. J Laparoendosc Adv Surg Tech A. 2006;16:422–4.
24. Simforoosh N, Nouri-Mahdavi K, Tabibi A. Laparoscopic Pyelopyelostomy for Retrocaval ureter without excision of the Retrocaval segment: first report of 6 cases. J Urol. 2006;175:2166–9.
25. Liu E, et al. Retroperitoneoscopic ureteroplasty for retrocaval ureter: report of nine cases and literature review. Scand J Urol. 2016;50:319–22.

Ureteral Reconstruction: An Overview of Appendiceal Interposition and Ureterocalicostomy

10

Sij Hemal, Anna Quian, and Robert J. Stein

Appendiceal Interposition

Appendiceal interposition is a surgery wherein the vermiform appendix is utilized as replacement for the ureter. This procedure was described as early as 1912 by Melnikoff [1]. Since then, several case studies in both pediatric [2–10] and adult [11–20] patients have been published, but the procedure is still rarely used. With regard to recent literature, most studies are limited to retrospective studies consisting of small sample sizes with variable success rates related to the heterogeneous criteria for following patency/adequacy of these repairs and different follow-up timelines. Many methods exist for ureteral reconstruction and repair following ureteral pathology such as ureteroureterostomy, psoas hitch, Boari flap, renal autotransplantation, ileal interposition, and buccal mucosa graft. In some cases, several of these aforementioned techniques may not be possible such as where the ureteral defect is too long to bridge and a simple end-to-end ureteroureterostomy may not be feasible. Similarly, if the ureteral defect is proximally located, both the psoas hitch and Boari flap techniques are not viable options. Renal autotransplantation is a complicated surgery relying on expertise in performing vascular anastomosis and is typically fraught with complications, which may make it a last resort effort in order to salvage the kidney. Ileal interposition

Supplementary Information The online version of this chapter (https://doi.org/10.1007/978-3-030-50196-9_10) contains supplementary material, which is available to authorized users.

S. Hemal · R. J. Stein (✉)
Department of Urology, Glickman Urological and Kidney Institute Cleveland Clinic, Cleveland, OH, USA
e-mail: steinr@ccf.org

A. Quian
Case Western Reserve School of Medicine, Cleveland, OH, USA

© Springer Nature Switzerland AG 2022
M. D. Stifelman et al. (eds.), *Techniques of Robotic Urinary Tract Reconstruction*, https://doi.org/10.1007/978-3-030-50196-9_10

is an excellent reconstructive option for complex, large ureteral defects or multiple strictures within the same ureter. The use of ileum may be more technically challenging and mandates the application of a bowel anastomosis in comparison with an appendiceal interposition. Furthermore, the appendix may offer advantages over small bowel in that the appendix's smaller lumen contains less mucosal surface dedicated to nutrient absorption and does not require tapering [9, 21]. On the other hand, ileal substitution is more likely to lead to metabolic acidosis and serum electrolyte abnormalities [8, 15]. Some theorize that the appendix may also have natural peristaltic capabilities that aid in urine movement although Estevao-Costa [9] and Komatz and Itoh [22] did not encounter complications with antiperistaltic interposition. However, there may be certain disadvantages to the use of the appendix such as the possibility of increased anastomotic stenosis or stricture formation due to the smaller lumen [8].

When to Do

Similar to other procedures, appendiceal interposition is indicated in the repair of complex ureteral defects in a kidney unit with salvageable renal function. It is most often used when other techniques are not feasible, often due to more proximal and mid ureteric locations or in cases where end-to-end anastomosis of the ureter is not possible as the defect may be too long to bridge [7]. A variety of deficits can cause urinary tract damage include but not limited to iatrogenic sequelae often from pelvic surgery, trauma, malignancy, congenital development, and radiation therapy. Stricture, stenosis, necrosis, obstruction, or other defects arising in the ureter from a prior medical condition, such as malignancy, or ureteral strictures secondary to recurrent nephrolithiasis are the most common indications for appendiceal interposition [7, 8, 23, 24]. When considering the appendix as an option, the appendiceal length and vascularization should be checked to ensure adequacy and minimize the risk of ischemia. The length needs to be sufficient to replace the length of the ureter to be replaced. The vascularization should be adequate when mobilizing the appendix toward the ureteral defect and prevent ischemia from torsion or twisting of the blood supply. Renal function and pyelograms should be checked before the procedure to assess the size and location of the ureteral defect. Several reports suggest the removal of an indwelling JJ stent 2 weeks prior to surgery in order to decrease ureteral edema and better delineate the ureteral defect or stricture intraoperatively at the time of surgery. Some authors have reported success with a preoperative renal function as low as 11% on a diuretic renogram [7]. At the time of the surgery, a retrograde pyelogram may be performed with cystoscopic stent placement. Postoperative imaging and renal function tests should be done to ensure that the interposition is performing successfully. Anterograde and retrograde pyelograms can be taken 8 weeks postoperatively along with a renal scan 6 months postoperatively to assess renal drainage and differential function of the affected kidney [11].

Techniques of Harvesting Appendix, Focus on Reproducible Method

The more recent reports in literature suggest that this procedure may be done roboti-cally or laparoscopically with good success. The technique described is based on a minimally invasive platform. The right lateral peritoneal fold over the right iliac fossa is incised using the harmonic scalpel. The appendix and the cecum are then mobilized medially. Careful dissection is used to identify the ureter and is dissected/mobilized in the area of pathology with care taken to preserve the periadventitial ureteral tissue. The exact proximal and distal limits of the ureteral pathology are defined grossly, and the area in between is incised. Mobilization of the two ends—the distal and proximal ends—may be further achieved, if necessary, with care taken to preserve the blood supply. The surgeon then makes the decision intraoperatively whether the defect is too long to be bridged via a simple end-to-end ureteroure-terostomy. Once the decision is made to proceed with an interposition, the appen-dix should be liberated along the anti-mesenteric border with care to preserve the integrity of the mesoappendix as well as the appendiceal artery. Using an endo GIA stapler, the appendix is transected off the cecum [14, 15]. Depending on the loca-tion of the appendix, liberating the cecum and colon may be helpful for positioning off tension. The appendix can then be ligated from the cecum by creating a small window at its base to place a stapling device. The tip of the appendix is then divided to expose the lumen. A 6Fr or 8Fr feeding tube is passed through the lumen to confirm the patency. Antiseptic solution should be used to irrigate the lumen of the appendix [12].

Preparing Ureter: Onlay Versus True Interposition

The targeted length of ureter should be liberated from its attachments and resected and debrided as needed. While true interposition requires a tubular section of the ureter to be completely resected, using the onlay technique will only require the ureter to be opened or partially resected. The onlay technique may be preferred as it preserves the ureteral plate in order to preserve blood supply and assists in anchor-ing the reconfigured appendix [16].

In the case of a true interposition, the proximal ureter is first spatulated and anas-tomosed to the base of the appendiceal lumen using interrupted 3–0 vicryl suture along one half of the circumference. A feeding tube is cut open with a guidewire passed through the lumen to facilitate the passage of the wire to the renal pelvis. Over this wire, a 6 Fr JJ stent is placed proximally up to the kidney. Alternatively, the placement of the stent may be combined with a retrograde pyelogram prior to beginning the procedure. To ensure patency of the ureter, a double-J ureteral stent can be placed over a wire from the bladder to the renal pelvis cystoscopically or in the surgical field. Proximal anastomosis is then completed in a running fashion. The distal ureter is then spatulated and anastomosed in a similar manner along half of the circumference. Once the stent is adequately visualized with good positioning, the remaining distal anastomosis is then completed. Keeping the cut ends of the suture long helps to provide traction and rotation of the ureter to allow for ureteral manipulation and proper placement of the next suture [12].

Tricks for Positioning off Tension

While the appendix is ideally situated for the repair of right ureteral defects, cases of left ureter repair have been described. In pediatric patients, the short distance between the appendix and the left ureter may promote the use of the appendix for left ureteral replacement [2, 5, 6, 25]. For adult patients, the appendix may be used for left ureteral procedures in specific cases, such as when forming an Indiana pouch as reported by Horwitz and Jarrard, in which they passed the appendix under the sigmoid mesentery to the left side of the retroperitoneum [26].

What to Do if Obliterated

If the appendix is inflamed, of inadequate length, or the patient has previous appendectomy, then alternative procedures must be resorted to. Alternatives include psoas hitch, Boari flap, ileal interposition, renal autotransplantation, or buccal mucosa graft.

Next Step if Fails or Needs Revision

Depending on the nature of the complications after the surgery, different techniques may be helpful to correct an appendiceal interposition. In some cases of stricture or stenosis, a stent may be adequate to restore flow. If the appendiceal interposition is no longer vascularized, ileum interposition or other uses of small bowel may be necessary [12]. In extreme cases when the kidney is no longer viable, nephrectomy may be indicated. Small leaks may self-correct with conservative stent placement or require surgical revision [18]. Common postoperative sequelae may include recurrent UTIs, urine leak with or without urinoma formation, ureteral stenosis, cecal leak, mucus based obstruction of the ureter, anastomotic stricture, and fistula [2, 3, 9, 10, 15]. Most case reports indicate good results with adequate drainage at 3–16 months on postoperative renal scans [2, 6, 7, 11, 12, 16, 25, 27, 28].

Long-term success rates with the appendiceal onlay or interposition are unknown, given the low number of cases reported in the literature. However, some studies have quoted failure rates of 5–15%. Depending on the length and severity of the recurrent stricture, treatment options include chronic ureteral stenting, endoureter-otomy, open reconstruction (e.g., ileal ureter, autotransplantation), or nephrectomy.

Ureterocalicostomy (UC)

The principle behind this form of surgical reconstruction is to provide a channel for unobstructed urinary flow by anastomosing the lower-pole renal calyx to the proximal ureter after excision of hydronephrotic lower-pole parenchyma. A uretero-calicostomy offers the benefit of completely excluding the renal pelvis and stenotic UPJ area and establishing urinary drainage from the lower calix directly into the ureter [29, 30].

Indications

Ureterocalicostomy is a reconstructive, salvage urologic procedure involving the direct anastomosis between a lower pole exposed renal calix with a healthy por-tion of the upper ureter [31]. This procedure was first reported by Neuwirt in 1947 as a potential treatment for patients with complicated ureteropelvic junction (UPJ) obstructions [32]. Since then, it has been described in the surgical management of a variety of pathologies involving the renal pelvis and the upper ureter. UC is clas-sically indicated for recurrent UPJ obstruction, failed pyeloplasty leading to dense fibrotic scar tissue formation or parapelvic inflammatory adhesions, high ureteral insertion, giant hydronephrosis, malrotated or horseshoe kidney, UPJ obstruction with unfavorable anatomy such as in an intrarenal pelvis, iatrogenic upper ureteral injury, or stricture formation secondary to pelvic surgery and radiation [29, 30, 33, 34].

Technique

The key steps include amputation of the lower pole of the renal parenchyma to enter the dependent portion of the lower-pole calix, preservation of the periureteral tissues along with its blood supply, reconstruction of a widely spatulated healthy ureter, and performance of a tension-free anastomosis with mucosa-to-mucosa apposition with adequate internal stenting [35, 36]. Typically, a guillotine amputation of the lower-pole parenchyma is done rather than doing a wedge resection to prevent the formation of anastomotic stricture [37]. An important aspect is the proper identifica-tion of the most dependent part of the lower-pole calyx within the collecting system and anastomosis of this portion with a widely spatulated proximal ureter. A tension-free anastomosis between the spatulated ureter and opened calyx is done with a 6–0 PDS suture, with care taken to ensure continuity between the urothelial lining of the ureteric lumen and surface of the opened calyx [33, 38].

Gill et al. described a laparoscopic technique using a transperitoneal approach wherein the UPJ is first dismembered and suture ligated, the cut end of the proximal ureter spatulated, the attenuated lower-pole renal parenchyma amputated, and finally a mucosa-to-mucosa ureterocaliceal anastomosis performed with running 4–0 absorbable suture over a stent. The robotic technique essentially mirrors the laparoscopic technique except for the use of a different platform and robotic instruments. Suturing may be facilitated using a robotic platform compared to laparoscopic intracorporeal suturing; however, both minimally invasive forms of reconstruction have been well described in literature [29, 32, 33].

Prior to beginning the procedure, a retrograde pyelogram is done to assess the length of the defect and delineate the anatomy of the UPJ. A ureteral stent insertion is then done cystoscopically into the lower pole calyx. The specific steps of the technique are discussed as follows [31, 33, 36]:

1. The patient is positioned in a modified flank position, and laparoscopic or robotic ports are inserted under direct vision.
2. The colon is mobilized and reflected medial, with adequate exposure of hilar vessels for en bloc clamping. Renal hilum must be dissected prior to lower-pole renal amputation if bleeding is encountered such that cross clamping of the renal vessels can be accomplished with relative ease.
3. The kidney is then mobilized with overlying Gerota's fascia, and the lower pole is identified.
4. The ureter with its periureteral tissue is also dissected cephalad toward UPJ from the surrounding fibrosis and inflammatory tissue.
5. An ultrasound probe should be used if needed to identify the lower pole calix. An approximately 2 cm circular rim of the tip of lower-pole renal parenchyma is amputated and excised using electrocautery (monopolar scissors in the case of robotic platform or sharp endo-shear scissors laparoscopically) and the lower-pole calix is subsequently entered.
6. Excess bleeding from the lower-pole parenchyma may be controlled by oversewing the bleeding parenchyma with an absorbable running suture while avoiding the incorporation of the calyceal opening.
7. The UPJ is then transected and the area of pathology excised following which a suture ligation of the open end of the UPJ is done.
8. The proximal ureter is then debrided to obtain a healthy lumen. Spatulation is done with care taken to avoid cutting the double-J stent.
9. An end-to-end ureterocaliceal anastomosis is performed with mucosa-to-mucosa apposition using two hemi-circular running sutures of 3–0 polyglactin (vicryl) on an RB-1 needle.
10. IV indigo carmine may be administered at the surgeon's discretion to confirm watertight repair, and a Jackson-Pratt drain is inserted to monitor for urine leak.

Postoperative Monitoring

Excretory urogram such as CT or MR with delayed phase along with a diuretic renogram may be obtained at 1–2 months and 6 months postoperative to assess for leak or obstruction and preservation of renal function in the affected renal unit. Postoperative ureteroscopy may also be done to ensure the adequacy of anastomotic site but should be done only if indicated on a retrograde pyelogram or CT urogram [29, 36, 39].

Current Literature

Literature surrounding UC is limited predominantly to case reports and series with the indications as discussed within the introduction section such as a difficult UPJ obstruction after failed pyeloplasty resulting in peripelvic fibrosis and scarring. The most common complications observed after this surgery is urinary tract infection noted in some series to be as high as 31% and urine leak with a rate of approximately 6% [30, 39]. Not surprisingly, several authors have also reported previous episodes of pyelonephritis, degree of scarring, inferior baseline renal function (GFR < 20), and cortical thinning (<5 mm) to be associated with inferior outcomes [30]. Most of these failures were evident within the first year after surgery with rates quoted to be approximately 66%, thus making it important to follow up these patients closely in the first year after surgery [30, 39]. Additionally, close monitoring of patients with repairs likely to fail based on poor prognostic indicators is warranted and also helps identify patients who may need additional salvage procedures.

Conclusion

Here, we describe two forms of ureteral repair that are not as frequently performed but offer excellent outcomes for reconstructing the ureter and salvaging function of the affected renal unit. In both forms of repair, good clinical judgment on part of the surgeon is needed both pre- and intraoperatively to assess surgical candidacy along with close attention to detail to optimize surgical outcomes.

References

1. Melnikoff A. Sur le replacement de l'uretere par anse isolee de l'intestine grele. Rev Clin Urol. 1912;1:601–3.
2. Cao H, Zhou H, Yang F, Ma L, Zhou X, Tao T, et al. Laparoscopic appendiceal interposition pyeloplasty for long ureteric strictures in children. J Pediatr Urol. Available from: http://www.sciencedirect.com/science/article/pii/S1477513118303607

3. Moscardi PRM, Blachman-Braun R, Labbie A, Castellan M. Staged ureteral reconstruction using the appendix in a complex pediatric patient. Urol Case Report. 2018;21:98–100.
4. Kumar P, Sarin YK. Use of appendix as neoureter – a ray of hope. J Neonatal Surg. 2017;6(3):64.
5. Obaidah A, Mane SB, Dhende NP, Acharya H, Goel N, Thakur AA, et al. Our experience of ureteral substitution in pediatric age group. Urology. 2010;75(6):1476–80.
6. Deyl RT, Averbeck MA, Almeida GL, Pioner GT, Souto CAV. Appendix interposition for total left ureteral reconstruction. J Pediatr Urol. 2009;5(3):237–9.
7. Dagash H, Sen S, Chacko J, Karl S, Ghosh D, Parag P, et al. The appendix as ureteral substitute: a report of 10 cases. J Pediatr Urol. 2008;4(1):14–9.
8. Richter F, Stock JA, Hanna MK. The appendix as right ureteral substitute in children. J Urol. 2000;163(6):1908–12.
9. Estevão-Costa J. Autotransplantation of the vermiform appendix for ureteral substitution. J Pediatr Surg. 1999;34(10):1521–3.
10. Martin LW. Use of the appendix to replace a ureter. Case Report J Pediatr Surg. 1981;16(6):799–800.
11. Gn M, Lee Z, Strauss D, Eun D. Robotic appendiceal interposition with right lower pole calycostomy, downward nephropexy, and psoas hitch for the Management of an Iatrogenic Near-complete Ureteral Avulsion. Urology. 2018;113:e9–10.
12. Yarlagadda VK, Nix JW, Benson DG, Selph JP. Feasibility of intracorporeal robotic-assisted laparoscopic appendiceal interposition for ureteral stricture disease: a case report. Urology. 2017;109:201–5.
13. Alcántara-Quispe C, Xavier JM, Atallah S, Romagnolo LGC, Melani AGF, Jorge E, et al. Laparoscopic left ureteral substitution using the cecal appendix after en-bloc rectosigmoidectomy: a case report and video demonstration. Tech Coloproctol. 2017;21(10):817–8.
14. Adani GL, Pravisani R, Baccarani U, Bolgeri M, Lorenzin D, Terrosu G, et al. Extended ureteral stricture corrected with appendiceal replacement in a kidney transplant recipient. Urology. 2015;86(4):840–3.
15. Duty BD, Kreshover JE, Richstone L, Kavoussi LR. Review of appendiceal onlay flap in the management of complex ureteric strictures in six patients. BJU Int. 2015;115(2):282–7.
16. Ordorica R, Wiegand LR, Webster JC, Lockhart JL. Ureteral replacement and onlay repair with reconfigured intestinal segments. J Urol. 2014;191(5):1301–6.
17. Antonelli A, Zani D, Dotti P, Tralce L, Simeone C, Cunico SC. Use of the appendix as ureteral substitute in a patient with a single kidney affected by relapsing upper urinary tract carcinoma. ScientificWorldJournal. 2005;5:276–9.
18. Jang TL, Matschke HM, Rubenstein JN, Gonzalez CM. Pyeloureterostomy with interposition of the appendix. J Urol. 2002;168(5):2106–7.
19. Medina JJ, Cummings JM, Parra RO. Repair of ureteral gunshot injury with appendiceal interposition. J Urol. 1999;161(5):1563.
20. Goldwasser B, Leibovitch I, Avigad I. Ureteral substitution using the isolated interposed vermiform appendix in a patient with a single kidney and transitional cell carcinoma of the ureter. Urology. 1994;44(3):437–40.
21. Global Burden of Disease Child and Adolescent Health Collaboration, Kassebaum N, Kyu HH, Zoeckler L, Olsen HE, Thomas K, et al. Child and adolescent health from 1990 to 2015: findings from the global burden of diseases, injuries, and risk factors 2015 study. JAMA Pediatr. 2017;171(6):573–92.
22. Komatz Y, Itoh H. A case of ureteral injury repaired with appendix. J Urol. 1990;144(1):132–3.
23. Okada Y, Ogura K, Ueda T, Kakehi Y, Terachi T, Arai Y, et al. Urinary reconstruction using appendix as a urinary and catheterizable conduit in 12 patients. Int J Urol. 1997;4(1):17–20.
24. Corbetta JP, Weller S, Bortagaray JI, Durán V, Burek C, Sager C, et al. Ureteral replacement with appendix in pediatric renal transplantation. Pediatr Transplant. 2012;16(3):235–8.
25. Springer A, Reck CA, Fartacek R, Horcher E. Appendix vermiformis as a left pyelo-ureteral substitute in a 6-month-old girl with solitary kidney. Afr J Paediatr Surg. 2011;8(2):218–20.

26. Horwitz GJ, Jarrard DF. Extension of a shortened ureter using the in situ appendix during Indiana pouch urinary diversion. Urology. 2004;63(1):167–9.
27. Thaker H, Patel N, García-Perdomo HA, Aron M. Open and robotic techniques for appendiceal interposition in ureteral stricture disease. Videourology. 2017;31(5). Available from: https://www.liebertpub.com/doi/full/10.1089/vid.2017.0011
28. Thomas A, Eng MM, Hagan C, Power RE, Little DM. Appendiceal substitution of the ureter in retroperitoneal fibrosis. J Urol. 2004;171(6 Pt 1):2378.
29. Matlaga BR, Shah OD, Singh D, Streem SB, Assimos DG. Ureterocalicostomy: a contemporary experience. Urology. 2005;65(1):42–4.
30. Srivastava D, Sureka SK, Yadav P, Bansal A, Gupta S, Kapoor R, et al. Ureterocalicostomy for reconstruction of complicated Ureteropelvic junction obstruction in adults: long-term outcome and factors predicting failure in a contemporary cohort. J Urol. 2017;198(6):1374–8.
31. Cherullo EE, Gill IS, Ponsky LE, Banks KLW, Desai MM, Kaouk JH, et al. Laparoscopic Ureterocalicostomy: a feasibility study. J Urol. 2003;169(6):2360–4.
32. Lobo S, Mushtaq I. Laparoscopic ureterocalicostomy in children: the technique and feasibility. J Pediatr Urol. 2018;14(4):358–9.
33. Korets R, Hyams ES, Shah OD, Stifelman MD. Robotic-assisted laparoscopic ureterocalicostomy. Urology. 2007;70(2):366–9.
34. Casale P, Patel RP, Kolon TF. Nerve sparing robotic extravesical ureteral reimplantation. J Urol. 2008;179(5):1987–90.
35. Raj A, Kudchadker S, Mittal V, Nunia S, Mandhani A. Importance of lower pole nephrectomy during ureterocalicostomy. Urology Annals. 2017;9(4):407.
36. Gill IS, Cherullo EE, Steinberg AP, Desai MM, Abreu SC, et al. Laparoscopic ureterocalicostomy: initial experience. J Urol. 2004;171(3):1227–30.
37. Jameson SG, McKinney JS, Rushton JF. Ureterocalyostomy: a new surgical procedure for correction of ureteropelvic stricture associated with an intrarenal pelvis. J Urol. 1957;77(2):135–43.
38. Ragoori D, Chiruvella M, Kondakindi PR, Bendigeri MT, Enganti B, Ghouse SM. Upper ureteric stricture secondary to celiac plexus block managed by robotic ureterocalicostomy. J Endourol Case Report. 2018;4(1):183–5.
39. Arap MA, Andrade H, Torricelli FCM, Denes FT, Mitre AI, Duarte RJ, et al. Laparoscopic ureterocalicostomy for complicated upper urinary tract obstruction: mid-term follow-up. Int Urol Nephrol. 2014;46(5):865–9.

Robotic Renal Autotransplantation and Ileal Ureter

11

Robert Steven Gerhard and Ronney Abaza

Introduction (Robotic Renal Autotransplantation)

Renal autotransplantation (RATx) was first described over 50 years ago by Hardy [1] for the treatment of severe proximal ureteral stricture. Since that time, RATx has been successfully used for several different conditions including complex ureteral injuries with significant ureteral loss, retroperitoneal fibrosis, loin pain-hematuria syndrome, severe nutcracker syndrome, and renal vascular anomalies.

Conventionally, RATx has been performed utilizing either a long midline incision from xiphoid to pubis or two separate incisions (flank incision for donor nephrectomy, pelvic incision for autotransplantation). Although excellent functional outcomes can be achieved, they are associated with significant incisional morbidity and extended recovery. As laparoscopic techniques improved, surgeons can now perform the auto-donor nephrectomy laparoscopically and then perform the conventional open pelvic incision for autotransplantation in the iliac fossa. Still, the ability to perform the operation with a completely minimally invasive intracorporeal approach was not technically feasible until the development of advanced robotic surgery.

The literature is limited with four cases reported to date specifically examining totally intracorporeal robotic RATx. In 2014, the first-ever completely intracorporeal robotic renal autotransplantation was performed and described in the literature by the author (RA) [2]. Since that time, surgeons in Canada [3], Japan [4], and most

Supplementary Information The online version of this chapter (https://doi.org/10.1007/978-3-030-50196-9_11) contains supplementary material, which is available to authorized users.

R. S. Gerhard · R. Abaza (✉)
OhioHealth Dublin Methodist Hospital, Dublin, OH, USA
e-mail: Robert.Gerhard@Ohiohealth.com; Ronney.Abaza@OhioHealth.com

© Springer Nature Switzerland AG 2022
M. D. Stifelman et al. (eds.), *Techniques of Robotic Urinary Tract Reconstruction*, https://doi.org/10.1007/978-3-030-50196-9_11

113

recently in Europe [5] have reported their experience with totally intracorporeal robotic RATx with similar techniques.

These studies have reported that totally intracorporeal robotic RATx is safe and feasible and results in a good functioning autotransplanted kidney in the well-selected patient and when performed by highly experienced surgeons. The robotic approach may be particularly advantageous as the graft is already intracorporeal allowing the operation to be performed with the longest incision being ~12 mm. With reduced overall morbidity from this entirely minimally invasive approach, there may be an opportunity to apply this technique more broadly within the field as a viable salvage option with acceptable morbidity when nephrectomy is being considered.

Preoperative Preparation and Planning

Preoperative Assessment

A standard preoperative assessment of the patient's medical and surgical history is completed. The ureteral anatomy should be examined by the surgeon to understand the location and extent of nonviable ureter utilizing cross-sectional imaging and fluoroscopic evaluation with antegrade and/or retrograde pyelography. Nuclear medicine renal scan should be obtained to ensure the kidney of interest has sufficient function to warrant RATx. These findings together with serum creatinine should be used to counsel the patient on treatment considerations. The surgeon may consider obtaining computed tomography angiography to obtain further detail of the vascular anatomy if any anomaly or concern is detected on standard imaging.

Operating Room Preparation, Positioning, and Instrumentation

The procedure is performed transperitoneally utilizing the da Vinci surgical system (Intuitive Surgical Inc., Sunnyvale, CA, USA). Antibiotic prophylaxis with second-generation cephalosporin is given, sequential compression devices are placed, and an orogastric tube is placed to decompress the stomach. A Foley catheter is placed. The patient should be positioned to allow access to both the renal and iliac fossae and also allow for intracorporeal renal hypothermic perfusion. An approach similar to robotic nephroureterectomy has been successfully utilized where the bed and robot are repositioned but the patient is not. This avoids the need for reestablishing a sterile field. The patient is placed supine on a bean bag with a gel roll bump under the kidney to slightly elevate the flank. The bean bag assists in securing the patient in the desired position. The legs are placed in Allen stirrups and spread in a scissor fashion to allow access between the legs for the robot to be positioned during the pelvic portion of the operation if utilizing the da Vinci S or Si robots, whereas this can be avoided if using the Xi robot with side docking. The arms are secured by the patient's side using foam padding. A foam-padded strap is also placed loosely around the chest to ensure the patient is secure and allow for changes in bed positioning. The bed is rotated during the nephrectomy portion of the operation to further elevate the flank (Fig. 11.1).

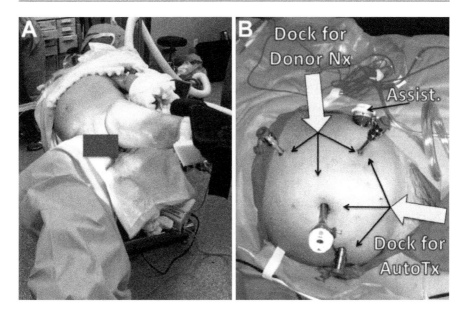

Fig. 11.1 Patient positioning (**a**) and port placement (**b**) for a left-sided RATx. This approach allows for the repositioning of the bed and robot rather than the patient to complete the operation. (Picture from Gordon et al. [2])

Surgical Technique

Step 1: Port Placement and Instruments

For left-sided operations, as few as five ports are utilized: (1) 12 mm periumbilical camera port (30° lens), (2) 8 mm left upper quadrant, (3) 8 mm left lower quadrant, (4) 8 mm right lower quadrant, and (5) 12 mm AirSeal assistant port far lateral left lower quadrant. For right-sided operations, the surgeon may also consider utilizing an additional port for liver retraction. For the nephrectomy portion of the operation, the author utilizes a three-arm approach with Maryland bipolar forceps in the 8 mm left upper quadrant port and monopolar scissors in the 8 mm left lower quadrant port. An additional 8 mm port can be placed for the use of the robotic fourth arm if preferred. For the autotransplanted pelvic portion of the operation, a 0° lens is used, and all three 8 mm ports are utilized with a ProGrasp placed in the upper quadrant port. During the anastomoses portion of the operation, large needle drivers and DeBakey forceps are utilized. For vessel ligation, the author (RA) utilizes the large robotic clip applier with large Hem-o-Lok® clips.

Step 2: Robotic Donor Nephrectomy

Left Kidney Harvest

The colon is medialized, and the hilar vessels are dissected circumferentially down to the aorta to allow for maximum vessel length. The venous branches of the left renal vein (gonadal, adrenal, lumbar) are ligated and divided using large Hem-o-Lok® clips placed by the surgeon with the robotic clip appliers. The kidney is entirely mobilized, and perinephric fat is removed except off the lower pole to preserve ureteral blood supply. The ureter is carefully dissected while preserving as much adventitial tissue as possible. The dissection is continued as distally as possible until the diseased ureteral segment is reached. The ureter is divided above the diseased area. Visual confirmation that the caliber and mucosa of the viable ureter are normal is adequate. Prior to renal vessel ligation, 10 mg of furosemide and 12.5 mg of mannitol are administered by the anesthesiologist. Preparations are then made to establish renal hypothermia after the vessels are divided.

Right Kidney Harvest
The positioning and technique for right-sided operation are similar to the left-sided operation. The primary consideration is the anatomic limitation of the short right renal vein. For this reason, it is imperative that the vein be ligated close to the vena cava to ensure as much length as possible. The renal artery can be taken at the aorta for additional length by accessing it in the interaortocaval space.

Protective Intracorporeal Renal Hypothermia
The equipment and instruments utilized for protective renal hypothermia during conventional donor transplant nephrectomy can be utilized readily intracorporeally (LifeShield Macrobore Extension Set, No. 12655-28). The perfusion cannula and tubing are introduced via the valveless AirSeal assistant port; 3000 units of heparin are administered, and the renal artery is ligated at the level of the aorta with robotic Hem-o-Lok® clips. It is critical to use more than one clip and to leave enough of an arterial stump to prevent dislodgement from the high blood pressure of the aorta. If this would require overly shortening the renal artery for the transplantation, an alternative would be to place one clip for expediency and then place a suture stick tie on the artery stump once the cold perfusion has begun and time is no longer a limitation. An alternative would be to use a TA stapler with the goal of maximizing the length of the vessels. The renal vein is ligated with clips and does not require any additional measures for control. The vessels are then divided above the clips. The perfusion cannula is then placed into the lumen of the renal artery, and the kidney is then perfused with ice-cold lactated ringer solution (or other solution) by gravity. Clear effluent should be seen from the renal vein. The cannula is secured to the renal artery cuff with a silk tie to keep it in place when the patient is repositioned and the kidney brought into the pelvis. Hemostasis is confirmed in the operative field, and the abdomen is then desufflated, and the robot is undocked. The bed and robot are repositioned for the pelvic portion of the operation.

Step 3: Vascular Anastomoses
The bed is flattened and then placed in Trendelenburg, and the robot is moved to between the legs for the pelvic portion of the operation. Importantly, this approach does not require the patient to be repositioned, and the sterile field is maintained.

The bladder is mobilized from the abdominal wall, and the space of Retzius is entered in similar fashion as in prostatectomy. The external iliac artery and vein are identified and circumferentially dissected away from surrounding tissue. Dissection should be continued until sufficient length is achieved to allow for clamping and the anastomosis. The kidney is placed into the pelvis and onto the bladder maintaining cold perfusion through the catheter at all times.

The external iliac vein (EIV) is clamped using laparoscopic bulldog clamps. A venotomy is made, and a running end-to-side anastomosis is performed between the EIV and renal vein utilizing a CV-6 GORE-TEX suture. Prior to completion, the lumen is irrigated with heparinized saline via a 5 French ureteral catheter. When the anastomosis is completed, a bulldog clamp is placed on the renal vein, and the clamps on the EIV are removed.

The perfusion cannula from the renal artery is removed, and the distal portion of the vessel is sharply trimmed where the silk ligature was used to secure the perfusion cannula. An end-to-side arterial anastomosis is then performed in the same fashion as described for venous anastomosis. There should now be three clamps in place: distal external iliac artery (EIA), proximal EIA, and the renal vein. The clamps are removed starting with the distal EIA to test for a leak, followed by the renal vein and finally the proximal EIA. With renal perfusion, the kidney should begin to produce urine and return to a pink appearance, and a laparoscopic Doppler ultrasound probe is used to confirm blood flow.

Step 4: Ureteral Reconstruction

The approach and technique for ureteral reconstruction will depend on the etiology of the patient's condition, status of the ureter and bladder, and surgeon preference. Similar principles used in other areas of reconstructive urology are utilized with the goal of achieving a watertight, tension-free repair with viable mucosa to mucosa approximation. Options for reconstruction include but are not limited to ureteroureterostomy if the ipsilateral distal ureteral segment is healthy, ureteroneocystostomy, and pyelocystostomy. The author (RA) uses two 3–0 Vicryl sutures in running fashion over an indwelling ureteral stent for ureteral reconstruction. The repair should be tested by filling the bladder with saline to ensure it is watertight.

After the desired ureteral reconstruction is completed, the kidney must be pexed to the abdominal wall. The author (RA) performs this by securing capsular fat on the anterior kidney to the peritoneum using robotic Hem-o-Lok® clips.

The entirety of the operative field including the vascular anastomoses are reexamined. The robotic instruments are then removed, 12 mm port sites are closed, and a drain is placed into the pelvis in proximity to the reconstructed ureter (Fig. 11.2).

Surgical Technique Discussion

There is limited experience reported in the literature regarding totally intracorporeal robotic RATx, and all were for long-segment proximal ureteral stricture disease. These cases utilized a similar surgical technique as described above. Lee et al. approached this operation in three separate stages rather than two with the primary

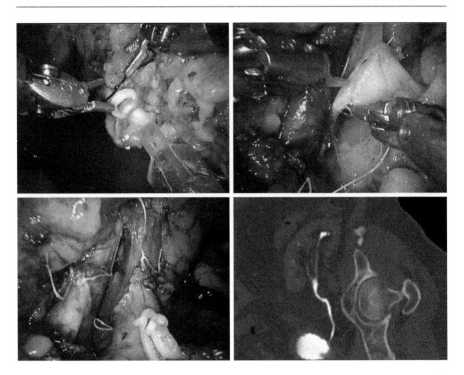

Fig. 11.2 Clockwise from upper left-arterial cannula for cold perfusion, venous anastomosis, completed vascular anastomoses, and CT scan of autotransplanted kidney

difference being an initial stage in the pelvis with the mobilization of the bladder and evaluation of the lower urinary tract and dissection of the iliac vessels to ensure the suitability of ultimate reconstruction prior to proceeding with nephrectomy. Decaestecker and colleagues developed a robotic surgical technique utilizing extracorporeal bench surgery for those patients with complex oncologic and urolithiasis cases as well as multiple vessel grafts and also when the contralateral iliac fossa is utilized because of pelvic vascular anatomy or for lower urinary tract reconstructive purposes. While this allows the surgeon to address certain complexities by extracting the kidney and then reintroducing it as in robotic living donor kidney transplantation, it requires a larger incision than the completely intracorporeal approach.

Postoperative Care

Postoperative care and criteria for discharge are similar to other major urologic robotic operations with an emphasis on early ambulation, narcotic avoidance, and diet as tolerated. The author utilizes intravenous ketorolac and oral acetaminophen assuming the patient has normal renal and liver function. The drain is removed prior to discharge if there is no concern for a urine leak. Doppler ultrasound of the autotransplant can be obtained on postoperative day one, and the serum creatinine is trended during hospitalization. If these studies show no abnormalities, then the patient can be considered for discharge as early as postoperative day one.

The patient is seen in routine postoperative follow-up. A mercaptoacetyltrigly-cine nuclear renogram can be obtained approximately 6 weeks after surgery with ureteral stent removal once the normal renal function is confirmed to avoid confusion over the potential that ureteral obstruction is present if renal function is compromised. A CT with contrast and delayed images can also be obtained to ensure prompt contrast excretion into the collecting system and to evaluate the ureteral and vascular anastomoses for patency.

Complications associated with this procedure include typical complications that could be seen in any minimally invasive or robotic procedure (e.g., access injury, bowel injury) as well as the potential complications associated with open or robotic allograft renal transplantation (e.g., arterial thrombosis, lymphocele, graft torsion) with the notable exception, of course, of graft rejection [6].

Introduction (Robotic Ileal Ureter)

Utilizing a portion of small bowel for ureteral substitution for the long-segment and complex ureteral disease was first reported in 1959 by Goodwin [6]. Ileal interposition has demonstrated good long-term outcomes in appropriately selected patients. Replicating the principles of open surgery, the procedure was first performed laparoscopically by Gill and colleagues in 2000 [7].

Wagner et al. reported the first totally intracorporeal robot-assisted laparoscopic ileal ureter in 2008 [8]. Since that time, several other authors have reported case reports [9–13]. The largest series to date was published in 2018 by Ubrig and colleagues [14]. The series included seven consecutive patients undergoing completely intracorporeal ileal interposition for ureteric replacement and represents the most recent and largest series to date.

Surgical Technique

Operating Room Preparation, Positioning, and Instrumentation
The patient is placed in a flank position utilizing a bean bag or towel rolls, and the bed is slightly flexed. Robotic instruments include monopolar scissors, vessel sealer, large needle driver, Cadiere forceps, fenestrated or Maryland bipolar forceps, and an Endo GIA stapler or alternatively the robotic stapler when available. A transperitoneal approach is used. A foley catheter is placed into the bladder on the operative field (Fig. 11.3).

Operative Steps
A four-arm approach with an assistant port is utilized. A 12 mm camera port is placed above the umbilicus, and a 30° down robotic camera is introduced. Two 8 mm robotic ports are placed in the same line at the costal margin and in the lower

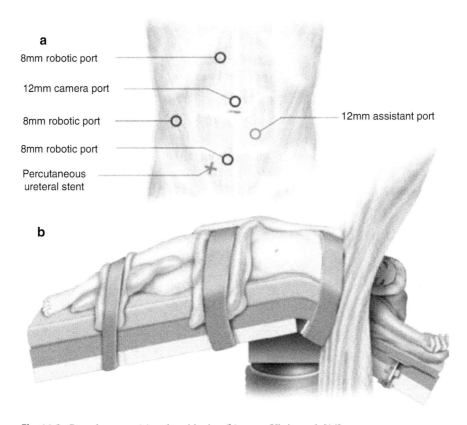

Fig. 11.3 Port placement (**a**) and positioning (**b**) as per Ubrig et al. [14]

quadrant which are used for the primary working left- and right-hand instruments. An additional 8 mm port is placed above the anterior superior iliac spine which is used for the fourth arm. An additional assistant port is placed generally between the camera and the lower quadrant 8 mm port.

The operation begins as in routine renal surgery where the intestine is medialized and the hilum and ureter are identified. The renal pelvis is mobilized and dissected free of surrounding tissue to allow for eventual anastomosis with the ileum. The entire length of the diseased ureter segment is mobilized down to the bladder. The bladder is then dissected free from the abdominal wall. If necessary, a psoas hitch is performed.

The ileum and the ileocecal valve are identified. Similar to an ileal conduit, an approximately 20 cm segment of the terminal ileum is preserved, and a suitable segment of ileum is identified. A known length of vessel loop can be used to assist in measurement. Once the desired portion of ileum is identified, it is transected utilizing an Endo GIA stapler. A marking suture is placed at the distal aspect of the ileal segment to be utilized. The bowel is placed back in continuity by performing a standard end-to-end anastomosis with the Endo GIA stapler or suture depending on surgeon preference. Ubrig et al. introduce a 14 French drain through the abdominal wall and under direct vision place the drain into the bladder which ultimately will be placed across the ileal anastomoses with the renal pelvis and bladder as a type of modified suprapubic tube. A separate 3 cm cystotomy is made at the superior aspect of the bladder where the ultimate ileovesical anastomosis will be performed.

The segment of ileum for interposition is then placed into a retroperitoneal position. On the right side, the segment has to be rotated to ensure the appropriate peristaltic direction for urine transport. On the left side, a window in the sigmoid and left colon mesentery is created for the ileal segment to be brought through. Next, utilizing the upper quadrant robotic arm, the previously placed a 14 French drain is brought out of the cystotomy at the superior aspect of the bladder where ileovesical anastomosis will occur and through the entire length of ileum and placed into the renal pelvis. The pyeloileal and ileovesical anastomosis are then completed with two running 4–0 PDS sutures in a semicircular fashion. The bladder is filled to ensure that these anastomoses are watertight. A surgical drain is placed near each anastomosis, and the operation is completed (Fig. 11.4).

Postoperative Care

The patient is admitted to the hospital for routine postoperative care. Ubrig and colleagues perform a fluoroscopic retrograde study of the 14 French percutaneous ileal ureter stent and the ureteral Foley catheter around postoperative day 10–12 prior to removal. The day after stent removal, renal ultrasound is obtained. Post-discharge follow-up includes routine renal ultrasonography to ensure no evidence of obstruction and routine renal function testing.

Potential complications associated with this procedure include any potential complications seen in laparoscopic or robotic surgery in general (e.g., access injury, port-site hernia) as well as complications particular to use of bowel segments and ureteral surgery. These could include urine leaks, stricture at anastomotic sites, bowel obstruction, reflux nephropathy, recurrent urinary tract infections (i.e., from reflux), and metabolic side effects of absorption from the bowel segment. Use of an

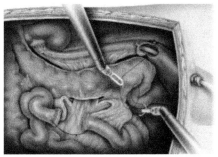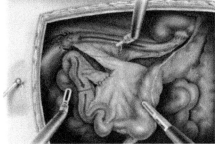

Figs. 11.4 Right and left ileal interposition from Ubrig et al. [14]

antirefluxing mechanism or antiperistaltic configuration has been associated with more complications, such that their role is uncertain [7, 15].

References

Introduction (Robotic Renal Autotransplantation)

1. Hardy JD, Eraslan S. Autotransplantation of the kidney for high ureteral injury. J Urol. 1963;90:563.
2. Gordon ZN, Angell J, Abaza R. Completely intracorporeal robotic renal autotransplantation. J Urol. 2014;192(5):1516–22.
3. Lee JY, Alzahrani T, Ordon M. Intra-corporeal robotic renal auto-transplantation. Can Urol Assoc J. 2015;9(9–10):E748.
4. Araki M, Wada K, Mitsui Y, Sadahira T, Kubota R, Nishimura S, et al. Robotic renal autotransplantation: first case outside of North America. Acta Med Okayama. 2017;71(4):351–5.
5. Decaestecker K, Van Parys B, Van Besien J, Doumerc N, Desender L, Randon C, et al. Robot-assisted kidney autotransplantation: a minimally invasive way to salvage kidneys. Eur Urol Focus. 2018;4(2):198–205.
6. Territo A, Mottrie A, Abaza R, Rogers C, Menon M, Bhandari M, Ahlawat R, Breda A. Robotic kidney transplantation: current status and future perspectives. Minerva Urol Nefrol. 2017;69(1):5–13.

Introduction (Robotic Ileal Ureter)

7. Goodwin WE, Winter CC, Turner RD. Replacement of the ureter by small intestine: clinical application and results of the ileal ureter. J Urol. 1959;81:406–18.
8. Gill IS, Savage SJ, Senagore AJ, et al. Laparoscopic ileal ureter. J Urol. 2000;163:1199–202.
9. Wagner JR, Schimpf MO, Cohen JL. Robot-assisted laparoscopic ileal ureter. JSLS. 2008;12:306–9.
10. Brandao LF, Autorino R, Zargar H, et al. Robotic ileal ureter: a completely intracorporeal technique. Urology. 2014;83:951–4.
11. Baumgarten AS, Shah BB, Patel TB, et al. Robotic ileal interposition for radiation-induced ureteral stricture disease. Urology. 2017; https://doi.org/10.1016/j.urology.2017.02.033.
12. Abhyankar N, Vendryes C, Deane LA. Totally intracorporeal robot-assisted laparoscopic reverse seven ileal ureteric reconstruction. Can J Urol. 2015;22:7748–51.
13. Sim A, Todenhöfer T, Mischinger J, et al. Intracorporeal ileal ureter replacement using laparoscopy and robotics. Cent Eur J Urol. 2014;67:420–3.
14. Ubrig B, Janusonis J, Paulics L, Boy A, Heiland M, Roosen A. Functional outcome of completely Intracorporeal robotic Ileal ureteric replacement. Urology. 2018;114:193–7.
15. Shokeir AA, Ghoneim MA. Further experience with the modified ileal ureter. J Urol. 1995;154(1):45–8.

Ureterolysis and Boari Flap

12

Nathan Cheng, Mutahar Ahmed, and Michael D. Stifelman

Indications for Ureterolysis

Ureterolysis is typically reserved to manage patients that have developed an extrinsic compression of the proximal/mid ureter. Causes may include infection, tumor, and most commonly retroperitoneal fibrosis (RPF). RPF is a rare disease (incidence 0.1–1.3 cases/100,000 people per year) characterized by fibrosis and chronic inflammation of the retroperitoneum frequently causing ureteral obstruction, usually stemming from periaortic and peri-iliac adventitia and their surrounding soft tissue. RPF is idiopathic in 70% of patients, currently thought to be a disease process on the spectrum of large vessel vasculitides, whereas the 30% with known causes can be traced back to medication adverse effects, especially of ergot alkaloids such as methysergide, radiation, malignancy, and infection. Over the past decade, the concept of idiopathic RPF belonging to the spectrum of IgG4-related disease has emerged, a disease process encompassing fibro-inflammatory disorders characterized by lymphoplasmacytic, fibrotic, and IgG4+ plasma cell infiltration of various organ systems (i.e., lymph nodes, pancreas, and biliary tree) [1].

Ureteral involvement is the most common complication related to RPF. It can be unilateral or bilateral; in cases of unilateral disease, contralateral disease may

Supplementary Information The online version of this chapter (https://doi.org/10.1007/978-3-030-50196-9_12) contains supplementary material, which is available to authorized users.

N. Cheng (✉)
Hackensack Meridian Health, Hackensack University Medical Center, Hackensack, NJ, USA

Hackensack Meridian School of Medicine, Nutley, NJ, USA

M. Ahmed
Hackensack Meridian Health, Hackensack University Medical Center, Hackensack, NJ, USA

M. D. Stifelman
Department of Urology, Hackensack Meridian Health School of Medicine, Nutley, NJ, USA

rarely progress weeks to years after the initial presentation [2]. Acute renal failure can be seen in RPF with ureteral involvement, more commonly in bilateral disease. Patients most commonly present with systemic symptoms such as fatigue, weight loss, anorexia, and ureteral colic.

Idiopathic RPF is associated with other autoimmune disorders such as rheumatoid arthritis, ankylosing spondylitis, systemic lupus erythematosus, and, most commonly, thyroiditis.

Workup

The etiology of a patient's retroperitoneal disease should be determined prior to surgical consideration. If believed to be idiopathic/autoimmune, many studies have suggested a trial of glucosteroids and/or immmunosuppresive therapies with a ureteral stent or nephrostomy tube placed to relieve obstruction, particularly in mild to moderate ureteral obstruction [3]. First-line medical therapy is prednisone with an initial dose of 0.75–1 mg/kg/day with a gradual taper to 5–7.5 mg/day within 6–9 months [4]. Commonly used immunosuppressants include mycophenolate mofetil and cyclophosphamide. Other studies have suggested a biopsy to confirm no evidence lymphoma or malignancy prior to definitive management [5–8]. For those that a biopsy is recommended or required, it has been suggested that a surgical excisional biopsy performed robotically may be performed in conjunction with a ureterolysis, assuming the frozen section biopsy rules out lymphoma or malignancy [9].

When medical therapy fails or the decision is made to perform a combined biopsy and ureterolysis as initial treatment, it is paramount to know the length and location of the diseased ureter. Imaging of the ureter includes either CT urogram or MRI urogram. MRI has been shown to have specific advantages in differentiating between lymphoma versus retroperitoneal fibrosis [10]. In patients where there is atrophy of the kidney or concern function, we recommend a diuretic renal scan to confirm adequate function for preservation, which we believe is >15% split function.

Cystoscopy with retrograde pyelography of the affected ureter should be performed at the time of surgery in order to identify the level and length of obstruction. Placement or exchange of ureteral stent should be performed preoperatively; this is an important step that will allow for intraoperatively ultrasound-guided identification of the ureter, protection of the ureter, and confirmation of inadvertent injury during dissection. In patients with complete ureteral obstruction where a nephrostomy tube has been placed, a simultaneous antegrade and retrograde pyelogram may be performed for better delineation. It is important to note we do not recommend doing a bilateral ureterolysis in patients with unilateral obstruction. Multiple studies have shown the risk of contralateral obstruction is small, and this is not required [8, 11, 12].

Patients require an extensive informed consent regarding all possibilities that may occur in complex ureteral reconstruction, including, but not limited to, ureterolysis, Boari flap, psoas hitch, ureteroureterostomy, transureteroureterostomy, ureterocalicostomy, ureteral reimplantation, nephrectomy, and even autotransplantation.

Robotic-Assisted Laparoscopic Ureterolysis and Omental Flap Surgical Technique

Unilateral

Patient Positioning

For unilateral ureterolysis with omental flap, the patient should be positioned in semilateral decubitus with modified low lithotomy, affected side up, similar to that of a robotic-assisted laparoscopic pyeloplasty. For female patients, we place both legs up in stirrups allowing for urethral access, intraoperative cystoscopic and/or retrograde procedures, and redocking of the robot to the foot of the bed if Boari flap or ureteral reimplantation became necessary.

Trocar Placement

When performing a multiport procedure, we prefer using all four arms of the da Vinci Xi system, as well as one additional 5 mm bedside assistant trocar. The 8 mm trocar for the camera port should be within or at the level of the umbilicus. The two working arms via 8 mm trocars should be along the ipsilateral lateral rectus line: one 2–3 cm below the costal margin and the other at the level of the iliac crest or caudal enough to be 8 cm from the camera port. The fourth arm of the robot will go through an 8 mm trocar inferolateral to the caudal working arm. The 5 mm bedside assistant trocar should be in the midline 8–10 cm inferior to the umbilicus. Trocar placement under direct visualization with the camera is recommended. After all trocars are placed in the appropriate positions, the robot will come in on the ipsilateral side for docking (Fig. 12.1).

Bilateral

Patient Positioning

We approach a bilateral ureterolysis with the setup similar to a robotic bilateral retroperitoneal lymph node dissection. The patient should be positioned supine and female patients in lithotomy to allow urethral access. The arms are padded appropriately and tucked to the side. The patient should be placed in slight Trendelenburg to allow for cephalad mobilization of the bowel. The template for port placements in bilateral retroperitoneal lymph node dissection has been referenced by many authors, most of which mimic to that of James Porter's, as detailed below [13, 14].

Trocar Placement

Again, all four arms of the da Vinci Xi systems are utilized with an assistant port. Pneumoperitoneum is achieved with a Veress needle at Palmer's point in the left

Fig. 12.1 **a**. Unilateral
(left-sided) robotic-assisted
laparoscopic ureterolysis
port placements. **b**.
Unilateral (left-sided)
robotic-assisted
laparoscopic ureterolysis
port placements

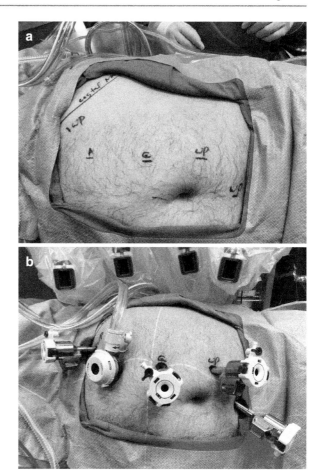

upper quadrant. The 8 mm camera trocar will be placed at midline about halfway
between the umbilicus and pubic symphysis. The remaining four trocars, including the two working ports, fourth arm, and 5 mm assistant port, are placed linearly
along the lower abdomen. 8 mm trocars should be placed on either side of the camera, and the 8 mm trocar for the fourth arm even more laterally. The 5 mm assistant
port is placed contralateral to the fourth arm. See the picture below (Fig. 12.2).

Retroperitoneal Exposure

The first step in the operation is to gain access to the retroperitoneum, and it is crucial to have adequate exposure of the entire length of the ureter. In a unilateral procedure, we rely on the assistance of gravity to help reflect the colon medially after
incising the white line of Toldt. On the right side, the entire ascending colon should
be reflected from the liver superiorly to the bladder inferiorly; on the left, the entire
descending colon should be reflected from the spleen to the bladder. For right-sided
procedures, the duodenum should be identified after reflecting the ascending colon;

Fig. 12.2 Bilateral
ureterolysis port
placements

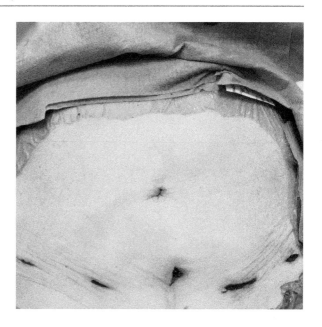

subsequently, Kocher maneuver should be performed in order to reflect small bowel medially and superiorly to adequately expose the right renal vein, inferior vena cava, and gonadal vessels. Raytec gauze may be used so the retraction arm is not directly touching delicate tissue.

When performing a bilateral ureterolysis, access to the retroperitoneum starts with mobilization of the cecum and ileum by incising the posterior peritoneum medial to the cecum up to the ligament of Treitz. The incised edge of the posterior peritoneum can then be tacked up to the anterior abdominal wall with V-lock sutures, Weck clips, or magnetic graspers in order to provide exposure to the retroperitoneum. The fourth arm is helpful to hold bowel cephalad.

Ureter Identification

Once the retroperitoneum is adequately visualized, the next step is to identify the ureter. This may be particularly challenging based on the degree of disease. The fibrotic rind encasing the ureter is often thick and may distort the normal location of the ureter to be more medial than expected, particularly on the left side. We always try to identify the normal ureter proximal or distal to the obstruction and work from known to unknown anteriorly. Some anatomic considerations include identifying the ureter distally at the crossing of the iliac vessels, looking for the ureter in the retroperitoneum more medial to normal anatomy, and following the medial umbilical ligament from the anterior abdominal wall into the pelvis where the ureter will be medial as it enters the bladder. When that is difficult, one can introduce an intraoperative robotic ultrasound probe to identify the stent placed in the ureter. One can also exchange the stent for a ureteroscope (URS) and use the light from URS to identify the location of the ureter which is enhanced on near-infrared imaging

(NIRF) modality. Also, if ICG is available, 5 cc diluted ICG can be given through a stent which will bind to the ureter and also be visible on NIRF. Once the location is confirmed, the first goal is to identify the anterior wall of the ureter and adventitia. Electrocautery should be sparingly used in this dissection, as risk for ischemia to ureteral tissue should be minimized in order to prevent delayed leak as a postoperative complication (Fig. 12.3).

Ureterolysis

Once ureteral adventitia is visualized, the curved scissors can be switched out for Potts scissors for finer dissection. Ureterolysis should be done systematically by exposing a segment of the anteriorureteral adventitia and then peeling back circumferentially to totally free the ureter from the posterior fibrosis. Once the segment of the ureter is completely freed posteriorly, a vessel loop should be introduced around the ureter to allow for traction. The direction of ureterolysis should be in the

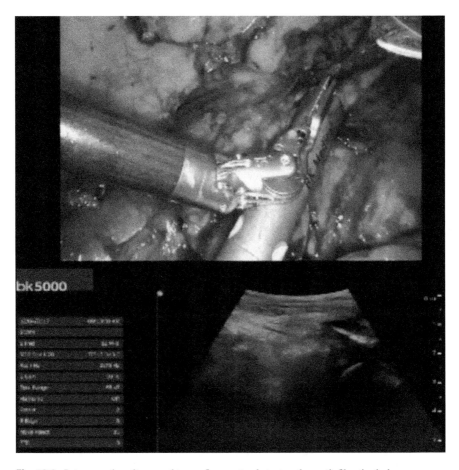

Fig. 12.3 Intraoperative ultrasound to confirm ureteral stent underneath fibrotic rind

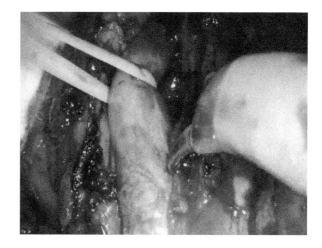

Fig. 12.4 Use of VessiLoop to help retract exposed ureter off fibrotic rind to allow for circumferential dissection distally

caudal direction for a unilateral repair and cephalad in a bilateral procedure. The vessel loop should freely slide in the direction of ureterolysis to assist in dissection. Usually, if the operator is in the correct plane, the fibrotic rind should not be difficult to peel off from the ureter. The distal and proximal extent of the ureterolysis is known when normal, healthy periureteral fat is seen (Fig. 12.4).

Biopsy Fibrotic Mass
After the ureter is completely freed from the sticky retroperitoneal mass, a biopsy of the mass should be sent for pathologic evaluation.

After freeing off the ureter, intravenous ICG of 2 mL may be given to assess the perfusion to the ureter in order to ensure good blood supply.

Stricturoplasty and Inadvertent Ureterotomy
It is not uncommon for certain segments of the ureter to be strictured due to extrinsic disease. If there are grossly strictured segments less than 1.5 cm or an inadvertent injury to the ureter, a stricturoplasty should be performed in the Heineke-Mikulicz fashion. A longitudinal, or vertical, ureterotomy is made along the strictured segment with Potts scissors. The longitudinal ureterotomy is then closed transversely, or horizontally, with a Vicryl suture. In longer segments, one should consider a buccal mucosa graft (BMG) ureteroplasty. BMG ureteroplasty, first pioneered in the mid-1990s, has been shown to be feasible robotically; Stifelman and Zhao described robotic onlay and augmented anastomotic ureteroplasty for strictures up to 6 cm in 2015 (Fig. 12.5) [15]. Subsequent reviews have shown BMG repairs in up to 11 cm diseased segments [16, 17]. These surgical principles prevent the area of the ureteral lumen to be decreased, lowering the risk for postoperative stricture.

Omental Wrap
After complete ureterolysis is performed, the healthy omentum should be used to encase the entire ureter length in order to prevent the recurrence of ureteral

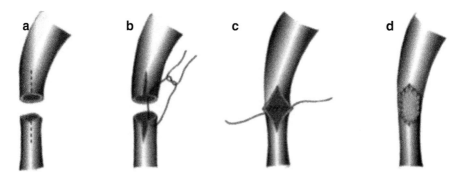

Fig. 12.5 Augmented anastomotic ureteroplasty. **a**. Strictured ureter segment excised and each end spatulated. **b**. Dorsal portion of transected renal pelvis and ureter anastomosed. **c**. Diamond-shaped ventral defect left. **d**. Defect covered with buccal mucosa graft

obstruction from fibrotic tissue and lateralize the ureter. The distal edge of the omentum is grasped and bifurcated with hot shears, bipolar electrocautery, and/or a vessel-sealing device toward the stomach. It is important to free enough omentum to wrap the entire length of the performed ureterolysis. If more length is needed, the omentum can be freed from the stomach by ligating the short gastric vessels; however, care must be taken to preserve the left and right gastroepiploic arteries, which provide the majority of the perfusion to the omentum. We like to give 2 cc of ICG intravenously to confirm good vascularity to the omentum. The wrap is performed by starting at the most distal aspect of the ureterolysis. The omentum should be brought around posterior to the ureter and tacked with securing an absorbable suture to the lateral wall. The medial aspect of the omental wrap is then placed anterior to ureter completing the wrap and retracting the ureter laterally along the entire length of the ureter. At the proximal extent of the omental wrap, the omentum may be tacked to the psoas fascia at kidney level (Figs. 12.6 and 12.7).

Peritonealizing the Ureter

Another method described, which we have little experience with, is to peritonealize the ureter to keep it away from the disease retroperitoneum. The peritoneal attachments of the colon are placed posterior to ureter; however, this does not provide for increased blood supply nor lateralization as does omental wrap, and it is the opinion of the authors to use only as a last resort.

Postoperative Course

There is no consensus for the need for a surgical drain documented in literature. Theoretically, if there was no need for stricturoplasty, ureteroureterostomy, or other necessary intraoperative maneuvers that open into ureteral lumen, there should be no risk for urine leakage. However, surgical drains are commonly placed near the omental wrap at the end of the procedure. A ureteral stent is left in place and removed in 4 weeks with follow-up symptom assessment, renal ultrasound, and MAG3 renal scan to evaluate for evidence of obstruction. The main two outcomes of interest post-ureterolysis are symptom and radiographic resolution of obstruction.

Fig. 12.6 Bifurcation of the omentum to prepare omental wrap

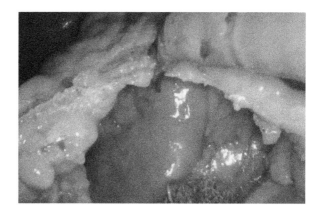

Fig. 12.7 ICG confirmation of adequately perfused ureter (foreground) and omentum wrap posteriorly (background)

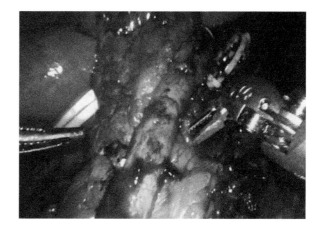

Complications

In addition to known perioperative complications including, but not limited to, thromboembolism, myocardial infarction, and those due to improper patient positioning, there are some robotic ureterolysis-specific considerations.

Failure to relieve ureteral obstruction is a known complication, suggested to be more common in salvage ureterolysis compared to primary ureterolysis [9]. Additional interventions may be required to alleviate the obstruction, including repeat robotic surgery (ureterolysis, ureteroureterostomy, ureteral reimplant) and endoureterotomy. Due to obscure anatomy as a result of fibrosis, iatrogenic injury to retroperitoneal structures can be inadvertent. As mentioned in the previous section, iatrogenic ureterotomy should be repaired immediately, leaving a ureteral stent.

Ureterolysis Outcomes

While RPF is rare and there has not been large prospective or randomized control studies with long-term follow-up on ureterolysis, there have been several studies touting its safety and efficacy. Open ureterolysis and omental wrap have been shown to have a GFR increase of 6% and a 94% stent-free rate at 12 months post-operation [18]. Kavoussi showed comparable outcomes between laparoscopic vs open ureterolysis with no significant difference in complications, estimated blood loss, and relief of obstruction, but with a markedly improved length of stay (3.41 vs. 10.88 days, $p < 0.001$) [19]. Finally, in the past decade, recent data has supported robotic ureterolysis. A study on 21 patients showed 100% radiographic and symptomatic success rates for both primary ($n = 11$) and salvage ($n = 10$) ureterolysis groups at last follow-up (mean 20.5 months) with the need for a secondary procedure to relieve obstruction in three patients of the salvage ureterolysis group [9]. A review of 40 patients showed 97% radiographic and 97% symptomatic success rate at last follow-up (mean 16.1 months), with 7 patients requiring a secondary procedure to relieve obstruction [20]. Most studies showed an average length of stay between 2 and 3 days.

Historically, in open ureterolysis, the contralateral ureter, even when uninvolved, was addressed in a prophylactic attempt to avoid reoperation should the contralateral ureter become diseased. Fugita and colleagues were the first to challenge this paradigm in 2002 by deferring contralateral operation in their laparoscopic ureterolysis study of 13 patients, reporting no RPF progression to the contralateral ureter [21]. Simone and colleagues showed the same lack of RPF progression to the contralateral ureter in their laparoscopic ureterolysis with omental wrapping series of six patients in 2008 [12]. Keehn and Stifelman demonstrated no contralateral ureteral RPF progression in 13 of their robotic unilateral ureterolysis patients in 2010 [9].

Robotic-Assisted Laparoscopic Refluxing Boari Flap Surgical Technique

Indications and Workup to Perform Boari Flap

A Boari flap should be considered when it is not possible to create a tension-free ureter-to-bladder anastomosis. This is most commonly seen in mid to distal ureteral strictures that occur iatrogenically, from pelvic radiation, or, in the case of retroperitoneal fibrosis, when the ureter is found to be unsalvageable due to long stricture, poor tissue, or poor perfusion. For any patient under consideration for a Boari flap, it is important to ensure that the patient's bladder capacity is within normal limits and has a normal bladder in compliance with preoperative cystogram and/or urodynamics prior to surgery. While there have been no published studies, to our best knowledge, describing the preoperative and postoperative urodynamics of bladders undergoing Boari flaps, patients who have poor bladder capacity and/or compliance due to various conditions including pelvic radiation or prior surgery may not be amenable to large Boari flaps. Urodynamics have also not been studied extensively in the psoas hitch, but a gynecologic study of 13 patients suggests that, with the exception of volume for first desire to void, which may actually be increased postoperatively, urodynamic parameters pre- and post-psoas hitch have no statistically significant difference [22]. In patients with poor capacity and/or compliance, a Boari flap may cause significant urinary symptoms such as frequency and urgency due to decreased bladder volume. In addition to this quality of life factor, a major concern for low bladder capacity and/or compliance is high resting and voiding pressures causing vesicoureteral reflux in both non-tunneled and tunneled systems. Patients with preoperative urodynamics showing low capacity or compliance may be better served with ileal ureter or augmentation cystoplasty, particularly those with underlying renal insufficiency or solitary kidney, in order to minimize the risk of kidney damage.

Patient Positioning

In the majority of cases where one is planning to do a Boari flap, from the onset, the male patient can be positioned in the supine position with the access to the urethra and the female patient in low lithotomy allowing access to the urethra. In cases where one is attempting a primary ureteral repair without reimplant and would be utilizing a Boari flap as a salvage procedure, we place patients in a modified flank position as described above (unilateral ureterolysis).

Trocar Placement

The trocar placement for Boari flap is similar to that of unilateral ureteral reimplant, with the ports more cephalad and the fourth arm contralateral to the Boari side to assist with retraction.

All four arms of the da Vinci Xi as well as one additional 5 mm bedside assistant trocar are used. The 8 mm trocar for the camera port should be a few centimeters superior to the umbilicus. The two working arms via 8 mm trocars should be several centimeters lateral to the camera port and a couple of centimeters caudal, with the contralateral working arm port cheating more caudally than the ipsilateral by a couple of centimeters. The fourth arm of the robot will go through an 8 mm trocar contralateral to the diseased ureter to better assist with exposure. The 5 mm bedside assistant trocar should be in the midline 8–10 cm inferior to the umbilicus. Trocar placement under direct visualization with the camera is recommended. After all trocars are placed in the appropriate positions, the robot will come in on the ipsilateral side for docking.

Retroperitoneal Exposure

When performing the case in a supine position with the patient in Trendelenburg, one just needs to incise the line of Toldt and medialize the colon from the lower pole of the kidney to the pelvis. We will often divide the gonadal to improve exposure.

Ureteral Identification and Dissection

Strategies for identifying the ureter are described in the previous ureterolysis section. The ureter should be traced as distally as possible to the area of obstruction, then clipped, and transected. We routinely send the obstructed ureter for frozen and permanent pathologic analysis to confirm no malignancy. We do not try to dissect out the diseased ureter as this is unnecessary and increases the risk of intraoperative complication, unless we are doing so for a known upper tract urothelial cell carcinoma and a distal ureterectomy is being performed. Confirming a healthy ureter for that anastomosis is crucial and can be done with white light and confirming the presence of pink, bleeding mucosa or the use of intravenous ICG with NIRF. The ureter is then spatulated posteriorly with scissors for approximately 15 mm. At this time, the distal tip of the spatulated ureter can be tagged with a suture and may be temporarily secured to the posterior wall in a tension-free fashion in order to estimate the length of Boari flap needed.

Caudalization of Kidney, as Needed

If one is trying to maximize ureteral length, the kidney can be mobilized and brought as caudally as possible without tension on the hilum. This can allow for an additional 3–4 cm. Securing sutures into the lower renal pole and psoas muscle can then be used to complete the caudal nephropexy (shown below) (Fig. 12.8).

This can only be accomplished if the initial position is lateral decubitus and is not able to be done when one starts in the supine position.

Bladder Mobilization and Psoas Hitch

As stated the majority of patients are placed in the supine position, allowing the bladder to be released in a similar fashion as in a transperitoneal prostatectomy.

Fig. 12.8 (Orientation, left is cephalad, and right is caudal) Downward nephropexy performed with two securing sutures through the lower pole of the kidney (left) to the psoas fascia

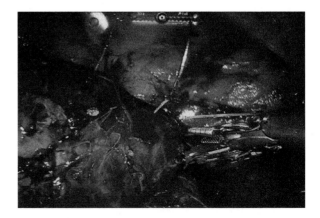

The peritoneum should be incised from just lateral to the medial umbilical ligament to the contralateral medial umbilical ligament. The urachus is then transected. The contralateral side of the bladder must be freed, but attention should be paid to the contralateral ureter when doing as to avoid inadvertent injury.

Once the bladder is thoroughly released and anterior bladder exposed, a psoas hitch should be performed with securing sutures into the bladder dome and the ipsilateral psoas muscle. For more proximal ureteral disease, it is important to maximize the length added with psoas hitch; it is okay for the bladder to be on tension to allow for a tension-free Boari flap anastomosis.

The bladder is then filled with 300–500 mL of saline in order to outline the flap with electrocautery. A flap length up to 10–15 cm can be developed if bladder capacity is adequate and careful construction of the flap is employed. It is crucial that the base of the flap be wide in order to minimize the risk of flap ischemia, often described to be at a minimum of 4 cm in width. As can be seen in the images below, the flap is wide at the base and tapers toward the bladder neck: the apex of the flap should be approximately so that when it is tubularized, the diameter is similar to that of the ureter it will be anastomosed to. If more length is required, the bladder flap can be made in a diagonal fashion across the anterior bladder. For example, when performing a right-sided Boari flap, the base of the flap is always at the right dome, and instead of the apex coming straight caudally to the right bladder neck, the surgeon angles toward the left bladder neck. Another technique shown to provide up to 20 cm in length is creating a "spiral" Boari flap with vascular pedicles (diagram shown below) (Fig. 12.9) [23].

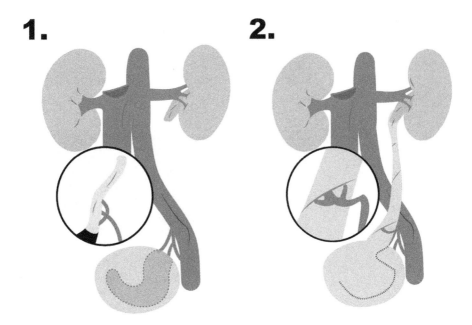

Fig. 12.9 Spiral Boari flap

After the appropriate Boari flap is outlined on the distended bladder, a full-thickness incision into the bladder is made sharply. The bladder is a very vascular organ, allowing for this healthy flap to be created. ICG can also be used later to reassure flap perfusion. The proximal aspect of the flap can also be tacked posteriorly to the psoas to further minimize tension (Figs. 12.10 and 12.11).

The flap is then brought up to the proximal ureteral stump, already spatulated posteriorly, and the anastomosis started posteriorly with interrupted full-thickness 4–0 Vicryl sutures to construct the posterior wall over the neoureter. A double-J stent should then be placed into the proximal ureteral stump at this time. The anastomosis should then be completed circumferentially with full-thickness sutures. It is imperative to ensure accurate urothelial mucosa to mucosa approximation in this anastomosis. The remainder of the flap should then be tubularized with running a 4–0 Vicryl suture down to the bladder in two layers: the first to approximate mucosa and the second to close detrusor. The bladder defect then should be closed with 3–0

Fig. 12.10 Marking Boari flap with electrocautery on a distended bladder

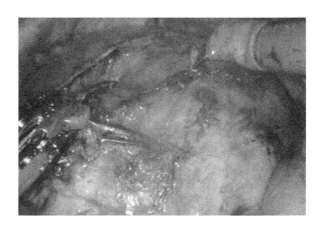

Fig. 12.11 Creation of Boari flap with a full-thickness incision. Note a wide flap base

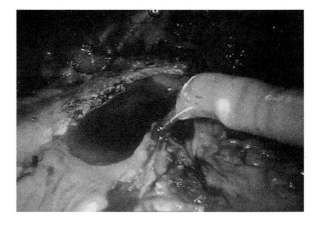

Vicryl in either one or two layers. A watertight seal should then be tested by instilling 300 mL of sterile saline via the Foley catheter (Figs. 12.12, 12.13, and 12.14).

If a nonrefluxing anastomosis is considered, the proximal ureteral stump is tunneled within the distal aspect of the Boari flap. To prevent vesicoureteral reflux, the tunneled ureteral length should exceed the ureteral diameter by a ratio of 4:1. This is performed by undermining the flap mucosa 3–4 cm, securing the ureteral stump to the submucosa while ensuring the distal edge communicates urothelium to urothelium with the flap, and closing the flap mucosa over the ureteral stump (as shown in the diagram below) [24]. For this approach, the ureter is spatulated anteriorly as outlined in the figure (Fig. 12.15).

Open and laparoscopic Boari flap has shown good long-term results, with expected shorter length of stay in the laparoscopic group [25, 26]. While outcomes for robotic-assisted approach have been limited to small sample-sized, single institutional studies, these also suggest that this approach has good obstruction relief outcomes [27, 28].

Fig. 12.12 Trimming the poorly perfused tissue from the Boari flap confirmed with ICG

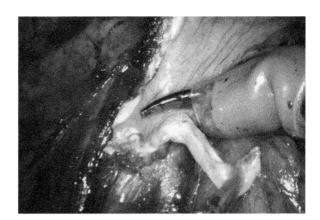

Fig. 12.13 First stitch in the ureter-Boari flap anastomosis posteriorly

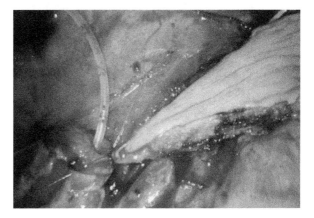

Fig. 12.14 Tubularization of the flap after the completion of ureteral stump-Boari flap anastomosis

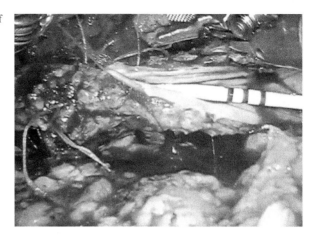

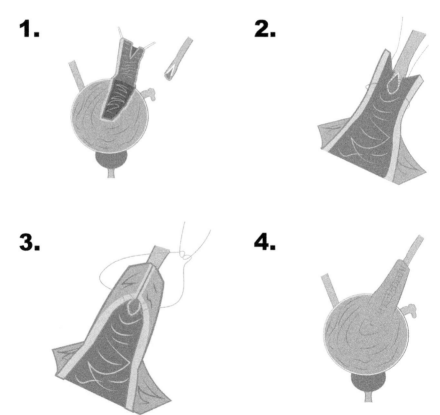

Fig. 12.15 Tunneled Boari flap

Complications and Management

If the patient continues to have ureteral obstruction postoperatively, this should be addressed with a retrograde pyelogram to identify stricture location.

If a wire can be advanced up the ureter to the level of the kidney in a retrograde fashion, the area that is strictured should be balloon dilated with a ureteral stent left for 4–5 weeks. A lot of patients who undergo this postoperative procedure do well, as it can take some dilation to break up a segment that was chronically fibrosed.

Balloon dilation and ureteral stents can be repeated multiple times if there continues to be recurrence, but at a certain point, further reconstruction should be considered. This includes buccal mucosa repair, transureteroureterostomy, ileal ureter, or even autotransplantation.

The Future: Single Port

Single-port (SP) robotic-assisted laparoscopic surgery was approved by the FDA for urologic surgery and clinically available in 2018. This new robotic system enables a camera and three separate instruments, with fully wristed motions, to be placed through a single 27 mm port. This system was designed to perform complex surgery in narrow deep spaces making it very suitable for complex urinary tract reconstruction surgery such Boari's flap and ureterolysis.

Access can be obtained via the umbilicus so that the SP cannula is positioned directly across from the target area. Selection of the initial incision must account for a minimum distance of 10–25 cm between the end of the cannula trocar and the target area or a Gelpoint and trocar "floating" Technique may be utilized. This allows for full deployment of the elbow and wristed joints of the robotic instruments and the ability to operate with the surgical field minimizing collisions. Another key advantage of the SP system is target relocation. This allows the surgeon to move the entire system from one area to another without the need for re-docking. In ureterolysis and Boari flap, one can work as proximal as the kidney and move down to the distal ureter without repositioning the robot. All of the same steps, considerations, and techniques may be used with this newer robotic platform as described above. Early experince with the SP demonstrates it to be safe and reproducible with equally excellent results [29].

References

1. Khosroshahi A, Carruthers MN, Stone JH, Shinagare S, Sainani N, Hasserjian RP, Deshpande V. Rethinking Ormond's disease: "idiopathic" retroperitoneal fibrosis in the era of IgG4-related disease. Medicine (Baltimore). 2013;92:82–91.
2. Kermani TA, Crowson CS, Achenbach SJ, Luthra HS. Idiopathic retroperitoneal fibrosis: a retrospective review of clinical presentation, treatment, and outcomes. Mayo. Clin Proc. 2011;86:297–303.
3. Scheel PJ Jr, Feeley N. Retroperitoneal fibrosis. Rheum Dis Clin N Am. 2013;39:365–81.
4. Vaglio A, Palmisano A, Alberici F, Maggiore U, Ferretti S, Cobelli R, Ferrozzi F, Corradi D, Salvarani C, Buzio C. Prednisone versus Tamoxifen in patients with idiopathic retroperitoneal fibrosis: an open-label randomized controlled trial. Lancet. 2011;378:338–46.

5. Drake M, Nixon P, Crew J. Druginduced bladder and urinary disorders: incidence, prevention and management. Drug Saf. 1998;19:45–55.
6. Drieskens O, Blockmans D, Van Den Bruel A, Mortelmans L. Riedel's thyroiditis and retroperitoneal fibrosis in multifocal fibrosclerosis: positron emission tomographic findings. Clin Nucl Med. 2002;27:413–5.
7. Kottra J, Dunnick N. Retroperitoneal fibrosis. Radiol Clin N Am. 1996;34:1259–75.
8. Vaglio A, Salvarani C, Buzio C. Retroperitoneal fibrosis. Lancet. 2006;367:241–51.
9. Keehn A, Mufarrij P, Stifelman M. Robotic ureterolysis for relief of ureteral obstruction from retroperitoneal fibrosis. Urology. 2010;77(6):1370–4.
10. Rosenkrantz AB, Spieler B, Seuss CR, Stifelman MD, Kim S. Utility of MRI features for differentiation of retroperitoneal fibrosis and lymphoma. Am J Roentgenol. 2012;199(1):118–26.
11. Baker LR, Mallinson WJ, Gregory MC, et al. Idiopathic retroperitoneal fibrosis. A retrospective analysis of 60 cases. Br J Urol. 1987;60:497–503.
12. Simone G, Leonardo C, Papalia R, et al. Laparoscopic ureterolysis and omental wrapping. Urology. 2008;72:853–8.
13. Stepanian S, Patel M, Porter J. Robot-assisted laparoscopic retroperitoneal lymph node dissection for testicular cancer: evolution of the technique. Eur Urol. 2016;70:661–7.
14. Klaassen Z, Hamilton R. The role of robotic retroperitoneal lymph node dissection for testis cancer. Urol Clin N Am. 2019;46:409–17.
15. Zhao L, Yamaguhi Y, Bryk D, Adelstein S, Stifelman M. Robot-assisted ureteral reconstruction using buccal mucosa. Urology. 2015;86(3):635–8.
16. Zhao L, Weinberg A, Lee Z, Ferretti M, Koo H, Metro M, Eun D, Stifelman M. Robotic ureteral reconstruction using buccal mucosa grafts: a multi-institutional experience. Eur Urol. 2018;73:419–26.
17. Lee Z, Keehn A, Sterling M, Metro M, Eun D. A review of buccal mucosa graft ureteroplasty. Curr Uro Rep. 2018;19:23.
18. O'Brien T, Fernando A. Contemporary role of ureterolysis in retroperitoneal fibrosis: treatment of last resort or first intent? An analysis of 50 cases. BJU Int. 2017;120:556–61.
19. Srinivasan A, Richstone L, Permpongkosol S, Kavoussi L. Comparison of laparoscopic with open approach for ureterolysis in patients with retroperitoneal fibrosis. J Urol. 2008;179:1875–8.
20. Marien T, Bjurlin M, Wynia B, Bilbily M, Rao G, Zhao L, Shah O, Stifelman M. Outcomes of robotic-assisted laparoscopic upper urinary tract reconstruction: 250 consecutive patients. BJU Int. 2015;116:604–11.
21. Fugita OE, Jarrett TW, Kavoussi P, et al. Laparoscopic treatment of retroperitoneal fibrosis. J Endourol. 2002;16:571–4.
22. Carmignani L, Ronchetti A, Amicarelli F, Vercellini P, Spinelli M, Fedele L. Bladder psoas hitch in hydronephrosis due to pelvic endometriosis: outcome of urodynamic parameters. Fertil Steril. 2009;92(35):40.
23. Li Y, Li C, Yang S, Song C, Liao W, Xiong Y. Reconstructing full-length ureteral defects using a spiral bladder muscle flap with vascular pedicles. Urology. 2014;83(5):1199–204.
24. Simmons M, Gill IS, Fergany A, Kaouk JH, Desai MM. Technical modifications to laparoscopic Boari flap. J Urol. 2007;69(1):175–80.
25. Fugita OE, Dinlenc C, Kavoussi L. The laparoscopic Boari flap. J Urol. 2001;166:51–3.
26. Mauck RJ, Hudak SJ, Terlecki RP, Morey AF. Central role of Boari bladder flap and downward nephropexy in upper ureteral reconstruction. J Urol. 2011;186:1345–9.
27. Yang C, Jones L, Rivera ME, Verlee G, Deane LA. Robotic-assisted ureteral reimplantation with Boari flap and psoas hitch: a single-institution experience. J Laparoendosc Adv Surg Tech. 2011;21(9):829–33.
28. Bansal A, Sinha RJ, Jhanwar A, Prakash G, Purkait B, Singh V. Laparoscopic ureteral reimplantation with Boari flap for the management of long-segment ureteral defect: a case series with review of literature. Turk J Urol. 2017;43:313–8.
29. Billah MS, Stifelman M, Munver R, Tsui J, Lovallo G, Ahmed M. Single port robotic assisted reconstructive urologic surgery-with the da Vinci SP surgical system. Transl Androl Urol. 2020;9(2):870–878. https://doi.org/10.21037/tau.2020.01.06. PMID: 32420202; PMCID: PMC7214978.

Proximal and Mid-Ureteral Reconstruction in the Pediatric Population

13

Jonathan S. Ellison and Courtney Rowe

Introduction

The continued advancement of robot-assisted laparoscopic surgical techniques has expanded the landscape for surgical treatment of pediatric urologic disease. Nowhere is this clearer than with the growing utilization of robotic ureteroureterostomy for the treatment of the complications of duplex kidneys. While heminephrectomy was the historical approach to these patients, ipsilateral ureterostomy is now seen as an increasingly appealing option to preserve nephrons and reduce complications.

As urologists increasingly choose minimally invasive approaches, so are gynecologists, colorectal surgeons, and vascular surgeons. Consequently, more iatrogenic ureteral injuries during robotic surgeries may be encountered. Thus, urologists should be prepared to evaluate and possibly treat these robotically as well, potentially alleviating the need for open conversion.

Supplementary Information The online version of this chapter (https://doi.org/10.1007/978-3-030-50196-9_13) contains supplementary material, which is available to authorized users.

J. S. Ellison (✉)
Children's Hospital of Wisconsin and Medical College of Wisconsin, Milwaukee, WI, USA
e-mail: JEllison@chw.org

C. Rowe
Pediatric Urology, Connecticut Children's Medical Center, Hartford, CT, USA
e-mail: CRowe@connecticutchildrens.org

Congenital Ureteral Anomalies

Ureteral Duplication

Ureteral duplication occurs in 0.8–1.8% of the population due to duplicate ureteral buds or early division of these buds [1, 2]. Complete duplication will typically follow the Weigert-Meyer law with an upper-pole ureter that is caudal, medial, and more commonly obstructed, ectopic, or associated with a ureterocele. Meanwhile, the lower-pole ureter in a complete duplication is lateral and more commonly refluxing [3]. Duplication can also be partial, resulting in a bifid renal pelvis with a distal confluence into a single ureter. There is a strong genetic link for this anatomic anomaly, with ureteral duplication found in 12% of screened siblings and parents of patients [4].

Ureteral duplication is often asymptomatic and discovered incidentally on ultrasonography. However, about half of patients have an associated anomaly including obstruction, ureterocele, or vesicoureteral reflux, with the risk of infection and renal parenchymal loss [5]. In females, ectopic upper-pole ureters can insert distal to the external urinary sphincter either within the urinary tract or to Mullerian structures such as the uterus or vagina. In these cases, the ureteral duplication will often present as continuous urinary incontinence or failure to toilet train [6]. In males, the ectopic ureter can drain proximal to the external sphincter into the urethra or into mesonephric structures such as the epididymis or prostate, presenting as recurrent epididymitis or remaining asymptomatic [7]. Obstruction arises from an abnormal ureteral insertion within the bladder, typically from a more medial insertion with a longer intramural tunnel, or an insertion into an ectopic location such as the bladder neck, proximal urethra, or vagina, in which case the opening may be stenotic owing to aberrant embryological development.

Mid-Ureteral Strictures

Congenital mid-ureteral strictures are found in 4–5% of pediatric hydronephrosis cases. The embryologic cause is unclear, but proposed mechanisms include ischemia, ureteral valves, and disorganized arrangement of ureteral muscle [8]. Mid-ureteral strictures are generally asymptomatic and are diagnosed using retrograde pyelography or MRI as ultrasound and nuclear medicine evaluation have poor sensitivity for this diagnosis [9].

Retrocaval Ureter

The retrocaval ureter should more accurately be referred to as the pre-ureteral vena cava. While the presentation is generally urologic, the embryologic cause is an abnormally anterior inferior vena cava due to failed atrophy of the posterior cardinal vein, resulting in extrinsic compression of the ureter [2]. Patients present with obstructive symptoms such as hydronephrosis or flank pain. Diagnosis is made due to a classic "fishhook" appearance to the ureter on IVP, retrograde pyelogram, nuclear medicine study, or CT scan [10, 11]. This anomaly can also be diagnosed intraoperatively, so surgeons planning renal and ureteral surgery should be prepared to correct this rare finding if encountered [12].

Ureteral Injuries

Iatrogenic

The most common cause of ureteral trauma in adults is iatrogenic injury, and the incidence in adults appears to be increasing along with the increased use of minimally invasive approaches for gynecologic, vascular, and colorectal procedures [13]. While iatrogenic ureteral injuries in children are rare, with increasing percutaneous, laparoscopic, and robotic approaches for pediatric surgery, one can expect the incidence of these injuries to increase [14, 15]. Meanwhile, while the urologic community is faced with an increase in pediatric nephrolithiasis, current published rates of ureteral stricture after ureteroscopy and percutaneous nephrolithotomy for stone treatment are quite low around 0.2% [16, 17].

Similar to adults, only about 40% of iatrogenic surgical ureteral injuries in pediatric patients are recognized intraoperatively after open or minimally invasive surgery [18, 19]. Unlike adults, pediatric patients have good outcomes after injury with low rates of strictures after either ureteroureterostomy or ureteroneocystostomy, where the iatrogenic ureteral injury in a patient resolved with stenting only [14, 20]. The main benefit of immediate diagnosis of an injury appears includes the avoidance of complications such as urinoma and a reduction in the number of procedures required [19].

Preoperative ureteral stenting has been used in adults in an attempt to reduce the rate of iatrogenic injury. Results have been mixed, with some studies finding benefit while others note that the small benefits are outweighed by complications from the stents themselves [21]. Preoperative stenting is not currently a common practice for pediatric surgical patients.

Traumatic

Ureteral injuries account for approximately 2.5% of all genitourinary trauma. While adult series report that only 38% of ureteral injuries occur after blunt trauma, children represent the majority of cases with ureteral rupture after road accidents [22, 23]. As with other urologic trauma, the key to diagnosing a ureteral injury is delayed

CT imaging to evaluate the urinary tract during the excretory phase. Though traumatic ureteral injuries are rare, if unrecognized, they can lead to urine leak, sepsis, or renal loss [24].

Preoperative Evaluation

All surgery in pediatric patients should be preceded by a complete history including prenatal and antenatal history, physical examination, and review of the available imaging. If considering a ureteroureterostomy, a voiding cystourethrogram (VCUG) is necessary to ensure there is no reflux to the recipient ureter. It is also reasonable to obtain a functional nuclear medicine study prior to surgery to document function and to assist in counseling families on expectations, though there is no evidence of increased complications after surgery on poorly functioning moieties [25]. A MAG-3 renogram is still the gold standard for the diagnosis of obstruction. Children should be at least 1 month of age for reliable results, though the kidney continues to mature through 6 months of age, and the results continue to be variable as late as 1 year of age due to the child's small size [26–28].

If the anatomy is unclear on ultrasound or MAG-3 scan, other imaging modalities can be used. MRI can be particularly helpful in identifying dysplastic renal moieties that are difficult to see with ultrasound or with MAG-3 renography. While MRI may be more sensitive than other modalities in identifying mid-ureteral strictures, there is a risk of false positives when evaluating ectopic ureters [9, 29, 30]. Both CT and MRI have been used to identify retrocaval ureters. It should be noted that most of these advanced imaging studies are performed with anesthesia in pediatric patients. Therefore, there may be instances in which it is preferable to use a cystoscopy with retrograde pyelogram immediately before the reconstructive ureteral surgery to appropriately define the anatomy without the need for a separate anesthetic for these advanced imaging modalities.

Intraoperative Consultation

When an iatrogenic injury is suspected intraoperatively, the gold standard for evaluation is cystoscopy and retrograde pyelogram [31]. Unfortunately, surgical positioning may preclude thorough fluoroscopy. There are a number of other options for the evaluation of ureteral injuries, none of which should be considered 100% sensitive. In the absence of indigo carmine, both intravenous sodium fluorescein and intravesical 10% dextrose have proven to be helpful adjuvants to the cystoscopic observation of ureteral jets [32]. An alternative is the retrograde placement of open-ended ureteral catheters either via cystoscopy or cystotomy; if these can be placed smoothly, an injury is unlikely. Because of the morbidity of a missed ureteral injury, if the above techniques are not available or not satisfactory, there should be a low threshold for direct and thorough open, laparoscopic or robotic evaluation of the ureters [33].

Surgical Approach

Open Versus Robotic

Robotic ureteral reconstruction appears to be safe and effective in pediatric patients. Operative time and blood loss are similar to the open approach, though the length of stay is one-half day shorter for the robot-assisted approach [34].

Extirpative Versus Reconstructive

The decision to perform reconstructive as opposed to extirpative surgery on a poorly functioning renal moiety depends on surgeon preference as there is no clear comparative data to guide this decision. Renal function loss appears to be less common after ureteroureterostomy than heminephrectomy, but the data is sparse [35, 36].

Proximal Versus Distal Anastomosis

Historically, ureteroureterostomy was performed proximally to avoid the hypothetical concern of "yo-yo" reflux resulting from a surgically created "y"-type duplication [37, 38]. More recently, trends have shifted toward performing the anastomosis at the pelvic brim as there appears to be little clinically relevant implications of "yo-yo" reflux in this setting [39]. The benefits of exposing the ureter at the pelvic brim include ease of exposure and avoidance of aberrant pathology at the renal hilum.

Surgical Technique

Setup and Positioning

Robotic ureteral reconstruction is typically performed transperitoneally [40, 41]. Benefits include easy access to the anatomy of interest, a large intra-abdominal working space (even in infants), and surgeon familiarity with the anatomy. Standard port placement typically triangulates over the area of the anticipated anastomosis, whether at the level of the renal pelvis or above the pelvic brim (Fig. 13.1). Recently, a modification of port placements using the Hidden-Incision Endoscopic Surgery (HIdES)[SM] technique has allowed for improved cosmetic outcomes by concealing all visible ports beneath the pants line by placing one port within the umbilicus and the remaining ports in a transverse position inferior to the umbilicus (Fig. 13.2). Docking for the HIdES technique is best accomplished over the ipsilateral shoulder to minimize the clashing of the robotic arms [42].

    The patient is positioned in a flank or modified flank position for exposure of the anatomical side of interest. Flexion of the table is not required for exposure of the retroperitoneal structures but may be helpful to aid in maximum mobility of the

Fig. 13.1 Port placement for robotic ureteroureterostomy, triangulated over the area of pathology. Camera port is indicated by the orange star

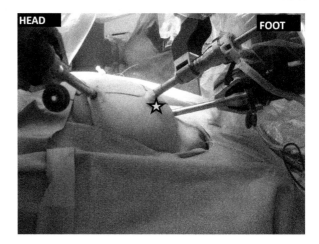

Fig. 13.2 Hidden incision port placement (HiDES) for a right upper tract reconstruction. Camera and robotic ports are triangulated over the area of pathology (blue arrow). Positioning of lower ports in a linear fashion beneath the belt line (white line) minimizes visual scars postoperatively

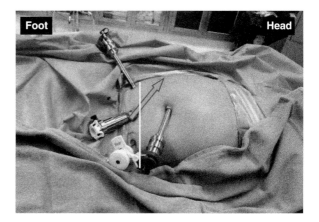

robotic arms away from the operating table. Trendelenburg positioning can aid with the reflection of the bowel, especially when operating near the pelvic brim.

Ipsilateral Ureteroureterostomy (for Ureteral Duplication)

Identifying the diseased ureter for transection and end-to-side anastomosis of the healthy ipsilateral ureter is *imperative* for the success of the operation. Even in instances of significant hydroureteronephrosis, the authors have found intraoperative identification of the diseased ureter by inspection alone to be challenging. For that reason, the authors recommend cystoscopy and retrograde placement of an indwelling ureteral stent or ureteral catheter into the healthy ipsilateral ureter at the onset of the operation.

After the patient is positioned and the robot is docked, the colon is reflected medially. The diseased ureter is identified and mobilized. The authors recommend performing the anastomosis at the pelvic brim for ease of exposure and to avoid renal vessels. Minimal dissection is required for the recipient ureter, which should be handled with care to avoid disruption of its fragile blood supply. This is especially true at the pelvic brim, which may represent a watershed area of vascular supply for the mid-ureter. Additionally, upward traction on the stented recipient ureter can dislodge the stent proximally. If the surgeon is concerned regarding possible stent migration, a plain film radiograph should be obtained at the end of the case to confirm distal stent placement.

A stay suture can be placed in a percutaneous fashion through the donor ureter to allow for traction and to aid with exposure. The authors use a 2–0 polydioxanone suture on an SH needle that has been straightened. The stay suture should be placed prior to the complete transection of the donor ureter to avoid cephalad retraction. Discrepancies in donor and recipient ureteral diameters do not appear to impact surgical success if an adequate ureterotomy was created to allow for a watertight and tension-free anastomosis [43]. The surgeon may determine the size of the ureterotomy necessary for an adequate anastomosis using either direct measurement with a ruler introduced via an assistant port or approximation of size gauged by comparison with the tips of the robotic instrument.

The distal ureteral stump is then resected. One benefit of the robotic platform is optimal visualization distally to allow maximal resection of the ureteral stump (Fig. 13.3). Complete resection may even be possible, though care must be taken to avoid injury to Wolffian or Mullerian structures as well as the bladder neck or sphincteric mechanism of the ureter [44]. The risk of complications from residual ureteral stump is quoted as up to 5–10% in the literature, although much of this data is from the era of open surgery and may not be applicable to the more extensive ureteral resections with the robotic approach [45]. In the absence of vesicoureteral reflux, the residual ureteral stump can be partially resected, leaving the back wall of the ureter and the shared distal blood supply intact and minimizing the risk of injury to the healthy recipient ureter.

Retrocaval Ureter

Management of a retrocaval ureter is approached in similar fashion to other upper tract ureteral reconstruction, though the duodenum often must be mobilized in order to gain adequate exposure [46]. The ureter is identified migrating medially and posterior to the vena cava. Dissection is carried out both proximally and distally in order to gain adequate visualization prior to the transection of the ureter, often performed proximal to the vena caval obstruction. Resection of the obstructed ureteral

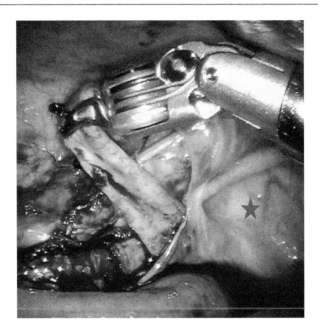

Fig. 13.3 Distal ureteral stump in a male with an obstructed, ectopic upper pole ureter. Key anatomical structures are identified. Vas deferens—blue highlight; bladder—red star

segment is optional and guided by direct visualization of the ureter to determine any intrinsic narrowing or segmental pathology [47]. The anastomosis and placement of the ureteral stent are then carried out similar to a robot-assisted laparoscopic pyeloplasty, with the transposition of the ureter anterior to the vena cava [48].

Ureteroureterostomy for Iatrogenic Injury

Surgical planning for ureteral reconstruction following an iatrogenic injury must involve an adequate assessment of the length of the diseased ureter as well as knowledge of the underlying mechanism of injury. Retrograde pyelograms are helpful in defining the location and length of ureteral injury. Avoiding a long-term preoperative ureteral stent, sometimes at the expense of a preoperative nephrostomy tube, can aid in adequate assessment of the transition between diseased and healthy ureter. All diseased ureteral tissue must be resected, and the anastomosis must be performed in a tension-free fashion for optimal success.

After defining the extent of ureteral injury, the ureter is exposed with caution. If possible, a retrograde stent placed at the time of the operation can be useful. It is important to understand the mechanism of injury. Bipolar electrocautery often results in thermal damage with at least 2 mm of lateral spread; care should be taken to cut back on the ureter accordingly. Primary ureteroureterostomy is typically limited to injuries or strictures less than 2–3 cm in length, given the need for adequate mobilization and avoidance of tension on the anastomosis [49]. Stay sutures as described above can provide additional traction and exposure. The anastomosis is completed following adequate ureteral spatulation both proximally and distally [50].

Advanced Techniques for Longer Ureteral Strictures

Because ureteroureterostomy is limited to shorter ureteral strictures, surgeons must be prepared for alternative reconstructive techniques in multifocal and/or longer-segment ureteral structures. Strategies for addressing these complex cases are based on stricture location and available tissue that is local or distant.

Boari flap: For distal ureteral strictures in patients with adequate bladder capacity, a Boari flap can be accomplished with robotic assistance. Stay sutures in the bladder may be useful for retraction in addition to a formal assistant port. Because the Boari flap is a random flap without a specific end-arterial blood supply, the width of the flap is vital for viability. A width-length ratio of at least 2:1 is recommended [51]. Boari flaps should be approached with caution in younger children with smaller bladder capacities.

Appendiceal interposition or onlay: The appendix is an option for ureteral interposition given its similar diameter to the ureter and proximity in the abdomen. It can be mobilized upon the mesoappendiceal pedicle to preserve blood supply and utilized as a complete interposition or an onlay graft. For left-sided repairs, the appendix should be passed in a retroperitoneal fashion through a peritoneal window in the descending colon mesocolon. Appendiceal interposition is accomplished by spatulation and anastomosis of the appendix to the proximal and distal ureter. While the appendix should ideally be positioned in an isoperistaltic fashion, with the distal appendix approximated to the distal ureter, this may not be necessary [52]. A recent case series reported good success with laparoscopic appendiceal interposition in four pediatric patients, with both isoperistaltic and antiperistaltic anastomoses used and both right and left ureters treated [53]. Appendiceal onlay techniques do not interpose the entire ureteral segment, but rather utilize a detubularized segment of the appendix as an onlay graft over a long-segment ureterotomy. Harvest of the appendix is similar to that of the appendiceal interposition, while the detubularization is created in an anti-mesenteric fashion [54].

Buccal graft ureteroplasty: The buccal mucosa is familiar to many urologists and has been successfully employed in ureteral stricture disease as dorsal or ventral onlay grafts. The buccal mucosa is harvested and introduced via the assistant port for grafting. The strictured segment of ureter is incised longitudinally both proximally and distally to normal, well-vascularized urothelium. Intracorporeal passage of a ureteroscope via the ureterotomy can sometimes be useful to confirm the incision adequately spans the entire length of unhealthy ureter. The graft is then sutured into place in a ventral or dorsal onlay fashion over the ureterotomy. In such cases, it is helpful to place the ureteral stent in a retrograde fashion prior to initiation of the laparoscopic or robotic portion of the case, in order to aid in ureteral identification as well as to support the anastomosis following the repair. Importantly, the buccal graft requires a flap for blood supply. This can be provided by the psoas muscle for dorsal onlay grafts or an omental flap for either dorsal or ventral onlay approaches. In the setting of a dorsal onlay, where the ureterotomy has been performed on the underside of the ureter, the psoas fascia can be opened and the graft secured to the psoas muscle following the anastomosis [55]. For ventral onlay procedures or the dorsal onlay procedures where the psoas may not be readily accessible at the site of the anastomosis, the omentum can be harvested as a flap and wrapped circumferentially around the grafted repair. This technique has been employed in the pediatric population in select situations with good short-term results. A small series of three patients showed continued patency at a median follow-up of 10 months. The median length of the stricture was 4.3 cm in these cases, and the median number of prior attempted repairs was two in the cohort [56]. Longer-term follow-up and larger pediatric series are needed to demonstrate the durability and further applicability of this approach.

Complications: Avoidance and Management

Urine Leak

Urine leak occurs in 1–5% of cases following upper tract urinary reconstruction in children [57, 58]. Extrapolating from the pyeloplasty data, ureteral stenting is associated with a lower risk of postoperative urinary diversion, though stent-free reconstruction is possible [59, 60]. Since higher rates of stent complications are seen in children with lower urinary tract dysfunction, the decision to place a stent should weigh these competing issues [61]. Modifiable risk factors should be addressed, though it is unclear if more aggressive bowel and bladder management can mitigate these risks. Meanwhile, a peri-anastomotic drain can help identify and manage a urinary leak if left in place postoperatively. If a urine leak is identified, initial management should include the replacement of the urethral catheter for 5–7 days to allow maximal bladder decompression. Upper tract decompression with a nephrostomy tube could be considered if the leak fails to seal conservatively.

Anastomotic Stricture

Short-term outcomes of robotic-assisted ureteroureterostomy in children are quite good [62]. Minimizing manipulation of the recipient ureter while ensuring adequate blood supply and a tension-free anastomosis are key in optimizing success. The longer-term reoperation-free success rates of these operations are not yet known. An anastomotic stricture could present with symptoms of renal colic, recurrent pyelonephritis, or asymptomatic hydronephrosis and should be evaluated with a nuclear medicine renogram as well as urography (either with cross-sectional imaging or retrograde studies) to further define the anatomy. Short strictures less than 1 cm can

Table 13.1 Tips and tricks for robotic-assisted ureteroureterostomy

Ureteroureterostomy: Tips and tricks
TIP 1: Retrograde stent placement for the identification of the healthy ipsilateral ureter. If this stent will not pass, consider intraoperative ureterotomy with retrograde catheterization and pyelography on the field to confirm ureteral anatomy.
TIP 2: Limit recipient ureteral dissection to the anterior surface to minimize ureteral trauma
TIP 3: Placement of a percutaneous stay suture prior to the transection of the donor ureter to prevent cephalad retraction
TIP 4: Use of Maryland bipolar grasper to estimate adequate recipient ureterotomy length for anastomosis
TIP 5: Triangulation of the port sites over the anticipated area of the inguinal canal to allow for both adequate exposure from the ureteral anastomosis at the pelvic brim and optimized visualization and maneuverability in the deep pelvis for resection of the ureteral stump.

be managed endoscopically, while longer strictures will likely require reoperative reconstruction.

Inadvertent Reverse Anastomosis

In children undergoing ureteroureterostomy for duplex pathology, correct identification of the donor and recipient ureters is imperative to avoid a reverse anastomosis. In cases where a ureteral stent or catheter cannot be inserted retrograde, the authors strongly suggest intraoperative imaging performed via a ureteral access catheter introduced via a ureterotomy to adequately define the anatomy (Table 13.1).

Conclusion

Pediatric urologic disease provides a prime opportunity for the expansion of the robotic platform, given the requirements of complex dissection and delicate suturing in a more confined abdomen. Novel port placement and instrumentation can improve cosmetic outcomes and surgeon efficiency. Outcomes for common applications such as upper to lower-pole ureteroureterostomy in the setting of upper-pole distal obstruction are excellent due to the improved motor control for suturing and optimal visualization for dissection and resection of the distal ureteral stump. The robotic platform allows for novel approaches in complex ureteral reconstructions while maintaining the benefits of minimally-invasive surgery.

References

1. Privett JT, Jeans WD, Roylance J. The incidence and importance of renal duplication. Clin Radiol. 1976;27:521–30.
2. Wein AJ, Kavoussi LR, Novick AC, Partin AW, Peters CA. Campbell-Walsh urology. St. Louis: Elsevier Health Sciences; 2011.

3. Meyer R. Normal and abnormal development of the ureter in the human embryo; a mechanistic consideration. Anat Rec. 1946;96:355–71.
4. Carter CO. The genetics of urinary tract malformations. J Genet Hum. 1984;32:23–9.
5. Doery AJ, Ang E, Ditchfield MR. Duplex kidney: not just a drooping lily. J Med Imaging Radiat Oncol. 2015;59:149–53.
6. Borer JG, et al. A single-system ectopic ureter draining an ectopic dysplastic kidney: delayed diagnosis in the young female with continuous urinary incontinence. Br J Urol. 1998;81:474–8.
7. Mohamed F, Jehangir S. Coexistent duplication of urethra and a refluxing ectopic ureter presenting as recurrent epididymo-orchitis in a child. BMJ Case Rep. 2017; https://doi.org/10.1136/bcr-2017-220278.
8. Hwang AH, et al. Congenital mid ureteral strictures. J Urol. 2005;174:1999–2002.
9. Arlen AM, et al. Magnetic resonance urography for diagnosis of pediatric ureteral stricture. J Pediatr Urol. 2014;10:792–8.
10. Hoffman CF, Dyer RB. The 'fish hook' sign of retrocaval ureter. Abdom Radiol (NY). 2018;43:755–7.
11. López González PA, et al. Retrocaval ureter in children. Case report and bibliographic review. Arch Esp Urol. 2011;64:461–4.
12. Junejo NN, et al. High retrocaval ureter: an unexpected intraoperative finding during robotic redo pyeloplasty. Urol Case Rep. 2018;20:19–21.
13. Palaniappa NC, Telem DA, Ranasinghe NE, Divino CM. Incidence of iatrogenic ureteral injury after laparoscopic colectomy. Arch Surg. 2012;147:267–71.
14. Chacko JK, Noh PS, Barthold JS, Figueroa TE, González R. Iatrogenic ureteral injury after laparoscopic cholecystectomy in a 13-year-old boy. J Pediatr Urol. 2008;4:322–4.
15. Ruatti S, Courvoisier A, Eid A, Griffet J. Ureteral injury after percutaneous iliosacral fixation: a case report and literature review. J Pediatr Surg. 2012;47:e13–6.
16. Ishii H, Griffin S, Somani BK. Ureteroscopy for stone disease in the paediatric population: a systematic review. BJU Int. 2015;115:867–73.
17. Onal B, et al. Factors affecting complication rates of percutaneous nephrolithotomy in children: results of a multi-institutional retrospective analysis by the Turkish pediatric urology society. J Urol. 2014;191:777–82.
18. Elliott SP, McAninch JW. Extraperitoneal bladder trauma: delayed surgical management can lead to prolonged convalescence. J Trauma. 2009;66:274–5.
19. Routh JC, Tollefson MK, Ashley RA, Husmann DA. Iatrogenic ureteral injury: can adult repair techniques be used on children? J Pediatr Urol. 2009;5:53–5.
20. Lu L, Bi Y, Wang X, Ruan S. Laparoscopic resection and end-to-end ureteroureterostomy for midureteral obstruction in children. J Laparoendosc Adv Surg Tech A. 2017;27:197–202.
21. Coakley KM, et al. Prophylactic ureteral catheters for colectomy: a national surgical quality improvement program-based analysis. Dis Colon Rectum. 2018;61:84–8.
22. Siram SM, et al. Ureteral trauma: patterns and mechanisms of injury of an uncommon condition. Am J Surg. 2010;199:566–70.
23. Kotkin L, Brock JW. Isolated ureteral injury caused by blunt trauma. Urology. 1996;47:111–3.
24. Helmy TE, Sarhan OM, Harraz AM, Dawaba M. Complexity of non-iatrogenic ureteral injuries in children: single-center experience. Int Urol Nephrol. 2011;43:1–5.
25. Kawal T, et al. Ipsilateral ureteroureterostomy: does function of the obstructed moiety matter? J Pediatr Urol. 2018; https://doi.org/10.1016/j.jpurol.2018.08.012.
26. Conway JJ, Maizels M. The 'well tempered' diuretic renogram: a standard method to examine the asymptomatic neonate with hydronephrosis or hydroureteronephrosis. A report from combined meetings of the Society for Fetal Urology and members of the Pediatric Nuclear Medicine Council – The Society of Nuclear Medicine. J Nucl Med. 1992;33:2047–51.
27. Ozcan Z, Anderson PJ, Gordon I. Robustness of estimation of differential renal function in infants and children with unilateral prenatal diagnosis of a hydronephrotic kidney on dynamic renography: how real is the supranormal kidney? Eur J Nucl Med Mol Imaging. 2006;33:738–44.

28. Brink A, Sámal M, Mann MD. The reproducibility of measurements of differential renal function in paediatric 99mTc-MAG3 renography. Nucl Med Commun. 2012;33:824–31.
29. Gylys-Morin VM, et al. Magnetic resonance imaging of the dysplastic renal moiety and ectopic ureter. J Urol. 2000;164:2034–9.
30. Figueroa VH, Chavhan GB, Oudjhane K, Farhat W. Utility of MR urography in children suspected of having ectopic ureter. Pediatr Radiol. 2014;44:956–62.
31. Elliott SP, McAninch JW. Ureteral injuries: external and iatrogenic. Urol Clin North Am. 2006;33:55–66, vi.
32. Espaillat-Rijo L, et al. Intraoperative cystoscopic evaluation of ureteral patency: a randomized controlled trial. Obstet Gynecol. 2016;128:1378–83.
33. Burks FN, Santucci RA. Management of iatrogenic ureteral injury. Ther Adv Urol. 2014;6:115–24.
34. Lee NG, et al. Bi-institutional comparison of robot-assisted laparoscopic versus open ureteroureterostomy in the pediatric population. J Endourol. 2015;29:1237–41.
35. Herz D, et al. Robot-assisted laparoscopic management of duplex renal anomaly: comparison of surgical outcomes to traditional pure laparoscopic and open surgery. J Pediatr Urol. 2016;12:44.e1–7.
36. Michaud JE, Akhavan A. Upper pole heminephrectomy versus lower pole Ureteroureterostomy for ectopic upper pole ureters. Curr Urol Rep. 2017;18:21.
37. Chacko JK, Koyle MA, Mingin GC, Furness PD. Ipsilateral ureteroureterostomy in the surgical management of the severely dilated ureter in ureteral duplication. J Urol. 2007;178:1689–92.
38. Husmann DA, Ewalt DH, Glenski WJ, Bernier PA. Ureterocele associated with ureteral duplication and a nonfunctioning upper pole segment: management by partial nephroureterectomy alone. J Urol. 1995;154:723–6.
39. Lashley DB, McAleer IM, Kaplan GW. Ipsilateral ureteroureterostomy for the treatment of vesicoureteral reflux or obstruction associated with complete ureteral duplication. J Urol. 2001;165:552–4.
40. Corbett ST, Burris MB, Herndon CDA. Pediatric robotic-assisted laparoscopic ipsilateral ureteroureterostomy in a duplicated collecting system. J Pediatr Urol. 2013;9:1239.e1–2.
41. Leavitt DA, Rambachan A, Haberman K, DeMarco R, Shukla AR. Robot-assisted laparoscopic ipsilateral ureteroureterostomy for ectopic ureters in children: description of technique. J Endourol. 2012;26:1279–83.
42. Gargollo PC. Hidden incision endoscopic surgery: description of technique, parental satisfaction and applications. J Urol. 2011;185:1425–31.
43. McLeod DJ, Alpert SA, Ural Z, Jayanthi VR. Ureteroureterostomy irrespective of ureteral size or upper pole function: a single center experience. J Pediatr Urol. 2014;10:616–9.
44. Biles MJ, Finkelstein JB, Silva MV, Lambert SM, Casale P. Innovation in robotics and pediatric urology: robotic ureteroureterostomy for duplex systems with ureteral ectopia. J Endourol. 2016;30:1041–8.
45. Ade-Ajayi N, Wilcox DT, Duffy PG, Ransley PG. Upper pole heminephrectomy: is complete ureterectomy necessary? BJU Int. 2001;88:77–9.
46. Hemal AK, Rao R, Sharma S, Clement RGE. Pure robotic retrocaval ureter repair. Int Braz J Urol. 2008;34:734–8.
47. Li H-Z, et al. Retroperitoneal laparoscopic ureteroureterostomy for retrocaval ureter: report of 10 cases and literature review. Urology. 2010;76:873–6.
48. Gundeti MS, Duffy PG, Mushtaq I. Robotic-assisted laparoscopic correction of pediatric retrocaval ureter. J Laparoendosc Adv Surg Tech A. 2006;16:422–4.
49. Marien T, et al. Outcomes of robotic-assisted laparoscopic upper urinary tract reconstruction: 250 consecutive patients. BJU Int. 2015;116:604–11.
50. Passerotti CC, et al. Robot-assisted laparoscopic ureteroureterostomy: description of technique. J. Endourol. 2008;22:581–4, discussion 585.
51. Musch M, et al. Robot-assisted reconstructive surgery of the distal ureter: single institution experience in 16 patients. BJU Int. 2013;111:773–83.

52. Yarlagadda VK, Nix JW, Benson DG, Selph JP. Feasibility of intracorporeal robotic-assisted laparoscopic appendiceal interposition for ureteral stricture disease: a case report. Urology. 2017;109:201–5.
53. Cao H, et al. Laparoscopic appendiceal interposition pyeloplasty for long ureteric strictures in children. J Pediatr Urol. 2018; https://doi.org/10.1016/j.jpurol.2018.06.017.
54. Duty BD, Kreshover JE, Richstone L, Kavoussi LR. Review of appendiceal onlay flap in the management of complex ureteric strictures in six patients. BJU Int. 2015;115:282–7.
55. Zhao LC, et al. Robotic ureteral reconstruction using buccal mucosa grafts: a multi-institutional experience. Eur Urol. 2017;73:419–26.
56. Ahn JJ, Shapiro ME, Ellison JS, Lendvay TS. Pediatric robot-assisted redo pyeloplasty with buccal mucosa graft: a novel technique. Urology. 2017;101:56–9.
57. Silay MS, et al. Global minimally invasive pyeloplasty study in children: results from the Pediatric Urology Expert Group of the European Association of Urology Young Academic Urologists working party. J Pediatr Urol. 2016;12:229.e1–7.
58. Avery DI, et al. Robot-assisted laparoscopic pyeloplasty: multi-institutional experience in infants. J Pediatr Urol. 2015;11:139.e1–5.
59. Sturm RM, Chandrasekar T, Durbin-Johnson B, Kurzrock EA. Urinary diversion during and after pediatric pyeloplasty: a population based analysis of more than 2,000 patients. J Urol. 2014; https://doi.org/10.1016/j.juro.2014.01.089.
60. Silva MV, Levy AC, Finkelstein JB, Van Batavia JP, Casale P. Is peri-operative urethral catheter drainage enough? The case for stentless pediatric robotic pyeloplasty. J Pediatr Urol. 2015;11:175.e1–5.
61. Chrzan R, et al. Short-term complications after pyeloplasty in children with lower urinary tract anomalies. Urology. 2017;100:198–202.
62. Ellison JS, Lendvay TS. Robot-assisted ureteroureterostomy in pediatric patients: current perspectives. RSRR. 2017;4:45–55.

Part V

Introduction for Distal Ureteral Reconstruction

Daniel D. Eun

In this section, we address robotic reconstructive techniques that address adult and pediatric drainage pathology of the distal ureter. Although both children and adult patients can have obstructive and reflux-related problems, ureteral reimplantation is commonly done for different reasons in both populations. Although the etiologies can differ, there are many common skills, tips, and tricks that can be shared among both the pediatric and adult surgeon. In addition, the expanded role of pelvic radiation to treat various urologic, gynecologic, and colorectal malignancies have created an ever-growing population of patients with challenging and devastating distal ureteral strictures and fistulas that have called many reconstructive and minimally invasive urologists to action. In this era, even the most challenging cases involving the distal ureter can be mediated by an experienced robotic surgeon. This section describes both traditional and modified robotic-assisted techniques that have evolved over the past two decades to treat the various distal ureteral reconstructive needs. I hope that you will not only draw from the experience of our authors as you read this section but also incorporate these skills into your surgical repertoire.

Diagnosis, Evaluation, and Preoperative Considerations in Distal Ureteral Reconstruction

14

Uzoamaka Nwoye and Andrew A. Wagner

Mechanism of Injury and Implications

Acute Ureteral Injuries

Intraoperative Ureteral Injury

Intraoperative ureteral injuries make up 80% of acute ureteral injuries, although the majority are not recognized at the time of surgery and present in a delayed fashion [1]. Of iatrogenic ureteral injuries, 50–82% occur in gynecologic surgeries, 11–30% in urologic surgeries, and 5–25% in general surgery (colorectal, pelvic, and vascular surgeries) [1–3].

Iatrogenic ureteral injury can occur by laceration, suture ligation, avulsion, crush injury, devascularization, or damage from an energy-related source. Laceration injuries tend to be clean cut with healthy edges and can be spatulated and repaired over an indwelling ureteral stent. Ligation, when noted early, can be untied and stented. Unlike laceration and ligation injuries, crush injury, devascularization, and injury from an energy-related source are associated with a devascularized or injured segment of the ureter. This should be resected to healthy tissue and bleeding edges before reconstruction. Thermal or devascularization injuries tend not to be apparent immediately. For this reason, if suspected, a clinician should evaluate intraoperatively, place a stent, and/or monitor closely for ureteral patency postoperatively [1, 2]. When a ureteral injury is managed conservatively with the placement of a stent, follow-up imaging with CT urogram or retrograde pyelogram should be obtained to evaluate for ureteral stricture and kidney viability.

Ureteral injury in the setting of open abdominal or pelvic surgery should be evaluated by direct exposure and evaluation of the ureteric segment in question.

U. Nwoye (✉) · A. A. Wagner
Division of Urology, Beth Israel Deaconess Medical Center, Boston, MA, USA
e-mail: awagner@bidmc.harvard.edu

© Springer Nature Switzerland AG 2022
M. D. Stifelman et al. (eds.), *Techniques of Robotic Urinary Tract Reconstruction*, https://doi.org/10.1007/978-3-030-50196-9_14

157

Methylene blue or indigo carmine can be injected intravenously or directly into the renal pelvis prior to visual inspection of the ureter to evaluate for extravasation or to determine the level of obstruction.

In laparoscopic or robotic cases, evaluation and repair can be attempted using the same approach depending on the comfort level and experience of the surgeon. In situations where a surgeon's experience precludes optimal minimally invasive ureteral reconstruction, he/she should not hesitate to convert to an open approach. Immediate repair within 24 hours is usually feasible and preferable to delayed ureteral reconstruction.

Access to the ureter is limited in transvaginal surgery. Therefore, the gold standard for evaluating the ureter in this situation is cystoscopy with retrograde pyelogram, and all effort should be made to obtain fluoroscopy to properly complete this evaluation. This also allows for intervention if indicated. When fluoroscopy is not available, intravenous injection of indigo carmine or methylene blue can at least document patency of the ureter if blue urine is seen emanating from the ureteral orifice.

Evaluation of the Ureter After a Trauma-Related or Iatrogenic Injury

Injuries from blunt trauma or stab wounds tend to involve a short segment of the ureter and are likely to be amenable to ureteral reimplantation or ureteroureterostomy. Ureteral injuries from gunshot wounds (GSW), electrocautery, cryoablation, or any other thermal device are likely to involve a longer segment of the ureter than can often be appreciated by visual inspection. In a study of ballistic injury in a military laboratory, Amato et al. showed that microvascular injury can be present in normal-appearing ureteral segment for up to 2 cm on either side past grossly injured ureteral segment [4]. For this reason, when assessing ureteral injuries from GSW or other thermal devices, the surgeon should resect the ureter widely and up to the bleeding edge prior to spatulation and repair over a ureteral stent using interrupted absorbable sutures.

In patients for whom ureteral reconstruction cannot be safely performed at the time of presentation because of other more pressing competing injuries or hemodynamic instability, the ureter should be ligated and the kidney drained using a nephrostomy tube as a temporizing measure with subsequent elective repair after the patient is stabilized. If ureteral reconstruction is performed in the setting of associated colon or pancreatic injury, an omental wrap is recommended to isolate the ureteral repair. This prevents periureteral adhesions and protects the repair from succus or pancreatic enzymes. As a last resort in an unstable patient with a normal contralateral kidney, a nephrectomy can be performed.

Ureteral injury may not present with hematuria. Hence, the mechanism and trajectory of injury should guide the decision on whether to evaluate the ureter for injury. The most recent AUA urotrauma guidelines support CT urogram for the evaluation of the ureter in blunt or penetrating trauma when a patient is stable enough to be transported to the CT scanner [5].

For penetrating trauma or any external violent trauma requiring immediate exploration, where a CT scan cannot be performed, consider an on-table intravenous pyelogram to verify the presence of the contralateral kidney. This is performed using 2 ml/kg of contrast medium as an IV bolus with a single fluoroscopy image after 10 minutes [6, 7].

Insidious Onset Distal Ureteral Disease

Ureteral injuries with more insidious onset present as ureteral stricture, urinoma, or fistula. The goal of the evaluation of a ureteral stricture or fistula is to determine the extent and nature of the diseased segment, rule out malignancy, evaluate for adjacent pathology, and determine the split renal function of the ipsilateral kidney.

CT urogram or MR urogram is usually necessary to evaluate the location of the stricture/fistula, presence of urinoma, and disease in adjacent organs. The presence of goblet sign, ureteral filling defects, or retroperitoneal or pelvic lymphadenopathy can indicate a malignant etiology. If this is suspected, ureteroscopy with ureteral brushing or ureteral biopsy can be performed. Additionally, retrograde and/or antegrade pyelogram is often required to determine the length of the diseased ureteral segment.

Diuretic renogram is used to evaluate split renal function in the ipsilateral kidney unit as well as diagnose ureteral obstruction. Traditionally, poorly functioning kidneys with split renal function less than 20% are thought to have a higher risk of failure after ureteral reconstruction. This was found in at least one review of endopyelotomy for the management of benign ureteral strictures where ureteral strictures in kidneys with less than 25% renal function uniformly failed endoscopic treatment [8]. However, retrospective studies looking at pyeloplasty in patients with split renal function of less than 25% found similar success rates when compared with pyeloplasty in patients with function greater than 25%. The latter studies are limited by relatively short duration of follow-up [9, 10]. In patients with poor split function, a risk to benefit calculation of undergoing an invasive surgery to preserve minimal renal function factors into the decision to proceed. It is reasonable to discuss with the patient the possibility of conservative management in asymptomatic patients with poor ipsilateral renal function or nephrectomy in symptomatic patients with adequate contralateral renal function and no significant comorbidities that put the solitary kidney at risk.

Indications for Reflux Versus Nonrefluxing Anastomoses

In the age of ureterosigmoidostomy, anti-refluxing anastomosis was performed to prevent the reflux of fecal contents and colonic air into the upper tracts from the high-pressure sigmoid colon. Although lower-pressure pouches and conduits circumvented the need for an anti-reflux mechanism, concern regarding adverse effects of reflux remained [11, 12]. Jorge Lockhart et al. helped resolve these concerns by demonstrating no increased rate of pyelonephritis or deterioration of renal function in refluxing vs anti-refluxing anastomosis groups [13]. Other studies have documented similar findings in bowel as well as bladder vesicoureteral anastomoses [14–16].

While the above findings are true of the adult population, the effects of vesicoureteral reflux in the pediatric population have been well documented [17]. There is, however, a subset of adults who benefit from the prevention of vesicoureteral reflux, in particular those adults with recurrent pyelonephritis [18]. This is especially important in women of childbearing age because of the increased risk of fetal morbidity and mortality associated with pyelonephritis in pregnancy [19, 20]. Hence, an anti-refluxing anastomosis should be considered when performing ureteral reimplantation in very young patients, women of childbearing age, and adults with history of recurrent pyelonephritis.

Assessing the Bladder

Bladder capacity should be assessed prior to performing a ureteral reimplantation, in particular, if a Boari flap is required for longer-length ureteral defects. This can be accomplished using simple cystometrogram or cystoscopy. A large bladder capacity allows for a flap base long enough to support vascularization and prevent ischemic stricture. Stolze recommended a capacity greater than 150 ml based on clinical experience [21]. Olsson et al. recommended a bladder capacity of over 400 ml [22]. There is little or no data evaluating optimal bladder capacity for Boari flap ureteral reconstruction; however, we believe that a capacity greater than 300 ml is adequate.

Timing of Repair: Early Versus Late

In the absence of significant infection, urinoma, or fistula, immediate definitive repair can be attempted. This repair should ideally be performed within 24 hours of the injury but can be attempted up to 7 days from the time of the initial surgery. After this time, the tissue planes are distorted by marked inflammation making repair technically challenging [23]. In patients in whom immediate reconstruction is not performed, attempted placement of a retrograde stent is successful 20–33% of the time with variable rates of spontaneous healing after 6 weeks without the need for definitive repair [24–26]. The majority will present with a ureteral stricture after stent removal, which may be amenable to endoscopic management. If stent placement is unsuccessful, a percutaneous nephrostomy tube may be placed to drain the kidney and delayed reconstruction performed after 1–3 months [23]. Though delayed repair is the current convention, some authors have described successful outcomes with immediate definitive repair after delayed diagnosis [27].

Preoperative Preparation

The following should be obtained in preoperative preparation:

- A complete preoperative history and physical exam.
- Laboratory studies to include complete blood count, basic metabolic panel, coagulation panel, urinalysis, and urine culture.
- Bowel prep: We do not formally bowel prep our patients; however, a fleet enema the night before surgery and a clear liquid diet the day before ensure a decompressed colon that is easier to retract out of the surgical field.
- Antibiotics prophylaxis: Per AUA best practice statement 2012, a first- or second-generation cephalosporin or aminoglycoside + flagyl/clindamycin is recommended for prophylaxis.
- DVT prophylaxis: Pneumoboots are recommended for DVT prophylaxis in low-risk patients. If a pelvic lymph node dissection is required for high-grade TCC, then additional DVT prophylaxis including low-molecular-weight heparin should be considered.
- Renal unit drainage preoperatively: long-term stent placement induces ureteral edema and inflammatory changes that often make dissection challenging. We have found that in select patients who can tolerate stent removal, removing the stent 1–2 weeks prior to surgery can reduce this inflammation making for an improved dissection and reconstruction.

Outcomes

There is significant experience with robot-assisted laparoscopic distal ureteral reconstruction. The table below summarizes studies with at least 10 patients (Table 14.1). These reports demonstrate generally high success rates with few complications.

Elsamra et al. [40], comparing open, laparoscopic and robotic ureteroneocystostomy in 130 patients, found operative times to be similar in all three groups; however, they noted less blood loss and shorter length of stay in the laparoscopic and robotic groups as compared to the open group. Isac et al. [41] reviewed their cohort of 66 patients and noted a shorter operative time for the open group but decreased hospital stay, less narcotic requirement, and less blood loss in the robotic group. The overall success rate was similar between the two groups. Koznin et al. [42] in a matched control retrospective study found that the robotic surgery group

Table 14.1 Published outcomes on robotic-assisted laparoscopic distal ureteral reconstruction

References	Year	N	Mean age	Surgery	Mean EBL (ml)	Mean OR time (min)	Mean LOS	Mean F/u mos	Success rate (%)	Study
Patil et al. [28]	2008	12	41	UNC + PH- 12	48	208	4.3	15.5	100	Retrospective
Baldie et al. [29]	2012	13	46	UNC- 4 + PH- 8 + BF- 1	187	266.7	2.77	4.46	100	Retrospective
Lee et al. [30]	2013	10	52.9	UNC- 4 +PH- 6	102.5	211.7	2.8	28.5	80	Retrospective
Musch et al. [31]	2013	14	61.8	UNC- 5 +PH- 4 + BF- 5	NR	261	11.3	10.8	92.8	Retrospective
Fifer et al. [32]	2014	55	(52)	UNC +/− PH- 45 BF- 9	(50)	(221)	1.6	6	94.7	Retrospective
Gelhaus et al. [33]	2014	22	52	UNC- 10 +PH- 11 +BF- 1	88	214	2.4	13.44	90.9	Retrospective
Marien et al. [34]	2015	31	62	UNC- 2 +PH- 26 +BF- 3	101.6	260.3	3	10.8	100	Retrospective
Slater et al. [35]	2015	13	40	UNC- 10 + BF- 3	40	286	2.3	20.7	100	Retrospective
Wason et al. [36]	2015	13	46	UNC- 6 +PH- 8	123	282	2.5	9.8	100	Retrospective
Schiavina et.al [37].	2016	12	39.4	UNC- 9 +PH- 3	47.2	185	7.6	25.6	92.3	Retrospective
Stolenburg et al. [38]	2016	11	49.9	PH+ BF- 11	155.5	166.8	NR	15.2	100	NR
Buffi et al. [39]	2017	21	43	UNC- 21	NR	165	8	30	93.3	Retrospective

Values in bracket are median values, not mean

EBL estimated blood loss, *OR* operating room, *LOS* length of stay, *F/u* follow-up, *UNC* ureteroneocystostomy, *PH* psoas hitch, *BF* Boari flap, *NR* not recorded

had decreased estimated blood loss, length of hospital stay, and narcotic requirement. There were no stricture recurrences at median follow-up of 30 months. Lastly, Packiam et al. [43] in an NSQIP database query compared outcomes in 512 patients undergoing open vs robotic ureteral reimplantation. Patients undergoing robotic ureteral reimplantation had a shorter hospital stay and overall lower complication rate. Readmission and reoperation rates were similar between the two groups.

These results, particularly operative time, continue to improve as surgeons gain more experience with minimally invasive surgery.

In summary, the nature of ureteral injuries, timing, and approach to repair are determined by several factors. When detected, the ureter should be thoroughly evaluated. Traditionally open and transvaginal approaches to repair were most commonly used. Today, more repairs are done using a minimally invasive approach with documented high success rates and few complications.

References

1. McAninch J, et al. Ureteral injuries: external and iatrogenic. Urol Clin N Am. 2006;33:55–66.
2. Delacroix SE Jr, Winters JC. Urinary tract injures: recognition and management. Clin Colon Rectal Surg. 2010;23:104–12.
3. Parpala-Sparman T, Paananen I, Santala M, et al. Increasing numbers of ureteric injuries after the introduction of laparoscopic surgery. Scand J Urol Nephrol. 2008;42:422–7.
4. Amato JJ, Billy LJ, Gruber RP, et al. Vascular injuries. An experimental study of high and low velocity missile wounds. Arch Surg. 1970;101(2):167–74.
5. Morey A, et al. Urotrauma guidelines. 2014, amended 2017. https://www.auanet.org/guidelines/urotrauma-(2014-amended-2017)
6. McAninch JW, et al. Ureteral injuries from external violence: the 25-year experience at San Francisco general hospital. J Urol. 2003;170(4 Pt 1):1213–6.
7. Morey AF, et al. Single shot intraoperative excretory urography for the immediate evaluation of renal trauma. J Urol. 1999;161:1088–92.
8. Clayman RV, et al. Long-term results of endoureterotomy for benign ureteral and ureteroenteric strictures. J Urol. 1997;158(3 Pt 1):759–64.
9. Iwamura M, et al. Improvement in renal function and symptoms of patients treated with laparoscopic pyeloplasty for ureteropelvic junction obstruction with less than 20% split renal function. J Endourol. 2016;30(11):1214–8.
10. Caddedu JA, et al. Poor split renal function and age in adult patients with ureteropelvic junction obstruction do not impact functional outcomes of pyeloplasty. Can J Urol. 2016;23(5):8457–64.
11. Goodwin WE, Harris AP, Kaufman JJ, Beal JM. Open transcolonic ureterointestinal anastomosis. A new approach. Surg Gynecol Obstet. 1953;97:295–300.
12. Leadbetter WF, Clark BG. Five years' experience with ureteroenterostomy by the 'combined' technique. J Urol. 1954;73:67–82.
13. Halal M, et al. Direct(non-tunnelled) ureterocolonic reimplantation in association with continent reservoirs. J Urol. 1993;150:835–7.
14. Pantuck AJ, et al. Ureteroenteric anastomosis in continent urinary diversion: Long-term results and complications of direct versus nonrefluxing techniques. J Urol. 2000;163:450–5.
15. Studer UE, et al. Antireflux nipples or afferent tubular segments in 70 patients with Ileal low pressure bladder substitutes: long-term results of a prospective randomized trial. J Urol. 1996;156:1913–7.
16. Stefanovic KB, et al. Non-anti reflux versus antireflux ureteroneocystotomy in adults. Br J Urol. 1991;67:263–6.

17. Elder JS, et al. Primary vesicoureteral reflux guidelines panel summary report on the management of primary vesicoureteral reflux in children. J Urol. 1997;157:1846–51.
18. Guthman DD, et al. Vesicoureteral reflux in the adult. V Unilateral disease. J Urol. 1991;146:21.
19. Farkash E, et al. Acute antepartum pyelonephritis in pregnancy: a critical analysis of risk factors and outcomes. Eur J Obstet Gynecol Reprod Biol. 2012;162(1):24–7.
20. Wing AD, et al. Acute pyelonephritis in pregnancy: an 18-year retrospective analysis. Am J Obstet Gynecol. 2014;210(3):219e1–6.
21. Stolze KJ. Board plastic operation and reflux. Int Urol Nephrol. 1972;4(1):21–4.
22. Olsson C, et al. The use of the board-flap and psoas-bladder hitch technique in the repair of high ureteric lesion: a case report. Scand J Urol Nephrol. 1985;20(3):233–4.
23. Santucci RA, et al. Ureteral trauma. Medscape. 11 Feb 2017. http://emedicine.medscape.com/article/440933-overview
24. Ghali AMA, et al. Ureteric injuries: diagnosis, management, and outcome. J Trauma. 1999;46:150–8.
25. Oh BR, et al. Late presentation of ureteral injury after laparoscopic surgery. Obstet Gynecol. 2000;95:337–9.
26. Selzman AA, et al. Iatrogenic ureteral injuries: a 20 year experience in treating 165 injuries. J Urol. 1996;155:878–81.
27. Hoch WH, et al. Early, aggressive management of intraoperative ureteral injuries. J Urol. 1975;114:530–2.
28. Patil NN, et al. Robotic-assisted laparoscopic ureteral reimplantation with psoas hitch: a multi-institutional, multinational evaluation. Urology. 2008;72:47–50.
29. Baldie K, et al. Robotic management of benign mid and distal ureteral strictures and comparison with laparoscopic approaches at a single institution. Urology. 2012;80:596–601.
30. Lee Z, et al. Single-surgeon experience with robot-assisted ureteroneocystostomy for distal ureteral pathologies in adults. Korean J Urol. 2013;54:516–21.
31. Musch M, et al. Robot-assisted reconstructive surgery of the distal ureter: single institution experience in 16 patients. BJU Int. 2013;111:773–83.
32. Fifer GL, et al. Robotic ureteral reconstruction distal to the ureteropelvic junction: a large single institution clinical series with short-term follow up. J Endourol. 2014;28:1424–8.
33. Gelhaus P, et al. Robotic management of genitourinary injuries from obstetric and gynaecological operations: a multi-institutional report of outcomes. BJU Int. 2014;115(3):430–6.
34. Marien T, et al. Outcomes of robotic-assisted laparoscopic upper urinary tract reconstruction: 250 consecutive patients. BJU Int. 2015;116(4):604–11.
35. Slater RC, et al. Contemporary series of robotic-assisted distal ureteral reconstruction utilizing side docking position. Int J Urol. 2015;41(6):1154–9.
36. Wason SE, et al. Robotic-assisted ureteral re-implantation: a case series. J Laparoendosc Adv Surg Tech A. 2015;25:503–7.
37. Svhiavina R, et al. Laparoscopic and robotic ureteral stenosis repair: a multi-institutional experience with a long-term follow-up. J Robot Surg. 2016;10(4):323–30.
38. Stolzenburg JU, et al. Robot-assisted technique for Boari flap ureteric reimplantation: replicating the techniques of open surgery in robotics. BJU Int. 2016;118(3):482–4.
39. Buffi NM, et al. Robot-assisted surgery for benign ureteral strictures: Experience and outcomes from four tertiary care institutions. Eur Urol. 2017;71(6):945–51.
40. Elsamra SE, et al. Open, laparoscopic and robotic ureteroneocystostomy for benign and malignant ureteral lesions: a comparison of over 100 minimally invasive cases. J Endourol. 2014;28:1455–9.
41. Isac W, et al. Open, laparoscopic, and robotic ureteroneocystostomy for benign and malignant ureteral lesions: a comparison of over 100 minimally invasive cases. J Endourol. 2014;28(12):1455–9.
42. Koznin SI, et al. Robotic versus open distal ureteral reconstruction and reimplantation for benign stricture disease. J Endourol. 2012;26(2):147–51.
43. Packiam VT, et al. Open vs minimally invasive adult ureteral reimplantation: analysis of 30-day outcomes in the National Surgical Quality Improvement Program (NSQIP) database. Urology. 2016;94:123–8.

Jan Lukas Hohenhorst, Michael Musch, Anne Vogel,
Heinrich Löwen, and Darko Kröpfl

Introduction and Objectives

This chapter focuses on the management of distal ureteral obstruction and/or distal ureteral malignancy managed by ureteral reimplantation. Open reconstructive surgery of the lower ureteric segment in adults requires large incisions, to allow for wide exposure and complex reconstruction. This is especially true for pre-operated and or pre-irradiated patients in whom adhesions are a major obstacle. It has been suggested and reported that suturing and tissue handling in the limited space of the pelvis can be more easily performed with the robot compared to conventional laparoscopy. Nevertheless, published experience on minimally invasive techniques in this challenging field still remains limited [1–4].

Minimally invasive da Vinci robot-assisted procedures allow precise identification of proper tissue planes and thereby avoidance of unnecessary tissue damage [1–4]. All these allow a consistent and easier application of the gold standards of open surgery in the deep small pelvis. We feel the steps presented here are the most important steps of robot-assisted distal ureteral reconstruction (RAURI) using the

Supplementary Information The online version of this chapter (https://doi.org/10.1007/978-3-030-50196-9_15) contains supplementary material, which is available to authorized users.

J. L. Hohenhorst
Department of Urology and Urologic Oncology, Alfried-Krupp Krankenhaus,
Essen, NRW, Germany
e-mail: jan.hohenhorst@krupp-krankenhaus.de

M. Musch · A. Vogel · H. Löwen · D. Kröpfl (✉)
Department of Urology, Urologic Oncology and Pediatric Urology, Kliniken Essen-Mitte,
Essen, Germany
e-mail: m.musch@kliniken-essen-mitte.de; h.lowen@kliniken-essen-mitte.de;
d.kroepfl@kliniken-essen-mitte.de

da Vinci robot. The results of our RAURI series were presented recently in one of the largest European single-institution series on robot-assisted reconstructive surgery (RARS) of the lower ureteric segments (LUS) [4]. This chapter is based on our own previous publications [5] and videos [6] and hitherto unpublished new data, all focusing on the operative technique of RAURI.

Materials and Methods

We briefly describe the patient characteristics and perioperative data, the incidence of 90-day postoperative complications, and the results of follow-up examinations. We then present in detail the operative technique used. Each procedure was recorded and could be analyzed for the purpose of this article. All data were collected retrospectively using the patients' records and standardized questionnaires sent to the patients and their referring urologists. The follow-up examinations were done at the discretion of the referring urologists. Descriptive statistics comprise median and range for continuous variables and frequencies and percentages for categorical variables.

Preoperative Diagnostic Workup

There are no defined algorithms for preoperative diagnostic workup in the case of distal ureteral obstruction. Most patients are symptomatic, or the dilated ureter is detected as an incidental finding of abdominal sonography, a CT scan, or MRI of the abdomen. A malignant tumor as the cause of a ureteric obstruction should always be considered and ruled out. Cystoscopy should follow, and in the case of a suspected vesical or extravesical malignancy, biopsies should be taken. Bullous edema of the bladder mucosa from the ipsilateral side strongly suggests an extravesical tumor. The next steps are retrograde pyelography and, if indicated, ureterorenoscopy and targeted biopsies (Figs. 15.1 and 15.2). During these procedures, we fill the bladder with a diluted, slightly warmed x-ray dye to measure the bladder capacity and its cranial extension and so estimate if the psoas hitch procedure alone or in combination with a Boari flap will be necessary. If malignancy is disclosed and reasonable ipsilateral function can be expected, the diseased ureter should be excised and reimplant considered if negative margincs and no proximal tumor is confirmed.

Results

Between October 2009 and December 2016, ureteric resection and reimplantation of the distal part of the ureter were performed in 38 patients. Resection of the distal ureter was necessary due to urothelial carcinoma in nine patients, ureteric stricture secondary to advanced prostate cancer seen in two patients, ureteric stricture caused by an inflammatory conglomerate tumor of the adnexa in one patient, ureteric

Fig. 15.1 Retrograde pyelography in a patient with the iatrogenic right-side distal ureter

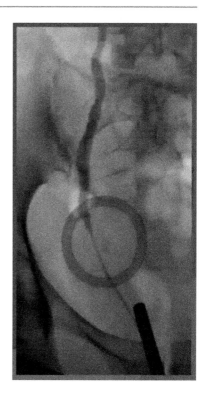

stricture of unknown cause in three patients, inflammation in one patient, ureteric stricture due to a B-cell lymphoma in one patient, and iatrogenic ureteric stricture following gynecologic or urologic surgery in eight patients.

RARS of the LUS comprised 26 cases of anti-refluxive ureteric reimplantation and psoas hitch technique with ($n = 13$) or without ($n = 13$) Boari flap. Furthermore, six cases of extravesical anti-refluxive ureteric reimplantation, two cases of intra-vesical anti-refluxive ($n = 1$) or refluxive ($n = 1$) ureteric reimplantation, three cases of ureteric stricture resection and end-to-end anastomosis, and one case of ureter-olysis with omentum wrap were necessary due to benign conditions. In all cases, we aimed to reduce traumatic handling of the ureter by using a vessel loop and the fourth robotic arm for traction (Fig. 15.3). In those cases where a urothelial carci-noma of the LUS was the underlying pathological condition, an ipsilateral pelvic lymphadenectomy was always performed. Furthermore, in order to avoid tumor cell spillage, the affected segment was isolated, clipped proximally and distally with Hem-o-Lok® clips and transected proximally (Fig. 15.4). Then, the bladder was filled with distilled water, a bladder cuff was resected along with the distal ureter, and directly thereafter, the specimen was collected in a retrieval bag. When ureteric reimplantation was done with a psoas hitch technique (+/− Boari flap), the ureteral neo hiatus (entry point of the ureter into the bladder wall) and the direction of the submucosal tunnel were built in line with the anatomic course of the ureter to avoid angulation of the ureter in different filling states of the bladder (Fig. 15.5). Such a

Fig. 15.2 Retrograde
pyelography in a patient
with left distal
ureteric tumor

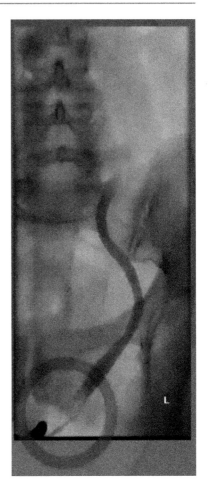

tunnel of adequate caliber should also allow uncomplicated ureteral catheterization or ureterorenoscopy (Fig. 15.6). End-to-end anastomosis of the distal ureter should certainly not be regarded as routine. However, in the cases presented here, it was considered because of a well-preserved blood supply of the generously spatulated ureteral ends and the possibility of an absolutely tension-free anastomosis between them. To prevent any kind of tension postoperatively, the surrounding scar tissue was partially left in situ and used as an anchor point in one case. Extravesical anti-refluxive ureteric reimplantation was necessary due to benign intramural strictures following urological surgery ($n = 3$) and persistent vesicoureteral reflux after endoscopic injection therapy ($n = 1$). Intravesical ureteric reimplantation was performed in one case following resection of an upper kidney pole megaureter and ureterocele and in another case following inadvertent bilateral ureteral transection of upper-pole ectopic ureters inserting into the prostatic urethra in a patient undergoing radical prostatectomy.

Fig. 15.3 Vessel loop to
put the ureter in position

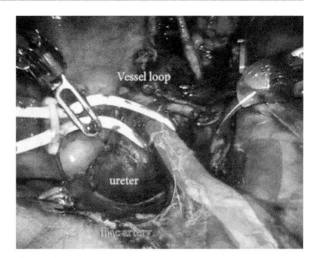

Fig. 15.4 Use of
Hem-o-Lok clips to
prevent tumor cell spillage

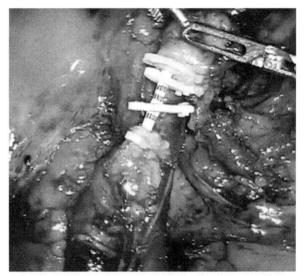

Fig. 15.5 Positioning of
the ureter to preserve the
natural course

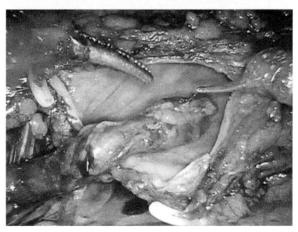

Fig. 15.6 Follow-up ureterorenoscopy in patients who underwent distal ureteric resection because of ureteric carcinoma

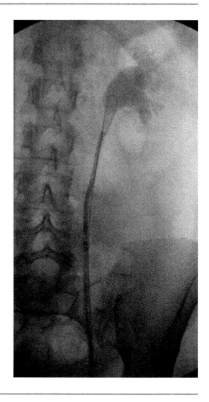

Robot Used

A standard four-arm da Vinci® surgical system (Intuitive Surgical Inc., Mountain View, CA, USA) was used at the beginning of the study, replaced from January 2011 with a da Vinci Si HD surgical system and an Xi HD surgical system in 2015.

RAURI

The principles of ureteric reconstruction and reimplantation that were applied here with robot assistance are generally accepted as the gold standard in open surgery and described in detail in Campbell-Walsh Urology in the chapter "Management of Upper Urinary Tract Obstruction" by Nakada and Hsu [7].

RAURI can be divided into the following important steps:

Positioning of the Patient on the Operating Table and Trocar Placement

After placing the patient in a steep Trendelenburg position, an 18-F Foley urethral catheter was inserted. Trocar positioning was as follows: a 12-mm robotic camera

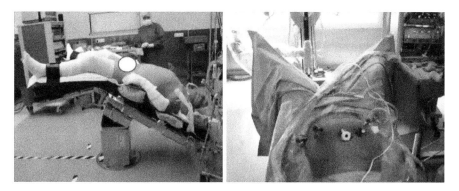

Fig. 15.7 Trendelenburg and trocar placement

port 5 cm above the umbilicus in the median line, two 8-mm robotic ports bilaterally along the midclavicular line at the level of the umbilicus, a fourth 8-mm robotic port on the contralateral side of the diseased ureter 10 cm lateral to the other ipsilateral 8-mm robotic port, and a 5-mm assistant port between the camera port and the 8-mm port.

The patients operated on with a standard, Si HD, or Xi robot were always put in a steep Trendelenburg position with the legs spread and slightly flexed at the knee (Fig. 15.7). In the patients operated on with a Xi robot, we routinely use side docking without flexing of the legs. In all three types of a robot, we used an abdominal pressure of 12 mmHg. All operations were performed using a four-arm robotic setting, with the fourth arm placed either on the left side of the patient or contralaterally to the operating field when possible. Careful padding of all conceivable pressure points was performed. In the case of severe arteriosclerosis, a pulse oximeter was placed on the toes of both legs and oxygen saturation measured continuously. Preoperative identification of high-pressure glaucoma is essential. The steep Trendelenburg position should be checked before starting the operation to make sure that the patient has not changed his position. This sounds banal, but a high number of patients can have positioning-related pain after steep Trendelenburg position, and some remain prescriptive and are partially disastrous [8] (Table 15.1).

Operative Procedure

The Steps of the Operation in a Case Where a Part of the Ureter Had to Be Resected

The principles and steps of the operation are shown in Table 15.2.

After resection of the diseased distal ureter, the bladder was mobilized as far as possible. Care was taken not to harm the bilateral vascular pedicles of the bladder, which is distinctly easier to do robotically than during an open procedure. Then, the bladder was filled with physiological saline until maximal capacity was reached. In the case of urothelial carcinoma of the ureter, the bladder is filled with air to avoid

Table 15.1 Patient characteristics

Procedure	Distal ureter resection and/or reconstruction
Patient no.	38
Localization (uni–/bilateral)	35/3
Gender (♀/♂)	19/19
Age (years) (median (range))	60 (25–86)
BMI (kg/m^2) (median (range))	26 (17.6–36.2)
Surgical time (min) (median (range))	225 (105–380)
Hospital stay (day) (median (range))	8 (5–35)
Postoperative complications	
Clavien grade IIIa-b	3
Clavien grade IVa-b	1
Clavien grade V	0
Follow-up (month)	17.3 (1.1–81.8)
(median (range))	Follow-up of 27 patients
No obstruction	26
	Follow-up of 27 patients
Asymptomatic	27
	Follow-up of 27 patients

Table 15.2 Principles of distal ureteric reconstruction and reimplantation used in the present series

1	Adequate mobilization of the distal ureter without traumatic tissue manipulation to preserve its blood supply
2	Gentle handling of the bladder to reduce postoperative hematuria and bladder spasms
3	Generous mobilization of the bladder with the preservation of its blood supply (dissection of the contralateral bladder pedicle only if necessary)
4	Fixation of the bladder on the psoas muscle carefully avoiding injuries to the genitofemoral or femoral nerves (Fig. 15.5)
5	Choosing the position of the neo-hiatus (entry point of the ureter into the bladder) and the direction of the submucosal tunnel to correspond well with the anatomical course of the ureter (Figs. 15.6 and 15.10)
6	Creation of a submucosal tunnel of adequate width and length and with sufficient muscular backing
7	Spatulation of the ureter
8	Anchoring sutures of the ureter
9	Meticulous suturing when creating the neo-orifice
10	Complete covering of the ureter with bladder mucosa to avoid fibrosis (Fig. 15.7)
11	Tension-free vesico-ureteric anastomosis
12	Meticulous watertight closure of the bladder
13	Adequate postoperative drainage is obligatory
14	Omentum majus wrap, if impaired blood supply is suspected

spillage of potentially contaminated urine. Thereafter, as said before, the decision should be made as to whether the anti-refluxive psoas hitch procedure will be enough to achieve a tension-free anastomosis between the bladder and the ureter or a

Boari-flap should be additionally used. In our opinion, an anti-reflux reimplantation should be done whenever possible because it is technically easier to perform, imitates the natural course of the ureter, and prevents an anastomotic stenosis (Fig. 15.8).

In cases where a psoas hitch procedure was judged sufficient for a tension-free anti-refluxive anastomosis, the bladder was dorsally detached from the overlying peritoneum in a meticulous fashion. If this was done properly, in our experience, it was not necessary in a single case to transect the ipsilateral or even the contralateral pedicle. The author of this text would prefer to use a Boari flap rather than transect the pedicles to mobilize the bladder. We feel that such a decision is most probably the result of the robot-assisted procedure which allows such precise preparation of functional tissue such as vessels and nerves that the pedicle resection is rendered obsolete. Then, two 2-0 polyglactin sutures with UR-5 needles were used to fix the spread posterior bladder wall to the psoas muscle on the side of the affected ureter (Fig. 15.9), carefully avoiding the genitofemoral and the femoral nerves. The

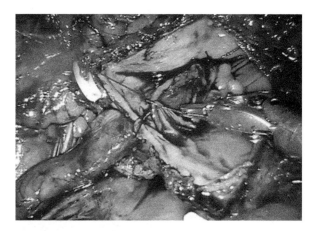

Fig. 15.8 Anti-reflux ureteric reimplantation of the left ureter

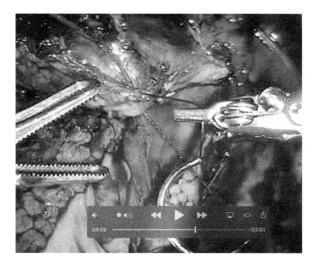

Fig. 15.9 Fixation of the bladder on the psoas muscle

bladder was filled again with physiological saline, and a longitudinal incision was made at the anterior bladder wall in the direction between the two fixing sutures to ensure an appropriate anatomic course of the ureter (Fig. 15.10). The sides of the incised bladder were then fixed to the surrounding tissue with Weck clips to facilitate further procedure (Fig. 15.5). Then, the ureter was spatulated, brought through a 3–4 cm-long submucosal tunnel into the bladder, and anchored in the detrusor with three 3-0 polyglactin sutures (Fig. 15.11). Using interrupted 5-0 polyglactin sutures, the reconstruction of the neo-orifice was completed (Fig. 15.12). Then, a 6-F JJ stent was passed into the reimplanted ureter via a guidewire through one of the assistance ports. If the creation of a Boari flap was necessary, it was fashioned

Fig. 15.10
Bladder opening

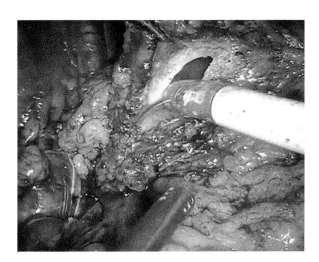

Fig. 15.11 Anchoring of the ureter

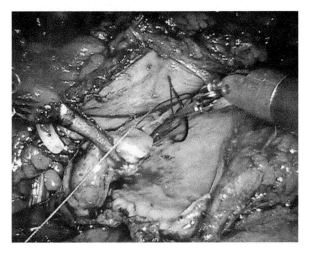

from the anterior wall of the bladder with a length-width ratio of 2:1 (e.g., 8 cm in length and 4 cm in width). The technique for anti-refluxive implantation of the ureter when a Boari flap is used is the same as described previously for the psoas hitch procedure. Implantation of the ureter in the flap was performed with the same technique as described previously for the psoas hitch procedure. Thereafter, the Boari flap was tubularized with 4-0 poliglecaprone sutures in two layers. If anti-refluxive reimplantation was not possible, a wide oval anastomosis between a spatulated ureter and Boari flap was performed with 5-0 and 4-0 polyglactin sutures in two layers (Fig. 15.13).

Fig. 15.12 Reconstruction of neo orifice

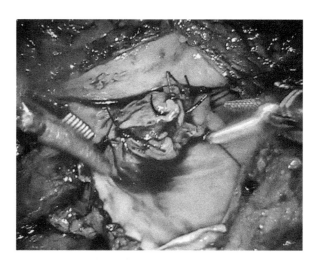

Fig. 15.13 DJ placement

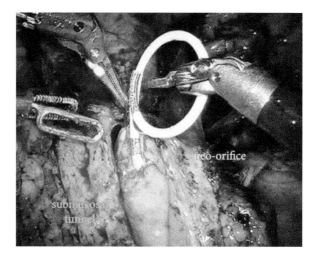

Extravesical Anti-Refluxive Ureteric Reimplantation

In some cases with short ureteral stenosis or symptomatic vesicorenal reflux where a psoas hitch was not necessary, there is an indication for a ureteric reimplantation on the anterolateral bladder wall [9].

The ureter is identified where it crosses the iliac vessels and followed caudally to its insertion into the bladder. Utmost care is necessary to avoid injury of the vesical nerve plexus and vascular pedicle, especially in cases with a bilateral stenosis or reflux. Based on the original position of ureteric insertion, the musculature of the bladder wall was incised on the anterolateral side of the filled bladder along a distance of 4–5 cm to avoid kinking of the ureter. The stenotic part was identified and resected. When the ureter was placed in proper position, its distal end was spatulated, and after finishing one half of the anastomosis, the JJ-stent was inserted over the guidewire and the neo-orifice reconstructed with 5 or 4.0 single Vicryl sutures. In the case of vesicorenal reflux, after creating a muscular incision leaving the intact, the detrusor is closed over the ureter taking care to avoid the creation of a too narrow tunnel (Fig. 15.14).

Ureteric End-to-End Anastomosis

There is no doubt that an end-to-end anastomosis of the ureter in the deep pelvis is very seldom indicated and should certainly not be propagated as routine procedure. But in a case presented here of a female patient with severe surrounding scarring, a wide tension-free anastomosis was judged to be possible. The left ureter was identified as it crossed the iliac vessels and followed caudally to its insertion into the bladder. In its distal course, the ureter was completely released from an encircling endometriosis focus. After ureteric stricture resection and before accomplishing an oval-shaped end-to-end anastomosis, the partially left surrounding scarred tissue

Fig. 15.14 Extravesical anti-refluxive ureteric reimplantation and creating a tunnel between bladder mucosa and bladder muscle

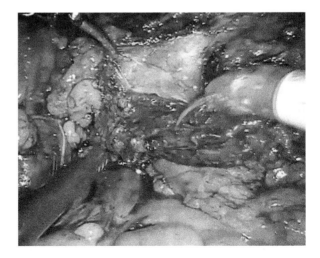

Fig. 15.15 Ureteric
end-to-end anastomosis

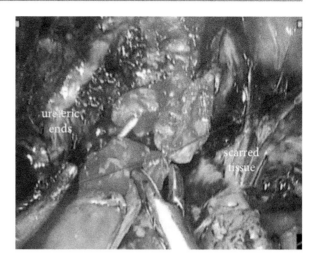

was used as an anchor point for approximation sutures of the ureteric ends to remove tension and create a tension-free spatulated ureteric end-to-end anastomosis. The left ureter was covered with a mobilized omentum majus wrap. The preoperatively implanted 6-F JJ stent was left in place for 4 weeks. The long-term follow-up was uneventful (Fig. 15.15).

In the case of a fresh accidental iatrogenic ureteric transection, we spatulate the ureter on both sides and put a stay suture on the cranial and distal parts of the spatulated ureter and run a 5.0 PDS suture in semicircular technique. The JJ stent is left for 4 weeks and the wound drained. In such a case, the use of indocyanine is probably very helpful to identify the viability of ureteral edges, but we have no personal experience of this to date.

Discussion

It has been reported that suturing and tissue handling in the limited space of the pelvis can be more easily performed with the robot compared with conventional laparoscopy [10]. Successful robot-assisted distal ureterectomy with psoas hitch and Boari flap reconstruction in patients with urothelial cancers has already been described [1, 11–14]. In this context, recently published studies suggest that a minimally invasive laparoscopic approach to upper tract urothelial carcinoma provides good oncological outcomes and does not result in a clinically significant increased risk of tumor spillage, provided that principles of oncological surgery are obeyed [15, 16].

As with urothelial carcinoma of the distal ureter, the use of robotics for surgery of benign distal ureteric defects or strictures is also still limited, probably due to the relative rarity of these conditions [1, 3, 13, 14, 17–19]. Furthermore, in almost all of these series, a refluxive ureteric reimplantation was performed. Only De Naeyer et al. [2] reported a robot-assisted anti-refluxive psoas hitch reimplantation in an early case report in 2007. In an evidence-based review, Tracey AT et al. analyzed 13 cases and showed the feasibility, safety, and success of robotic ureteral reconstruction in reconstruction of the ureter as well as the usefulness of fluorescence imaging and the use of buccal mucosa in ureteral reconstruction [20]. Our experience with robot-assisted treatment of ureteric injuries is limited but good, with successful outcomes in all patients thus treated.

Robot-assisted laparoscopic extravesical ureteral reimplantation is a minimally invasive alternative to open surgery in vesicorenal reflux or anomalies such as a ureterocele or megaureter in children and adults. In the meantime, this technique has been adopted by a substantial number of surgeons and has shown low complication rates and good results in long-term follow-up [21].

Prospective long-term analysis of nerve-sparing extravesical robotic-assisted laparoscopic ureteral reimplantation is needed.

We feel that an anti-refluxing reimplantation of the ureter regardless of whether performed extra- or intravesically, by open surgery or robot-assisted laparoscopy, has some advantages. If the position of the ureteric neo-hiatus (entry point of the ureter into the bladder wall) and the direction of the submucosal tunnel are in line with the anatomical course of the ureter, angulation of the ureter in different filling states of the bladder should be more easily avoided. Furthermore, such a tunnel of adequate caliber should also allow uncomplicated ureteric catheterization or ureterorenoscopy. In the context of ureteric reimplantation, it is also important to mention that we avoided long-term ureteric stenting before surgery whenever possible, in order to prevent alterations such as ureteric wall thickening complicating surgical reconstruction [22].

In patients with extrinsic endometriosis, ureterolysis alone may be sufficient to correct ureteric obstruction [23]. Following the surgical technique in retroperitoneal fibrosis, we additionally placed an omental wrap around the diseased ureter to prevent entrapment of the ureter in forming scars [24].

An incidentally encountered ectopic ureter in a man undergoing radical prostatectomy (RP) is a rare condition that has only been reported in a few case reports [25, 26]. To our knowledge, the present description of bilateral robot-assisted intravesical reimplantation of upper-pole ectopic ureters inserting into the prostatic urethra in a patient undergoing RP is the only case published to date.

Our experience with robotics in ureteric reconstruction for defects of the distal ureter is largely concordant with the still-limited worldwide experience. The present study has shown that robot-assisted reconstructive surgery of the distal ureter is feasible and can be performed without compromising the generally accepted principles of open surgical procedures. The functional outcome was good in short-term follow-up. The incidence of minor complications was high, but the number of severe complications was low, thus not discouraging. It is the personal opinion of the senior author that in the future, robotics will replace conventional laparoscopy in reconstructive surgery of the distal ureter and even come to challenge open surgery.

Acknowledgments We would like to thank Ms. H. Coleman for the revision of the English manuscript and Mr. Basheck for his help with the data processing.

References

1. Mufarrij PW, Shah OD, Berger AD, Stifelman MD. Robotic reconstruction of the upper urinary tract. J Urol. 2007;178:2002–5.
2. De Naeyer G, Van Migem P, Schatteman P, Carpentier P, Fonteyne E, Mottrie AM. Case report: pure robot-assisted psoas hitch ureteral reimplantation for distal-ureteral stenosis. J Endourol. 2007;21:618–20.
3. Patil NN, Mottrie A, Sundaram B, Patel VR. Robotic-assisted laparoscopic ureteral reimplantation with psoas hitch: a multi-institutional, multinational evaluation. Urology. 2008;72:47–50.
4. Musch M, Hohenhorst L, Pailliart A, Löwen H, Davoudi Y, Kroepfl D. Robot-assisted reconstructive surgery of the distal ureter: single institution experience in 16 patients. BJU Int. 2013;111(5):773–83.
5. Hohenhorst JL, Pailliart A, Musch M, Janowski M, Vanberg M, Kroepfl D. Robot-assisted ureteral reimplantation with the psoas hitch technique – important surgical steps. J Urol. 2014;191(4S):e551.
6. Hohenhorst L, Kunz I, Yanovskiy M, Pailliart A, Vanberg M, Musch M, Kröpfl D. Roboterassistierte Harnleiterneueinpflanzung in Psoas Hitch Technik – Wichtige operative Schritte. DGU 2012 – 1. Price Best Video.
7. Nakada SY, Hsu THS. Management of upper urinary tract obstruction. In: Wein AJ, Kavoussi LR, Novick AC, Partin AW, Peters CA, editors. Campbell-Walsh urology, Chap. 41, vol. II. 10th ed. Philadelphia: Saunders; 2012. p. 1122–68.
8. Rosevear HM, Lightfoot AJ, Zahs M, Waxman SW, Winfield HN. Lessons learned from a case of calf compartment syndrome after robot-assisted laparoscopic prostatectomy. J Endourol. 2010;24(10):1597–601. https://doi.org/10.1089/end.2009.0666.
9. Röhl L, Ziegler M. Uretero-neocystostomy in kidney transplantation. Urologe. 1969;8(3):116–9.
10. Rassweiler J, Pini G, Gözen AS, Klein J, Teber D. Role of laparoscopy in reconstructive surgery. Curr Opin Urol. 2010;20:471–82.
11. Allaparthi S, Ramanathan R, Balaji KC. Robotic distal ureterectomy with Boari flap reconstruction for distal ureteral urothelial cancers: a single institutional pilot experience. J Laparoendosc Adv Surg Tech A. 2010;20:165–71.
12. Singh I, Kader K, Hemal AK. Robotic distal ureterectomy with reimplantation in malignancy: technical nuances. Can J Urol. 2009;16:4671–6.
13. Uberoi J, Harnisch B, Sethi AS, Babayan RK, Wang DS. Robot-assisted laparoscopic distal ureterectomy and ureteral reimplantation with psoas hitch. J Endourol. 2007;21:368–73.
14. Hemal AK, Nayyar R, Gupta NP, Dorairajan LN. Experience with robot assisted laparoscopic surgery for upper and lower benign and malignant ureteral pathologies. Urology. 2010;76:1387–93.
15. Phé V, Cussenot O, Bitker MO, Rouprêt M. Does the surgical technique for management of the distal ureter influence the outcome after nephroureterectomy? BJU Int. 2011;108:130–8.
16. Eandi JA, Nelson RA, Wilson TG, Josephson DY. Oncologic outcomes for complete robot-assisted laparoscopic management of upper-tract transitional cell carcinoma. J Endourol. 2010;24:969–75.
17. Yang C, Jones L, Rivera ME, Verlee GT, Deane LA. Robotic-assisted ureteral reimplantation with Boari flap and psoas hitch: a single-institution experience. J Laparoendosc Adv Surg Tech A. 2011;21:829–33.
18. Schimpf MO, Wagner JR. Robot-assisted laparoscopic distal ureteral surgery. JSLS. 2009;13:44–9.
19. Kozinn SI, Canes D, Sorcini A, Moinzadeh A. Robotic versus open distal ureteral reconstruction and reimplantation for benign stricture disease. J Endourol. 2012;26:147–51.
20. Tracey AT, Eun DD, Stifelman MD, Hemal AK, Stein RJ, Mottrie A, et al. Robotic-assisted laparoscopic repair of ureteral injury: an evidence-based review of techniques and outcomes. Minerva Urol Nefrol. 2018;70(3):231–41. https://doi.org/10.23736/S0393-2249.18.03137-5. Epub 2018 Mar 28

21. Kasturi S, Sehgal SS, Christman MS, Lambert SM, Casale P. Prospective long-term analysis of nerve-sparing extravesical robotic-assisted laparoscopic ureteral reimplantation. Urology. 2012;79(3):680–3. https://doi.org/10.1016/j.urology.2011.10.052. Epub 2011 Dec 23
22. Ramsay JW, Payne SR, Gosling PT, Whitfield HN, Wickham JE, Levison DA. The effects of double J stenting on unobstructed ureters. An experimental and clinical study. Br J Urol. 1985;57:630–4.
23. Watanabe Y, Ozawa H, Uematsu K, Kawasaki K, Nishi H, Kobashi Y. Hydronephrosis due to ureteral endometriosis treated by transperitoneal laparoscopic ureterolysis. Int J Urol. 2004;11:560–2.
24. Keehn AY, Mufarrij PW, Stifelman MD. Robotic ureterolysis for relief of ureteral obstruction from retroperitoneal fibrosis. Urology. 2011;77:1370–4.
25. Funahashi Y, Kamihira O, Kasugai S, Kimura K, Fukatsu A, Matsuura O. Radical prostatectomy for prostate carcinoma with ectopic ureter: a case report. Nihon Hinyokika Gakkai Zasshi. 2007;98:580–2. Japanese
26. Marien TP, Shapiro E, Melamed J, Taouli B, Stifelman MD, Lepor H. Management of localized prostate cancer and an incidental ureteral duplication with upper pole ectopic ureter inserting into the prostatic urethra. Rev Urol. 2008;10:297–303.

Distal Ureteral Injury and Repair in Children

16

Christina Kim

Mechanism of Injury and Implications

Ureteral injuries account for <1% of all urologic external trauma. This is largely due to the ureteral location in the retroperitoneum, between the spinal vertebra and major muscle groups. Blunt trauma leading to ureteral injury typically entails extreme force to the entire body (e.g., falling from a large height or a high-speed motor-vehicle accident). Rapid deceleration can strain the ureters in its fixed locations (e.g., ureterovesical and ureteropelvic junctions).

More commonly ureteral injuries are iatrogenic and related to difficult abdominopelvic surgeries. Overall incidence of ureteral injuries ranges from 1% to 8% [28–31]. The majority of ureteral injuries involve the distal ureter (91%). The mid and proximal ureters are less commonly involved (7% and 2%, respectively) [1, 2].

Most common sites of injuries for open surgery are the ovarian vascular pedicle, the ureteral course adjacent to the uterine artery, vaginal fornices, and lateral rectal pedicles. During laparoscopy, the ureter is at risk near the adnexa and cardinal ligaments.

The most common surgeries associated with ureteral injuries are hysterectomy, colorectal procedures, and ovarian tumor removal. Factors that increase the chance of ureteral injury are uncontrolled bleeding in the pelvis. In addition, distorted anatomy can exist due to a large uterus, endometriosis, and prior surgery. If ureteral injuries go unrecognized, there are significant sequelae with the need for subsequent surgery. This is different than the hydronephrosis that develops in 12–20% of aortoiliac and aortofemoral bypass surgery. In these cases, the outcome for that

Supplementary Information The online version of this chapter (https://doi.org/10.1007/978-3-030-50196-9_16) contains supplementary material, which is available to authorized users.

C. Kim (✉)
Department of Urology, University of Wisconsin-Madison, Madison, WI, USA
e-mail: ckim@urology.wisc.edu

manipulated ureter is typically benign. Risk factors for ureteral injury from intra-abdominal vascular surgery are reoperation, placement of a graft anterior to the ureter, and retroperitoneal inflammation from dilated aneurysms.

Over the years, the incidence of ureteral injury due to laparoscopy has increased. One report of 1300 laparoscopic cases reported ureteral injuries in 0.8% of the cases [3]. The overall risk of ureteral injury from colorectal surgery was 0.24–5% [4–6].

Ideally, ureteral injuries are identified and treated immediately. If the injury is missed, the primary goal is urinary diversion until formal reparative surgery can be performed. Diversion will decrease the incidence of retroperitoneal fibrosis, sepsis, and infection.

Ureteral injuries from open procedures are recognized 1/3 of the time. Unfortunately, recognition of ureteral injury is less common in laparoscopic cases. Ureters may be injured by transections, crushing from clamps, thermal energy, and kinking after prolapse procedures. Known complications of a ureteral injury include urinoma, ureteral stricture, abscess, and fistula. A high index of suspicion is the best defense because delayed diagnosis has been associated with a higher rate of prolonged hospital stays and nephrectomy.

If there is a delayed diagnosis of a ureteral injury, most often a retrograde stent placement will be attempted. If a stent does not pass, a percutaneous nephrostomy tube can be placed with antegrade stent placement attempted 7–14 days later. If a stent cannot be placed, the area is left alone for approximately 6 weeks. At that time, an open or robot-assisted laparoscopic repair can be considered.

Indications for Refluxing Versus Non-refluxing Repairs

When the distal ureter is injured, a ureteroneocystostomy can often repair the issue.

The ureteral vascularity runs in the adventitia of the outer ureter. If ureteral injury is below the pelvic brim, the vascularity may be compromised, and an extravesical reimplantation is preferred.

To prevent reflux, an extravesical or intravesical approach can be done. Ideally, a non-refluxing technique is preferred. To prevent reflux, the detrusor tunnel is typically made 3–4 times longer than the width of the ureter [7, 8]. If there is insufficient length of the ureter or concern for postoperative stenosis, a non-refluxing reimplantation can be done.

If there is tension on the reimplantation, a psoas hitch can be done for injuries to the lower third of the ureter. A psoas hitch has a high success rate of 97–100% [9]. A psoas hitch can add 6–10 cm of length required for the procedure. The detrusor muscle is attached to the psoas muscle tendon. During the repair, one should carefully avoid the genitofemoral nerve as it crosses the psoas muscle [10].

If a ureteral injury involves the lower 2/3 of the ureter, a psoas hitch may not adequately suffice. Raising a flap of bladder in a cephalad direction (i.e., a Boari flap) can extend a longer distance than a psoas hitch (12–15 cm of length). This may be needed if the bladder is fixed in the pelvis due to adhesions or prior radiation. For a Boari flap, the bladder is incised anteriorly to create a flap. This flap is turned cranially and tubularized. Then the ureter is reimplanted in a non-refluxing fashion. The flap needs a ratio of length to width of at least 3:2 [11].

These types of repairs have been performed with open, laparoscopic, and robotic approaches. Initial data suggests excellent results with the minimally invasive approaches [12, 13].

Evaluation of Injury

The majority of injuries are identified postoperatively (>65%). When recognized, a cystoscopy and retrograde pyelogram is highly sensitive to diagnose the injury and has the added benefit of facilitating placement of a retrograde stent. The most reliable test for ureteral injury is a retrograde pyelogram [14]. Although this requires general anesthesia, it does allow simultaneous therapeutic manipulation of the ureter with stent placement.

Antegrade stent placement is rarely used in the setting of a ureteral injury. This may be employed if a retrograde approach is unsuccessful.

In regard to imaging techniques, CT urogram is the gold standard to identify a ureteral injury. It is important to remember that patients with a ureteral injury and two normal kidneys can have a normal creatinine level [15, 16].

Up to 70% of ureteral injuries are discovered relatively late [17]. If suspicion is high during an operation, injection of methylene blue can help identify the location of the ureteral injury. If there is direct access to the renal pelvis, the dye can be injected directly into the renal pelvis with a 27-gauge needle.

Other options to confirm a ureteral injury is a one-shot IVP that can provide nonspecific findings, such as ureteral dilation and ureteral deviation. As a result, delayed diagnosis can occur 8–20% of the time with a one shot IVP [1, 18, 19].

CT scans can miss ureteral injuries for a variety of reasons (e.g., the leak may be small and contained in Gerota's fascia). Many helical CT scans obtain images before contrast has been excreted in the urine. Therefore, it is important to obtain delayed images 5–20 minutes after the injection of intravenous contrast. This should minimize the chance of missing extravasation of contrast. Contrast in the ureter should be tracked throughout the course of the ureter.

Surgical Repair

Some minor ureteral contusions can be managed with an internal ureteral stent. However, the ureter's external appearance is not a reliable reflection of the severity. If microvascular injury is significant, it can lead to delayed ureteral stricture. Therefore, a low threshold for excision and primary ureteroureterostomy should be considered.

If there has been ligation of the ureter, the ligature needs to be removed. Then the ureter is observed (for peristalsis and appearance of vascularity). There should be a low threshold to cleanly excise any devascularized segment and reapproximate healthy ureteral tissue in a primary fashion. This is usually done by a ureteroureterostomy or a ureteroneocystostomy.

Stenting after ureteral repair reduces postoperative complications in both animal models and clinical series [17].

Minor ureteral injuries are best managed with a primary ureteroureterostomy. This has a success rate of 90% [20]. Primary surgical principles include the following:

1. Mobilization of the ureter with minimal manipulation of the adventitia (to avoid devascularization).
2. Debridement of ureteral ends to clean, healthy, well-vascularized tissue.
3. Perform anastomosis with spatulated ends. The repair should be watertight, tension-free, and stented. Consideration of a retroperitoneal drain is recommended.
4. Reapproximate the peritoneum to replace the ureter in the retroperitoneum.
5. If there is severe damage, consider an omental wrap. This increases the vascularity to the ureteral repair.

If the injury is above the pelvic brim and involving <50% of the ureteral circumference, then a primary repair can be done over a stent with absorbable sutures. But if more extensive injury is suspected, full mobilization with a spatulated end to end anastomosis is preferred.

For bladder level repairs, stay sutures are placed in the bladder before making a cystotomy to approximate the spatulated ureter in place. The cystostomy should be wide enough to allow a mucosa-to-mucosa anastomosis without tension.

Bowel transposition is reserved for long ureteral defects. The most common substitute is the ileum. This was first described in 1901 and gained popularity in the 1950s. When performed, a 15–20 cm segment of ileum is tubularized and anastomosed in an isoperistaltic fashion [21]. This has long-term success rates of >80% [9, 22]. Complication rates are low with a 3% stricture and 6% fistula rate [23]. Secondary malignancy rates are low: 0.8% at mean follow-up of 20.2 years [24].

Autotransplantation is typically a last resort option before nephrectomy. This is done when there is a severe ureteral deficit or multiple failed attempts to fix the issue. When done, the kidney is harvested and the renal vessels are sewn to the iliac vessels [21].

Transureteroureterostomy is occasionally considered for mid ureteral strictures. If done, this can lead to many challenges (e.g., cannulating the affected ureter across the midline). When performed, the donor ureter is passed through the posterior peritoneum anterior to the bifurcation of the vessels. The donor ureter is then anastomosed to the contralateral, recipient ureter.

Both transureteroureterostomy and autotransplantation are typically reserved for the rare cases when bowel transposition is not possible (e.g., Crohn's disease, prior radiation treatment).

Simple ligation with nephrostomy tube placement is reserved for unstable patients who require swift intervention to the injury. Tissue transposition with omentum and peritoneum is typically reserved for situations with questionable tissue viability (e.g., poor nutrition status, prior radiation and chemotherapy).

When delayed diagnosis and intervention is pursued, a typical waiting period for surgery is 6 weeks to 3 months. This delay allows for a decrease in inflammation, fibrosis, tissue edema, and adhesion formation [1].

Preoperative Preparation

Many surgeons place a ureteral stent to identify the ureter during complex procedures. However, placement of a ureteral stent has not been shown to decrease the incidence of ureteral injury [1, 25]. Some studies show stent placement can make the ureter more challenging to work around due to movement from its normal location and increased rigidity. But stents have also been associated with a higher chance of immediate, intraoperative recognition of the injury [1]. Concerning postoperative symptoms include fever, leukocytosis, and peritonitis [26].

One should consider stent placement for any traumatic injury of the ureter that is immediately repaired.

After the stent is removed, follow up is paramount to check for stricture formation and fistula formation.

Different techniques have been employed to identify the ureter during abdominopelvic surgery such as light emission and dye excretion in the ureter. However, issues such as difficulty passing a catheter and ureteral spasms can hamper the success of such techniques.

One option is placement of a lighted ureteral catheter [27]. This can be very useful when significant scar tissue exists and tactile sensation is limited. However, if there is no lumen, then the lighted catheter will impede urine flow [28].

During robotic surgery, use of Firefly with indocyanine green can highlight the ureter for these cases.

Mahalingam et al. describe a novel technique using near-infrared fluorescent dye (Uroglow) that is injected systemically and secreted by kidneys to allow ureteral visualization with a NIR fluorescence camera [29].

Review of Outcomes Data

Most literature reviewing the success of ureteral repairs from iatrogenic injury are in the adult literature. Considerations are similar: site, mechanism of injury, and the timing of identification of the injury are pertinent.

The pelvic plexus sits about 1.5 cm dorsomedial to the ureterovesical junction. Dissection around the efferent fibers to the pelvic plexus puts the bladder at risk for urinary retention after distal ureteral dissection [30]. Additionally, there are afferent fibers that run proximal to the obliterated umbilical ligament [5].

Results for these repairs are variable. Some have shown lower success rates with more complex ureteral repairs [31]. However, a study reviewing ureteral repairs after iatrogenic surgical injuries showed no difference in success based on complexity of repair (Boari flap vs. primary anastomosis) ($p = 0.768$). Multiple studies have shown higher success rates and lower morbidity when ureteral injuries are identified and treated early [32, 33].

Routh et al. reviewed 10 ureteral injuries over 20 years. The median ureteral defect length was 4 cm. The diagnosis of the injuries were made early in only four patients. For those with delayed recognition, the median time to diagnosis was 21 days. In these six patients, five underwent kidney drainage with a percutaneous nephrostomy tube and one with an internal ureteral stent. Delayed repair usually took place 1–3 months after the injury. Although the ultimate surgical success was comparable in the delayed group, their morbidity was higher, such as the higher urinoma rate. And on average, the delayed diagnosis patients required two additional surgeries [34].

In the adult literature, ureteral injuries <2.5 cm are often treated with stent placement for 2–6 weeks. Success rates have been estimated at 75–78%. However, these short-term results may not translate into pediatric injuries.

In a prior retrospective review, the results of refluxing and non-refluxing repairs were not significantly different [35].

In the adult literature, transureteroureterostomy had short-term complications 23.8% of the time. However, the long-term success rate was noted to be 96.4% [36].

Minimally invasive techniques (robotic and laparoscopic) have been used to repair ureteral injuries. The most commonly reported procedure has been uretero-ureterostomy. Success rates have been favorable at >90% [37, 38].

Some articles have questioned the cost efficacy of additional surgical procedures to identify the ureter. However, the average litigation costs associated with ureteral injuries range from $600,000 to several million dollars [39].

Conclusion

Ureteral injuries and strictures are most commonly iatrogenic. The majority of injuries involve the distal ureter. Early detection can decrease morbidity for the patient. Once recognized, the success rates for repair are favorable. Most distal injuries are managed with ureteroneocystostomy. When additional length is needed, a psoas hitch can frequently aid the reimplantation, while mid and proximal injuries are often managed by ureteroureterostomy or a Boari flap.

Although there is a high success rate, ileal substitution for long repairs is rarely required.

Most of the outcomes data in the literature are from the open approach, but minimally invasive techniques including robotic-assisted laparoscopic surgery have shown encouraging results so far.

References

1. Brandes S, Coburn M, Armenakas N, McAninch J. Diagnosis and management of ureteric injury: an evidence-based analysis. BJU Int. 2004;94(3):277–89.
2. Routh JC, Tollefson MK, Ashley RA, Husmann DA. Iatrogenic ureteral injury: can adult repair techniques be used on children? J Pediatr Urol. 2009;5(1):53–5.

3. Vallancien G, Cathelineau X, Baumert H, Doublet JD, Guillonneau B. Complications of trans-peritoneal laparoscopic surgery in urology: review of 1,311 procedures at a single center. J Urol. 2002;168(1):23–6.
4. Coburn M. Damage control for urologic injuries. Surg Clin North Am. 1997;77(4):821–34.
5. Leissner J, Allhoff EP, Wolff W, Feja C, Hockel M, Black P, et al. The pelvic plexus and anti-reflux surgery: topographical findings and clinical consequences. J Urol. 2001;165(5):1652–5.
6. McAchran SE, Palmer JS. Bilateral extravesical ureteral reimplantation in toilet trained children: is 1-day hospitalization without urinary retention possible? J Urol. 2005;174(5):1991–3; discussion 3
7. Riedmiller H, Becht E, Hertle L, Jacobi G, Hohenfellner R. Psoas-hitch ureteroneocystos-tomy: experience with 181 cases. Eur Urol. 1984;10(3):145–50.
8. Riedmiller H, Gerharz EW. Antireflux surgery: lich-Gregoir extravesical ureteric tunnelling. BJU Int. 2008;101(11):1467–82.
9. Armatys SA, Mellon MJ, Beck SD, Koch MO, Foster RS, Bihrle R. Use of ileum as ureteral replacement in urological reconstruction. J Urol. 2009;181(1):177–81.
10. Steffens J, Stark E, Haben B, Treiyer A. Politano-Leadbetter ureteric reimplantation. BJU Int. 2006;98(3):695–712.
11. Warwick RT, Worth PH. The psoas bladder-hitch procedure for the replacement of the lower third of the ureter. Br J Urol. 1969;41(6):701–9.
12. Ahn M, Loughlin KR. Psoas hitch ureteral reimplantation in adults--analysis of a modified technique and timing of repair. Urology. 2001;58(2):184–7.
13. Schimpf MO, Wagner JR. Robot-assisted laparoscopic distal ureteral surgery. JSLS. 2009;13(1):44–9.
14. Palmer LS, Rosenbaum RR, Gershbaum MD, Kreutzer ER. Penetrating ureteral trauma at an urban trauma center: 10-year experience. Urology. 1999;54(1):34–6.
15. Burks FN, Santucci RA. Management of iatrogenic ureteral injury. Ther Adv Urol. 2014;6(3):115–24.
16. Selzman AA, Spirnak JP. Iatrogenic ureteral injuries: a 20-year experience in treating 165 injuries. J Urol. 1996;155(3):878–81.
17. Kunkle DA, Kansas BT, Pathak A, Goldberg AJ, Mydlo JH. Delayed diagnosis of traumatic ureteral injuries. J Urol. 2006;176(6 Pt 1):2503–7.
18. Grainger DA, Soderstrom RM, Schiff SF, Glickman MG, DeCherney AH, Diamond MP. Ureteral injuries at laparoscopy: insights into diagnosis, management, and prevention. Obstet Gynecol. 1990;75(5):839–43.
19. Presti JC Jr, Carroll PR, McAninch JW. Ureteral and renal pelvic injuries from external trauma: diagnosis and management. J Trauma. 1989;29(3):370–4.
20. Campbell EW Jr, Filderman PS, Jacobs SC. Ureteral injury due to blunt and penetrating trauma. Urology. 1992;40(3):216–20.
21. Meng MV, Freise CE, Stoller ML. Expanded experience with laparoscopic nephrectomy and autotransplantation for severe ureteral injury. J Urol. 2003;169(4):1363–7.
22. Goodwin WE, Winter CC, Turner RD. Replacement of the ureter by small intestine: clinical application and results of the ileal ureter. J Urol. 1959;81(3):406–18.
23. Carlton CE Jr, Scott R Jr, Guthrie AG. The initial management of ureteral injuries: a report of 78 cases. J Urol. 1971;105(3):335–40.
24. Verduyckt FJ, Heesakkers JP, Debruyne FM. Long-term results of ileum interposition for ureteral obstruction. Eur Urol. 2002;42(2):181–7.
25. Eswara JR, Raup VT, Potretzke AM, Hunt SR, Brandes SB. Outcomes of iatrogenic genitourinary injuries during colorectal surgery. Urology. 2015;86(6):1228–33.
26. Leff EI, Groff W, Rubin RJ, Eisenstat TE, Salvati EP. Use of ureteral catheters in colonic and rectal surgery. Dis Colon Rectum. 1982;25(5):457–60.
27. Piaggio LA, Gonzalez R. Laparoscopic transureteroureterostomy: a novel approach. J Urol. 2007;177(6):2311–4.
28. Keveligan E, Jarvis GJ. Medico-legal aspects of ureteric damage during abdominal hysterectomy. Br J Obstet Gynaecol. 1998;105(1):127.

29. Kaestner L. Management of urological injury at the time of urogynaecology surgery. Best Pract Res Clin Obstet Gynaecol. 2019;54:2–11.
30. Mahalingam SM, Dip F, Castillo M, Roy M, Wexner SD, Rosenthal RJ, et al. Intraoperative ureter visualization using a novel near-infrared fluorescent dye. Mol Pharm. 2018;15(8):3442–7.
31. Roder JD, Siewert JR. Incidence, prevention and therapy of ureteral injury in colorectal surgery. Zentralblatt fur Chirurgie. 1991;116(9):581–5.
32. Mahendran HA, Praveen S, Ho C, Goh EH, Tan GH, Zuklifli MZ. Iatrogenic ureter injuries: eleven years experience in a tertiary hospital. Med J Malaysia. 2012;67(2):169–72.
33. Pokala N, Delaney CP, Kiran RP, Bast J, Angermeier K, Fazio VW. A randomized controlled trial comparing simultaneous intra-operative vs sequential prophylactic ureteric catheter insertion in re-operative and complicated colorectal surgery. Int J Color Dis. 2007;22(6):683–7.
34. Elliott SP, McAninch JW. Ureteral injuries: external and iatrogenic. Urol Clin North Am. 2006;33(1):55–66. vi
35. Gil Vernet JM. Ureterovesicoplasty under mucous membrane. (modifications of Boari's technic). Journal d'urologie medicale et chirurgicale. 1959;65:504–8.
36. Stefanovic KB, Bukurov NS, Marinkovic JM. Non-antireflux versus antireflux ureteroneocystostomy in adults. Br J Urol. 1991;67(3):263–6.
37. Ali-El-Dein B, El-Tabey N, Abdel-Latif M, Abdel-Rahim M, El-Bahnasawy MS. Late uroileal cancer after incorporation of ileum into the urinary tract. J Urol. 2002;167(1):84–8.
38. De Cicco C, Ret Davalos ML, Van Cleynenbreugel B, Verguts J, Koninckx PR. Iatrogenic ureteral lesions and repair: a review for gynecologists. J Minim Invasive Gynecol. 2007;14(4):428–35.
39. Ostrzenski A, Radolinski B, Ostrzenska KM. A review of laparoscopic ureteral injury in pelvic surgery. Obstet Gynecol Surv. 2003;58(12):794–9.

Distal Ureteral Reconstruction in Children

Aylin N. Bilgutay and Andrew J. Kirsch

Preoperative Considerations

Distal ureteral anomalies are usually diagnosed during evaluation of hydroure-teronephrosis and/or febrile urinary tract infections (fUTIs). Hydronephrosis with or without hydroureter is often diagnosed antenatally during routine ultrasound. The recommended initial postnatal study is a renal bladder ultrasound (RBUS), which should be obtained when the child is at least 48 hours old and well hydrated. Dehydration is nearly universally present in the first 1–2 days of life, and this can cause underestimation of hydronephrosis [1]. If significant hydronephrosis (Society for Fetal Urology (SFU) grade > 2) is identified or there is any evidence of signifi-cant hydroureter, additional studies are indicated to evaluate for vesicoureteral reflux (VUR) and/or obstruction [2]. Both possibilities should be explored, as a dilated system may be (1) refluxing and nonobstructed, (2) nonrefluxing and obstructed, (3) both refluxing and obstructed, or (4) neither refluxing nor obstructed.

Voiding cystourethrography (VCUG), nuclear cystography, or contrast-enhanced RBUS may be performed to evaluate for VUR. A VCUG is also indicated in patients with fUTIs, regardless of the presence or degree of hydronephrosis. It is our prac-tice to start continuous antibiotic prophylaxis upon ordering a test to evaluate for VUR. Prophylactic antibiotics can be discontinued if the test is negative. All patients with VUR should be assessed for bowel and bladder dysfunction, and if present, this should be addressed with conservative measures prior to any operative intervention. An asymptomatic patient with mild hydronephrosis (SFU ≤ 2) may be followed with serial RBUS.

Supplementary Information The online version of this chapter (https://doi.org/10.1007/978-3-030-50196-9_17) contains supplementary material, which is available to authorized users.

A. N. Bilgutay · A. J. Kirsch (✉)
Pediatric Urology, Children's Healthcare of Atlanta and Emory University, Atlanta, GA, USA

A 99m-technetium mercaptoacetyltriglycine (MAG 3) nuclear Lasix renogram or magnetic resonance urography (MRU) may be obtained to evaluate for obstruction. Ureterovesical junction (UVJ) obstruction can be diagnosed by MAG 3 if the appropriate areas of interest are chosen. However, MRU provides the most anatomic detail and is therefore our preferred study in the setting of complex anatomy including suspected duplication anomalies, megaureter, and/or ectopic ureter (Fig. 17.1). If an ectopic ureter is suspected based on preoperative imaging, cystourethroscopy (and vaginoscopy in a female patient if indicated) may be performed at the beginning of the case at the time of definitive reconstruction. This may allow for identification of the ureteral orifices and better understanding of the relevant anatomy.

When considering robotic reconstruction in a patient with distal ureteral anomalies, one must consider all options along with their associated risks and benefits. For VUR, other management options include continuous antibiotic prophylaxis, Deflux™, and open ureteral reimplantation. Open ureteral reconstruction is also

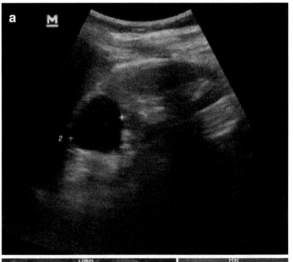

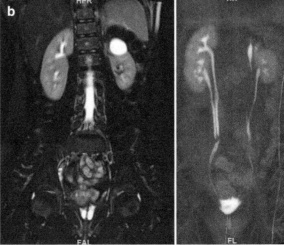

Fig. 17.1 a. Ultrasound of the left kidney showing a cystic dilation in the upper pole concerning for possible duplication anomaly in a healthy 10-year-old girl with persistent urinary incontinence. The patient was toilet trained at age 2–3 years without issues and remained dry for several years before developing symptoms at age 7 years including urinary urgency, post-void dribbling, and nocturnal enuresis every night. She did not have any UTIs. **b**. MRU of the same patient, showing bilateral duplication anomalies with a poorly functioning hydronephrotic left upper moiety draining ectopically into the vagina. VCUG (not shown) was negative. Surgical options in such a patient include left upper moiety ureteral reimplantation, left upper to lower distal or proximal UU, and left upper moiety nephrectomy. The patient underwent RAL left upper to lower distal UU performed just above the level of the iliac vessels

a consideration in cases of UVJ obstruction or ectopic ureter. The age and size of the child needs to be taken into account when weighing risks versus benefits of each treatment option. One might anticipate more *clashing* during robotic surgery in smaller children, especially with the use of the Si (as opposed to the Xi) da Vinci® robot. This may increase surgical complexity and operative time. In our experience, the benefits of robotic surgery as compared with open surgery are more pronounced in older children. Younger children tend to recover quite rapidly after open repair via Pfannenstiel incision, and these incisions are cosmetic and hidden. Pfannenstiel incisions may even be considered more cosmetically appealing than standard laparoscopic or robotic port scars by some patients and patient families [3].

Extravesical Ureteral Reimplantation for VUR

Extravesical ureteral reimplantation is the most common RAL distal ureteral surgery. This procedure is based on the open technique originally described by Lich and Gregoir in the 1960s [4, 5]. When performing RAL extravesical ureteral reimplantation with the Si robot, the patient is typically positioned in lithotomy, with the robot docked between the patient's legs. The same arrangement may be used for all distal ureteral procedures. A single prep and drape may therefore be used for cystoscopy if desired at the start of the case and the robotic portion. Side-docking is another alternative, allowing the patient to be supine. This works particularly well with the Xi robot.

Intraperitoneal access may be achieved with open Hasson or Veress needle technique, depending on surgeon preference. The ports are then placed, starting with the camera port. We use an 8.5 mm Si robotic camera port at the umbilicus. A 10 or 12 mm port such as the AutoSuture® balloon trocar may also be implemented as an Si camera port [6]. In contrast, the Xi camera port is identical to its working ports. The working ports are placed next, either below the umbilicus on either side to create a triangular working field (for the Si) or in line with the camera port (for the Xi); 8 and 5 mm working ports are available for the Si robot, while the Xi robot only uses 8 mm ports and instruments. Port placement as described above results in scars that are visible when wearing undergarments or a swimsuit. The alterative hidden incision endoscopic surgery (HIdES) port placement technique, described by Gargollo et al., places the working ports at or below the level of a Pfannenstiel incision in order to prevent visible scars (Fig. 17.2) [7]. If desired, one may place additional ports, such as an assistant port and/or third robotic working arm. We do not usually find it necessary to utilize more than three ports total. It is mandatory to adjust table height and position (e.g., degree of Trendelenburg) prior to docking unless using the Xi with Trumpf Medical's TruSystem® 7000dV OR table.

The first step after docking is to identify and mobilize the ureter, while taking care to preserve its blood supply. The peritoneum must be opened in order to allow mobilization of the ureter (Fig. 17.3). The ureter is then dissected distally to the UVJ. In a male patient, one must identify and preserve the vas deferens. The uterine arteries are a potential source of bleeding in a female patient; it is best to identify

a   b

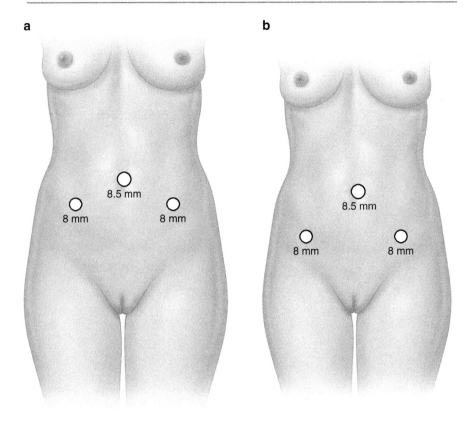

Fig. 17.2 a. Example of standard port placement for RAL ureteral reimplantation with the Si robot. The camera port is at the umbilicus. **b**. Example of HIdES port placement for RAL ureteral reimplantation with the Si robot. The camera port is at the umbilicus. The skin incisions for the two working ports are lower than in the standard port placement, so that they are at or below the level of a Pfannenstiel incision. The fascial entry sites for the working ports may be placed higher than the skin incisions in order to increase working space within the pelvis. This is achieved by applying cephalad traction during port placement

and preserve these arteries if possible. We recommend the use of an assistant port to provide greater control of bleeding risk seen with the increased vasculature seen in pubertal patients, especially young women.

We generally do not find hitch stitches necessary. However, if the bladder is floppy and the UVJ is not easily visible, hitch stitch placement may be of benefit. This is achieved by having the assistant or scrub tech straighten out the SH needle of a 4-0 Vicryl and pass this directly through the abdominal wall. The surgeon then passes the stitch through the posterior bladder wall cephalad to the UVJs and finally back out through the abdominal wall, where the assistant can adjust the tension as desired and snap the suture tails in place to maintain steady tension. A variation of this technique involves taking multiple bites of the bladder prior to

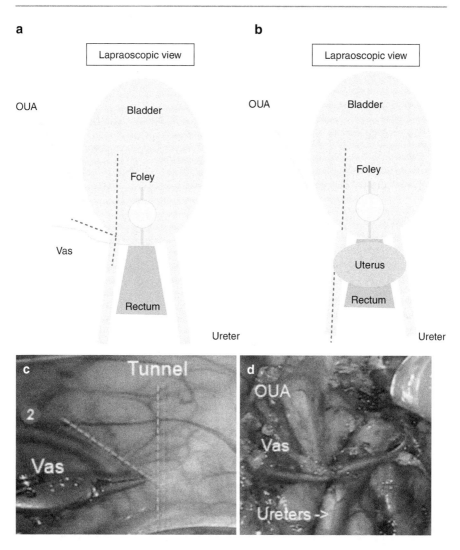

Fig. 17.3 a, b. Schematic showing sites for opening the peritoneum (---) during RAL ureteral reimplantation. The peritoneum may be opened in line with proposed detrusor tunnel or transversely for wider exposure. "V" flap (**a**) recommended for adequately exposing vas deferens in boys. One may open the peritoneum further cephalad along the ureter to allow for additional ureteral mobilization (**b**), especially in peri- or postpubertal girls or in otherwise complex cases. OUA = obliterated umbilical artery. **c, d**. Intraoperative view prior to (**c**) and after (**d**) opening peritoneum in a male patient. OUA = obliterated umbilical artery

exiting back out through the abdominal wall. This distributes the tension and flattens the posterior bladder wall.

Next, a detrusor tunnel of adequate length is created using the monopolar scissors. Rarely, a CO_2 laser may be used for this purpose [8]. The classical description of adequate tunnel length is 5:1 compared to ureteral diameter [9]. We have found that a hitch stitch may distort the anatomy and make it more difficult to appreciate the appropriate tunnel trajectory. In this case, the hitch stitch may be intermittently relaxed, while mapping out and creating the tunnel to avoid any ureteral kinking within the tunnel.

To prevent obstruction, flaps are developed on either side of the tunnel. The tunnel is then closed over the ureter. Closure may be performed with various suture types, in a running or interrupted fashion and starting distally or proximally, depending on surgeon preference. We prefer a running 3-0 V-Loc starting distally, having found this to be the most efficient and straightforward closure method.

Postoperative care typically involves observation overnight in the hospital with or without a Foley catheter in place. The catheter may be removed on postoperative day 1, and the child may be discharged home once voiding spontaneously. In the setting of postoperative urinary retention, a Foley catheter may be replaced prior to patient discharge with subsequent voiding trial in the clinic 1–2 weeks later. In patients with a history of bowel bladder dysfunction, it is prudent to leave a catheter for up to a week postoperatively to avoid urinary retention.

Several relatively small series have reported VUR resolution rates following RAL extravesical ureteral reimplantation, with reported rates ranging widely from 66.7% to 100% and an overall pooled success rate of 91% [10–21]. A large multi-institutional retrospective review published in 2017 found an 87.9% radiographic resolution rate in 280 ureters [22]. Even more recently, a prospective multicenter study on RAL extravesical ureteral reimplantation found radiographic resolution in 93.8% of 145 ureters [23]. These success rates are similar to those reported following open surgery.

There is concern that bilateral dissection of the posterior bladder may injure the pelvic nerve plexus, resulting in increased rates of postoperative urinary retention. Indeed, Boysen et al. reported that 7.1% of patients undergoing bilateral RAL extravesical ureteral reimplantation experienced transient urinary retention, compared to none of those undergoing a unilateral procedure [23]. In an attempt to reduce this complication, nerve-sparing techniques have been described [24]. Casale et al. reported a 97.6% success rate in 41 patients after RAL bilateral nerve-sparing extravesical ureteral reimplantation, with no complications or episodes or urinary retention [12]. Herz et al. more recently reported a 91.7% success rate after unilateral RAL extravesical reimplantation [25]. Success was much lower in bilateral cases (77.8% of ureters, 72.2% of children), whereas complications (including urinary retention, ureteral obstruction, and readmission) were higher. Of note, a nerve-sparing technique was not utilized in this series. While nerve sparing appears to offer a tangible benefit, identification of the pelvic nerve plexus may be challenging.

Periureteral diverticula, if present, may be reduced or excised at time of reimplantation [26]. Good outcomes have been reported following RAL common sheath reimplantation in duplex systems [27]. If only one ureter refluxes and the ureters are widely spaced, one may perform reimplantation of the refluxing ureter alone rather than a common sheath. In this case, it would be imperative to identify the ureters correctly (e.g., with cystourethroscopy and temporary stenting of one ureter at the start of the case). However, this would be less common, as duplex ureters are usually intimately associated that an attempted separation would potentially compromise vascularity. In the setting of a refluxing, nonobstructed megaureter, excisional tailoring while maintaining the native UVJ has been described [28].

Extravesical Ureteral Reimplantation for UVJ Obstruction/ Obstructed Megaureter

For the obstructed megaureter, RAL extravesical dismembered ureteral reimplantation with or without tapering may be performed [29, 30]. This approach, which may be used for orthotopic or ectopic ureters, requires division of the obstructed UVJ and creation of a new ureteroneocystostomy. The nonrefluxing mechanism is then created as described above. In theory, a refluxing anastomosis could be performed, which simply eliminates the tunneling portion of the procedure. However, a refluxing anastomosis is usually only indicated in neonates whose bladders are considered to be too small for creation of a tunnel, and these patients are generally not robotic candidates. Examples of the intraoperative view during RAL repair of an obstructed megaureter are shown in Fig. 17.4. If tapering is necessary, we prefer to keep the ureter attached to the bladder while tapering and dismember afterward (Fig. 17.4c–f). This allows maintenance of tension during the tapering process and is similar to the technique described by Khan et al. [31]. The steps for repair of an obstructed megaureter with a relatively long stenotic segment are shown in Fig. 17.5a. The Heineke-Mikulicz principle may also be used for obstructed megaureter repair in appropriate cases (Fig. 17.5b), obviating the need for complete dismemberment and creation of neoureterocystostomy [32]. This technique generally works well in the setting of a relatively short stenotic segment.

A retrospective study by Arlen et al. in 2015 evaluated outcomes of complex RALUR versus open extravesical ureteral reimplantation, with similar success and complication rates found in the two cohorts [33]. Reimplantation was considered

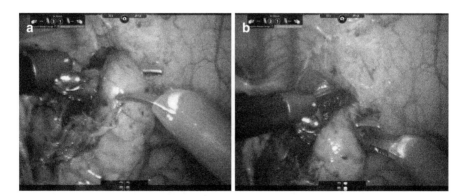

Fig. 17.4 **a**. Intraoperative view during robotic repair of an obstructed left megaureter. The ureter has been mobilized circumferentially without devascularizing it. **b**. The distally narrowed and obstructed segment is apparent in the view from above. **c**. A longitudinal ureterotomy has been created to allow for tapering. In this view, the ureter is still attached at the UVJ in order to maintain traction during tapering. **d**. The ureter is scored to demarcate excess tissue for excisional tapering. **e, f**. After excision of excess tissue, the ureter is closed/tapered using fine absorbable suture (5-0 Vicryl in the case above) over a 10 Fr catheter. The next steps include dismemberment at the UVJ, creation of ureteroneocystostomy, and creation of a detrusor tunnel to achieve a nonobstructed, nonrefluxing reimplantation

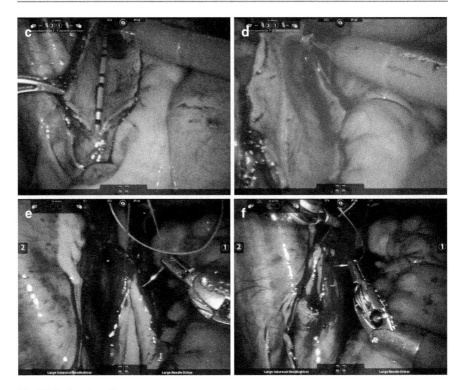

Fig. 17.4 (continued)

complex if the patient had undergone prior anti-reflux surgery, required tapering
and/or dismembering, or had an associated duplication or diverticulum. Patients
undergoing reimplantation for VUR and/or obstruction were included. Children
undergoing robotic surgery were significantly older than those undergoing open
surgery (9.3 ± 3.7 versus 3.1 ± 2.7 years, $p < 0.001$). All robotic patients went home
on postoperative day 1, while open patients were hospitalized for 1.3 ± 0.7 days
($p = 0.03$). Analgesic use was similar between the two groups.

It is common practice to leave a double J ureteral stent in place for 4–6 weeks
after any dismembered or partially dismembered ureteral reimplantation. The
patient is typically observed overnight in the hospital with a Foley catheter in place.
The catheter may be removed on postoperative day 1 in most cases, and the child
may be discharged home once voiding spontaneously or with a temporary indwelling catheter replaced if needed for retention.

A cystogram may be performed intraoperatively immediately after stent removal.
Although this would not include a voiding phase, it could potentially rule out clinically significant VUR during bladder filling and obviate the need for additional
radiation exposure and morbidity of an awake study in selected patients. Initial

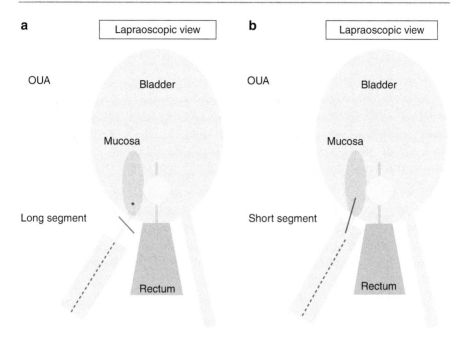

Fig. 17.5 a. Schematic showing repair of obstructed megaureter with a long segment of stenotic UVJ. Steps: (i) keep ureter attached, (ii) taper megaureter (·---), (iii) ligate UVJ (—), (iv) dismember ureter, (v) anastomosis at new site (*), with stent placement and optional peritoneal closure. OUA = obliterated umbilical artery. **b.** Repair of obstructed megaureter with a short stenotic UVJ segment. Steps: (i) keep ureter attached, (ii) taper megaureter (·---), (iii) partially dismember (—), (iv) in situ Heineke-Mikulicz anastomosis with stent placement and optional peritoneal closure. OUA = obliterated umbilical artery

postoperative imaging would then involve a RBUS approximately 1 month after stent removal, with additional imaging as clinically indicated thereafter.

Ureteral Reimplantation: Transvesical

Minimally invasive ureteral reimplantation has also been described using an extra-peritoneal transvesical technique with pneumovesicum, based on the open Cohen cross-trigonal approach. In this setting, ports are placed directly into the bladder under cystoscopic guidance. Reported success rates using this technique to treat VUR range from 83% to 96% [34–37]. This method does not require dissection of the posterior bladder wall near the pelvic nerve plexus, with the possible benefit of decreased risk of postoperative urinary retention. However, most minimally invasive surgeons (including those in our group) have had very little or no experience with this approach, which is currently only utilized at select institutions. The literature is correspondingly limited.

Distal Ureteroureterostomy in Duplex Systems

In duplex systems, minimally invasive definitive reconstruction may also be achieved with a distal ureteroureterostomy (UU) [27]. Preoperative evaluation, patient positioning, and docking of the robot would be performed as described above for other distal ureteral and pelvic cases. An upper to lower UU would be indicated in the setting of an obstructed upper moiety in the absence of lower moiety VUR, whereas a lower to upper UU would be indicated in a patient with lower moiety VUR and no upper moiety obstruction. While a proximal UU may also be performed in these cases depending on surgeon preference, we generally prefer the distal approach, as we find it to be more straightforward and with minimal associated risk compared to dissection near the hilar structures. It is, of course, imperative to correctly identify which ureter is associated with which moiety when considering a UU. This can be achieved by performing cystourethroscopy with temporary stenting of one of the moieties at the start of the case. We have found it helpful in some cases to perform the ureteral anastomosis cephalad to the iliac vessels. With this approach, it is generally easier to visualize both ureters with little dissection, while avoiding the vascular complexes along the posterior bladder (and uterus in girls). A holding suture is placed below both ureters with upward (ventral) traction. This allows both ureters to remain adjacent to each other during the end-to-side anastomosis. The posterior peritoneum may be closed to compartmentalize potential urine extravasation.

It is our practice to leave a double J ureteral stent in place across the anastomosis at the conclusion of the case. This is removed in the OR 4–6 weeks postoperatively. If the initial procedure was performed for VUR, a cystogram can be performed intraoperatively immediately after stent removal to rule out significant reflux during bladder filling, as described above after megaureter repair. A RBUS is then performed approximately 1 month after stent removal, with additional imaging as clinically indicated thereafter.

Conclusion

RAL surgery is a safe, effective, minimally invasive technique with multiple applications for distal ureteral reconstruction in the pediatric population. Conditions including VUR and/or obstruction in a single, duplex, or ectopic system may be addressed with RAL surgery. The magnified three-dimensional view and multiple degrees of freedom with wristed movements make the robotic approach eminently suitable for these delicate reconstructive surgeries. RAL surgery provides several additional potential benefits including smaller incisions and faster recovery, accounting for its continued rising popularity among pediatric urologists and patients alike.

References

1. Paliwalla M, Park K. A practical guide to urinary tract ultrasound in a child: pearls and pitfalls. Ultrasound. 2014;22(4):213–22.
2. Riccabona M. Assessment and management of newborn hydronephrosis. World J Urol. 2004;22(2):73–8.
3. Garcia-Roig ML, Travers C, McCracken C, Cerwinka W, Kirsch JM, Kirsch AJ. Surgical scar location preference for pediatric kidney and pelvic surgery: a crowdsourced survey. J Urol. 2017;197(3 Pt 2):911–9.
4. Gregoir W. The surgical treatment of congenital vesico-ureteral reflux. Acta Chir Belg. 1964;63:431–9.
5. Lich R Jr, Howerton L, Davis LA. Recurrent urosepsis in children. J Urol. 1961;86:554.
6. Chang C, Steinberg Z, Shah A, Gundeti MS. Patient positioning and port placement for robot-assisted surgery. J Endourol. 2014;28(6):631–8.
7. Gargollo PC. Hidden incision endoscopic surgery: description of technique, parental satisfaction and applications. J Urol. 2011;185(4):1425–31.
8. Diaz EC, Lindgren BW, Gong EM. Carbon dioxide laser for detrusor tunnel creation in robot-assisted laparoscopic extravesical ureteral reimplant. J Pediatr Urol. 2014;10(6):1283 e1281–2.
9. Wein AJ, Kavoussi LR, Campbell MF. Campbell-Walsh urology. Editor-in-chief, Alan J. Wein (editors, Louis R. Kavoussi, et al.) 10th ed. Philadelphia: Elsevier Saunders; 2012.
10. Chan KW, Lee KH, Tam YH, Sihoe JD. Early experience of robotic-assisted reconstructive operations in pediatric urology. J Laparoendosc Adv Surg Tech A. 2010;20(4):379–82.
11. Lee RS, Sethi AS, Passerotti CC, Peters CA. Robot-assisted laparoscopic nephrectomy and contralateral ureteral reimplantation in children. J Endourol. 2010;24(1):123–8.
12. Casale P, Patel RP, Kolon TF. Nerve sparing robotic extravesical ureteral reimplantation. J Urol. 2008;179(5):1987–9; discussion 1990
13. Marchini GS, Hong YK, Minnillo BJ, et al. Robotic assisted laparoscopic ureteral reimplantation in children: case matched comparative study with open surgical approach. J Urol. 2011;185(5):1870–5.
14. Smith RP, Oliver JL, Peters CA. Pediatric robotic extravesical ureteral reimplantation: comparison with open surgery. J Urol. 2011;185(5):1876–81.
15. Chalmers D, Herbst K, Kim C. Robotic-assisted laparoscopic extravesical ureteral reimplantation: an initial experience. J Pediatr Urol. 2012;8(3):268–71.
16. Kasturi S, Sehgal SS, Christman MS, Lambert SM, Casale P. Prospective long-term analysis of nerve-sparing extravesical robotic-assisted laparoscopic ureteral reimplantation. Urology. 2012;79(3):680–3.
17. Callewaert PR, Biallosterski BT, Rahnama'i MS, Van Kerrebroeck PE. Robotic extravesical anti-reflux operations in complex cases: technical considerations and preliminary results. Urol Int. 2012;88(1):6–11.
18. Gundeti MS, Kojima Y, Haga N, Kiriluk K. Robotic-assisted laparoscopic reconstructive surgery in the lower urinary tract. Curr Urol Rep. 2013;14(4):333–41.
19. Schomburg JL, Haberman K, Willihnganz-Lawson KH, Shukla AR. Robot-assisted laparoscopic ureteral reimplantation: a single surgeon comparison to open surgery. J Pediatr Urol. 2014;10(5):875–9.
20. Akhavan A, Avery D, Lendvay TS. Robot-assisted extravesical ureteral reimplantation: outcomes and conclusions from 78 ureters. J Pediatr Urol. 2014;10(5):864–8.
21. Grimsby GM, Dwyer ME, Jacobs MA, et al. Multi-institutional review of outcomes of robot-assisted laparoscopic extravesical ureteral reimplantation. J Urol. 2015;193(5 Suppl):1791–5.

22. Boysen WR, Ellison JS, Kim C, et al. Multi-institutional review of outcomes and complications of robot-assisted laparoscopic extravesical ureteral reimplantation for treatment of primary vesicoureteral reflux in children. J Urol. 2017;197(6):1555–61.
23. Boysen WR, Akhavan A, Ko J, et al. Prospective multicenter study on robot-assisted laparoscopic extravesical ureteral reimplantation (RALUR-EV): outcomes and complications. J Pediatr Urol. 2018;14(3):262 e261–6.
24. David S, Kelly C, Poppas DP. Nerve sparing extravesical repair of bilateral vesicoureteral reflux: description of technique and evaluation of urinary retention. J Urol. 2004;172(4 Pt 2):1617–20; discussion 1620
25. Herz D, Fuchs M, Todd A, McLeod D, Smith J. Robot-assisted laparoscopic extravesical ureteral reimplant: a critical look at surgical outcomes. J Pediatr Urol. 2016;12(6):402 e401–402 e409.
26. Noh PH, Bansal D. Pediatric robotic assisted laparoscopy for paraureteral bladder diverticulum excision with ureteral reimplantation. J Pediatr Urol. 2013;9(1):e28–30.
27. Herz D, Smith J, McLeod D, Schober M, Preece J, Merguerian P. Robot-assisted laparoscopic management of duplex renal anomaly: comparison of surgical outcomes to traditional pure laparoscopic and open surgery. J Pediatr Urol. 2016;12(1):44 e41–7.
28. Faasse MA, Lindgren BW, Gong EM. Robot-assisted laparoscopic ureteral reimplantation with excisional tailoring for refluxing megaureter. J Pediatr Urol. 2014;10(4):773 e771–2.
29. Fu W, Zhang X, Zhang X, et al. Pure laparoscopic and robot-assisted laparoscopic reconstructive surgery in congenital megaureter: a single institution experience. PLoS One. 2014;9(6):e99777.
30. Hemal AK, Nayyar R, Rao R. Robotic repair of primary symptomatic obstructive megaureter with intracorporeal or extracorporeal ureteric tapering and ureteroneocystostomy. J Endourol. 2009;23(12):2041–6.
31. Khan A, Rahiman M, Verma A, Bhargava R. Novel technique of laparoscopic extravesical ureteric reimplantation in primary obstructive megaureter. Urol Ann. 2017;9(2):150–2.
32. Landa-Juarez S, Guerra-Rivas A, Salgado-Sangri R, Castillo-Fernandez AM, de la Cruz-Yanez H, Garcia-Hernandez C. Laparoscopic ureterovesical repair for megaureter treatment. Cir Cir. 2017;85(3):196–200.
33. Arlen AM, Broderick KM, Travers C, Smith EA, Elmore JM, Kirsch AJ. Outcomes of complex robot-assisted extravesical ureteral reimplantation in the pediatric population. J Pediatr Urol. 2016;12(3):169 e161–6.
34. Yeung CK, Sihoe JD, Borzi PA. Endoscopic cross-trigonal ureteral reimplantation under carbon dioxide bladder insufflation: a novel technique. J Endourol. 2005;19(3):295–9.
35. Peters CA, Woo R. Intravesical robotically assisted bilateral ureteral reimplantation. J Endourol. 2005;19(6):618–21; discussion 621-612
36. Jayanthi V, Patel A. Vesicoscopic ureteral reimplantation: a minimally invasive technique for the definitive repair of vesicoureteral reflux. Adv Urol. 2008; https://doi.org/10.1155/2008/973616.
37. Kutikov A, Guzzo TJ, Canter DJ, Casale P. Initial experience with laparoscopic transvesical ureteral reimplantation at the Children's Hospital of Philadelphia. J Urol. 2006;176(5):2222–5; discussion 2225-2226

Part VI

Bladder

Chester J. Koh

In this section of the book, we encounter some of the most complex robotic reconstructive procedures since they involve the bladder. One of the advantages of robotic surgery is the facilitated ability to suture with minimally invasive instruments, and especially with surgical procedures that involve the bladder. As a result, procedures that were traditionally performed with large incisions can now be performed via keyhole incisions.

Drs. Johnson Tsui, Bethany Desroches, and Ravi Munver describe the minimally invasive options for partial cystectomy for a variety of conditions with the primary goal of preserving as much bladder as possible.

Drs. Rana Kumar and Mohan Gundeti describe the use of their pioneering work to utilize robotic surgery for bladder augmentation / ileocystoplasty and Mitrofanoff appendicovesicostomy which now has been performed completely intra-peritoneally at select centers.

Drs. Jonathan Gerber and Chester Koh describe the use of robotic surgery for benign bladder conditions, such as bladder diverticula, urachal anomalies, and bladder stones in children. While these are less common procedures, robot-assisted laparoscopic techniques offer a minimally invasive treatment option as an alternative to open surgery for these benign conditions in children.

Adult Bladder Diverticulectomy and Partial Cystectomy

18

Johnson Tsui, Bethany Desroches, and Ravi Munver

Indications

Bladder diverticulectomy can be performed for oncological cause as well as benign etiologies. As diverticula are outpouchings that form from weakness in the bladder wall, they lack the backing of a muscle wall and often do not empty appropriately. In patients with a large, symptomatic diverticulum that does not appropriately drain resulting in bladder calculi, cancer, recurrent infections, or ureteral reflux or obstruction, bladder diverticulectomy may be indicated [1]. Reduction cystoplasty may also be of benefit in carefully selected men with impaired detrusor contractility [2]. Bladder diverticulectomy using laparoscopic and robot-assisted laparoscopic approaches has been demonstrated to be feasible and safe [3].

In the setting of muscle-invasive urothelial carcinoma of the bladder, bladder cancer with high risk of progression, or treatment failure with high-grade disease, radical cystectomy is considered standard of care [4, 5]. However, in an optimized candidate who wishes to avoid the morbidity associated with radical cystectomy, partial cystectomy is an option when considering bladder preservation therapy in the management of a first-time occurrence of a solitary tumor [6, 7]. A concomitant bilateral pelvic lymph node dissection should also be performed if partial cystectomy

Supplementary Information The online version of this chapter (https://doi.org/10.1007/978-3-030-50196-9_18) contains supplementary material, which is available to authorized users.

J. Tsui · B. Desroches
Department of Urology, Hackensack University Medical Center, Hackensack, NJ, USA
e-mail: Bethany.Desroches@HackensackMeridian.org

R. Munver (✉)
Department of Urology, Hackensack University Medical Center, Hackensack, NJ, USA

Hackensack Meridian School of Medicine, Nutley, NJ, USA
e-mail: Ravi.Munver@HackensackMeridian.org

© Springer Nature Switzerland AG 2022
M. D. Stifelman et al. (eds.), *Techniques of Robotic Urinary Tract Reconstruction*, https://doi.org/10.1007/978-3-030-50196-9_18

is being performed for urothelial carcinoma, given its clear benefit in patients undergoing radical cystectomy [8, 9]. Partial cystectomy is also indicated in patients with urachal adenocarcinoma that involves the bladder dome [10]. Feasibility using both laparoscopic and robot-assisted approaches has been demonstrated through a number of studies and reports [11–13].

Preoperative Evaluation Requirements

Preoperative testing should include basic labs such as a complete blood count, comprehensive metabolic panel, anticoagulation panel, and if nutritional status is a concern, albumin and prealbumin. The identification of anemia, electrolyte abnormalities, and any blood dyscrasias may help reduce these known independent risk factors for postoperative mortality and morbidity [14]. Cardiovascular testing should be performed as per American Heart Association/American College of Cardiology (AHA/ACC) guidelines [15]. Special considerations for laparoscopic surgery include pulmonary function testing and assessment of hypoxia baseline hypercarbia, as the patient will be in a steep Trendelenburg position during the surgery. Obesity is not a contraindication for laparoscopic surgery, but may necessitate the use of extra-long trocars.

When considering partial cystectomy, an important part of the preoperative evaluation is excluding the diagnosis of carcinoma in situ. This can be done by obtaining multiple bladder biopsies to rule out multifocal disease, which is a contraindication to partial cystectomy. As chronic bladder outlet obstruction can contribute to the formation of bladder diverticula, any existing obstruction should be addressed prior to performing diverticulectomy. Addressing the obstructive issue after diverticulectomy can unduly stress the bladder repair [16].

Procedure/Technique

Patient Positioning

Patient should be placed in the low lithotomy position with all pressure points padded and the arms, legs, and chest secured to the operating table. The hips can be hyperextended and the table tilted to a low-to-steep Trendelenburg position (Fig. 18.1).

Trocar Placement

Initial access and insufflation can be achieved using the Veress or Hasson technique. With both conventional laparoscopic and robot-assisted laparoscopic surgery, a five- or six-port configuration may be used with port placement similar to that used for laparoscopic or robotic radical prostatectomy. The third arm of the robotic surgical system can be placed on either the right or the left, depending upon surgeon

Fig. 18.1 Patient
positioning in steep
Trendelenburg position

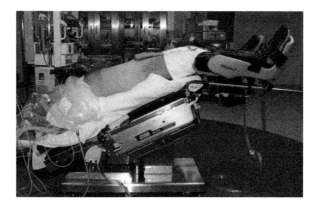

Fig. 18.2 Robotic trocar
template

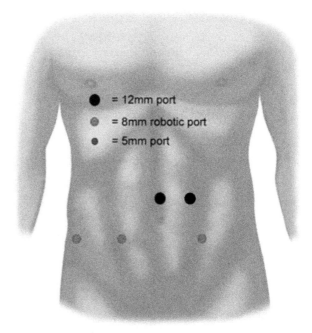

preference. At least one assistant port (12 mm trocar) is needed for entry and exit of sutures and suctioning. The camera port is placed in a supraumbilical position. For patients undergoing surgery for urachal cancer, the camera port should be placed 3–5 cm cephalad to the umbilicus. Trocar placement should also take into consideration any prior abdominal surgeries (Fig. 18.2).

Special Considerations

When performing partial cystectomy, on initial insertion of the laparoscope after trocar placement, the abdomen should be inspected for any abnormal findings or unusual anatomy. Any small or large bowel adhesions to the bladder or sidewall, or other adhesions that could impede surgery, should be released. To release the bladder further, the peritoneum can be incised lateral to the medial umbilical ligaments, which are then divided close to the urachus and dissected down to the pubis. In the case of urothelial carcinoma, bilateral pelvic lymphadenectomy should be performed either after the partial cystectomy and cystorrhaphy have been completed or prior to performing partial cystectomy. The technique for pelvic lymph node dissection is the same as that which would be performed during radical cystectomy.

A variety of methods can then be employed for intraperitoneal identification of the diverticulum. Bladder diverticulectomy can be performed via an extravesical or transvesical approach [16]. The transvesical approach involves using cystoscopy and a Collins knife to score the diverticulum neck circumferentially, with an adequate margin, under laparoscopic visualization [17]. This maneuver can be supervised robotically using the TilePro feature of the robotic surgical system. There are several techniques for extravesical diverticulectomy. The most straightforward and our preferred method to identify the diverticulum is detailed below under procedural steps and involves using a flexible cystoscope to transilluminate the bladder wall (Fig. 18.3). Turning off the light of the laparoscope and using white light cystoscopy or near-infrared fluorescence imaging will assist in demonstrating the location of the diverticulum. Another technique that can be employed involves placement of a urethral catheter into the diverticulum with inflation of the catheter balloon that is

Fig. 18.3 Transillumination of the bladder via a flexible cystoscope assists in localizing the area of interest

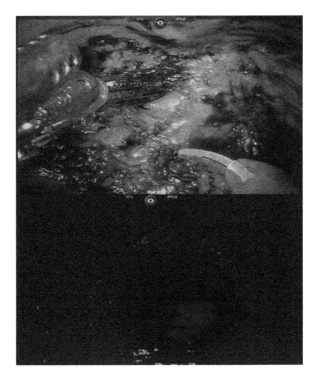

located within the diverticulum [18]. In this instance, we recommend placement of a council tip urethral catheter over a guidewire to direct the tip of the catheter into the diverticulum. This technique can be augmented by injecting methylene blue into the diverticulum to delineate its extent [19, 20]. Depending on the size of the diverticulum neck, it is also possible to insert an angiocatheter into the diverticulum to hydrodistend the diverticulum for ease of identification [21]. An additional review of several techniques for identification and robotic management of bladder diverticula is provided by Eyraud et al. [22].

Procedural Steps

Once the bladder has been adequately identified, we prefer transillumination with a flexible cystoscope that is inserted transurethrally to identify the precise location of the bladder diverticulum or site of the bladder tumor (Fig. 18.3).

The peritoneum overlying the desired site of the bladder is then incised (Fig. 18.4).

Dissection should be performed using systematic approach to traverse the perivesical tissues. The portion of the bladder or bladder diverticulum can be retracted with the third arm of the robotic system as the dissection is continued to ensure an adequate margin from the diverticulum neck or the bladder tumor site (Fig. 18.5).

The bladder detrusor and mucosal layers are then entered (Fig. 18.6).

A flexible cystoscope is utilized to confirm the entry point and is used to direct the dissection further to ensure an adequate margin. The bladder wall is excised circumferentially until the final attachment is reached and similarly excised. This maneuver is performed via an assistant that performs flexible cystoscopy as the robotic console surgeon use the TilePro mode to guide the dissection.

Should the partial cystectomy be performed for urachal adenocarcinoma, the resection should not only be wide but also include the urachal remnant. The portion of the bladder or bladder diverticulum is inspected and is placed in a specimen retrieval bag for subsequent extraction prior to incision closure.

The bladder defect is closed in a two-layer fashion with an absorbable suture. We prefer using a 2-0 absorbable braided suture with an SH needle; however with

Fig. 18.4 Peritoneal incision in the area of the bladder diverticulum or tumor site

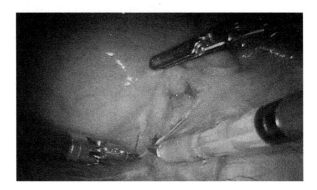

Fig. 18.5 The bladder
diverticulum is dissected
from the surrounding
perivesical tissue
and bladder

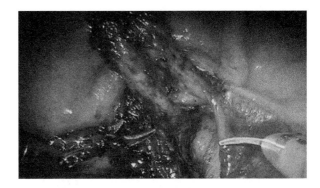

Fig. 18.6 Entry into the
bladder away from the
bladder tumor site or
diverticulum neck

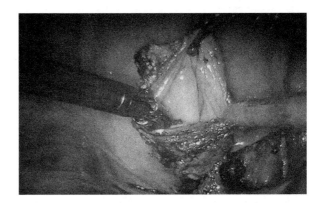

Fig. 18.7 Bladder mucosa
closure with a 2-0
absorbable suture

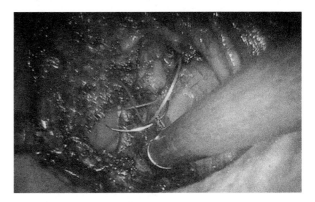

the advent of barbed suture, 2-0 V-Loc suture on an SH needle can also be used. We close the bladder using a continuous running suture technique. Based on surgeon preference, closure can also be performed using an interrupted suturing technique (Fig. 18.7).

The mucosa is closed until a watertight closure is achieved. The detrusor and serosa are similarly closed in a second layer, to ensure a watertight closure (Fig. 18.8).

Fig. 18.8 The detrusor
and serosa are closed in a
watertight fashion with 2-0
absorbable suture

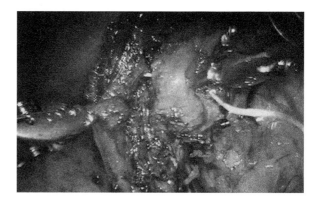

Fig. 18.9 The peritoneum
is closed in a running
fashion with
absorbable suture

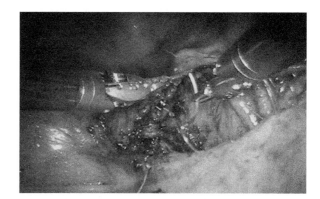

Fig. 18.10 Completed
peritoneal closure

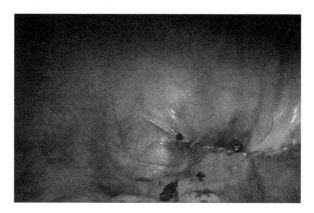

    Once the cystorrhaphy has been completed, the bladder is distended with 200 cc
of sterile saline via a urethral catheter to evaluate the integrity of the closure. Any
evidence of leaks can be reinforced with interrupted 2-0 absorbable sutures. The
peritoneum is then closed in a running fashion with 2-0 absorbable suture (Figs. 18.9
and 18.10).

Drainage Considerations

Drain and Catheter Placement

A pelvic drain is placed to assess for postoperative bleeding or urine leak. An indwelling urethral catheter is maintained for 7–10 days, and based on surgeon preference, a cystogram may be performed to confirm the absence of contrast extravasation from the bladder prior to urethral catheter removal and trial of void.

Ureteral Stenting

Ureteral stenting may be performed at the time of surgery. If the portion of the bladder that is to be excised is in close proximity to the ureteric orifice, we recommend early cystoscopic placement of an internal ureteral stent to aid in the identification of the ureter and to prevent iatrogenic ureteral injury [19]. This pre-placed stent can also ensure upper tract drainage, should extensive ureteral or bladder dissection be required during the procedure [3, 19]. The stent can be removed at the end of the procedure or be left indwelling in the case of extensive ureteral dissection. An indwelling stent can subsequently be removed in an outpatient setting at the time of urethral catheter removal. In certain instances, ureteral reimplantation may be necessary due to the proximity of the ureter to a large bladder diverticulum [23].

Adjunctive Procedures

Considerations in Benign Disease

A common etiology for bladder diverticula is chronic bladder outlet obstruction from an enlarged prostate or from other causes. It is therefore important to identify any cause of bladder outlet obstruction, and surgery to address the bladder outlet obstruction should be performed prior to bladder diverticulectomy. This may involve performing a transurethral prostate procedure or other minimally invasive bladder outlet surgery. In women, it is also important to address bladder and pelvic floor function prior to bladder diverticulectomy. While it is important to achieve adequate margins in particular for partial cystectomy, it is equally important to avoid excess excision of the normal bladder wall to reduce the risk of postoperative voiding dysfunction.

Considerations in Malignancy

There is scant literature on partial cystectomy for oncological control due to partial cystectomy's rare use and utility in the management of muscle invasive urothelial carcinoma. In 2004, Holzbeierlein et al. published their 6-year experience with 58 patients that demonstrated that in highly selected patients, partial cystectomy offers acceptable outcomes with an overall 5-year survival of 69%. They noted CIS and multifocality to be related to superficial recurrence and lymph node involvement and positive surgical margin related to advanced recurrence [24]. In 2006 Kassouf et al. published their 21-year experience with 37 patients that demonstrated similar outcomes with an overall 5-year survival of 67%, disease-specific survival of 87%, and recurrence-free survival of 39% [25]. Other studies since have also demonstrated that in appropriately selected patients, partial cystectomy does not undermine cancer control [7, 26–28].

Bilateral pelvic lymphadenectomy is an integral component of radical cystectomy in the extirpative management of urothelial carcinoma of the bladder. Although the benefit of pelvic lymphadenectomy has not been defined as an adjunct to partial cystectomy, in the role of radical cystectomy when an extended template is used, it not only allows for adequate staging of disease but also offers a survival benefit [3]. The feasibility of laparoscopic pelvic lymph node dissection using an extended template has been demonstrated [29–32]. When performing the lymph node dissection, care must be taken due to the proximity to blood vessels and nerves that can be easily injured. Cautery and hemostatic clips should also be used judiciously to minimize small vessel bleeding, maintain good surgical visualization, and reduce occurrence of lymphoceles [3].

The use of neoadjuvant chemotherapy in patients undergoing partial cystectomy has not been extensively documented. However, in a small series of 21 patients, the use of neoadjuvant chemotherapy has been demonstrated to provide oncologic outcomes in highly selected patients with 5-year recurrence-free survival, advanced disease recurrence-free survival, and overall survival of 28%, 51%, and 63%, respectively [33]. To highlight the need for high selectivity when considering a patient with muscle invasive urothelial carcinoma for partial cystectomy, a study of 101 patients demonstrated that among patients with muscle invasive bladder cancer, positive pelvic lymph nodes, prior history of urothelial carcinoma, ureteral reimplantation, and lymphovascular invasion were predictive of poor outcomes following partial cystectomy [34].

Complications

With robot-assisted laparoscopic bladder diverticulectomy and partial cystectomy, just as with any laparoscopic procedure, complications of laparoscopic access such as surrounding organ injury or gas embolism are possible and should be recognized in a timely fashion. Injury rates during laparoscopic access are relatively low, ranging from 0.05% to 0.3% [35]. Vascular injury is the most concerning type of injury and is one of the leading causes of death from laparoscopic access. Bowel injury is an ever-present concern with laparoscopic access and carries a mortality rate of 2.5–5.0% [35, 36]. Occurrence of bowel injury can be reduced by placement of an orogastric tube and Foley catheter prior to obtaining access, inserting trocars under visualization, taking extra care when placing trocars in patients with abdominal wall laxity, and temporarily increasing insufflation pressure during tro-car insertion. This complication is sometimes not recognized intraoperatively, and diagnosis occurs in a delayed fashion. Identifying bowel injury as early as possible is important in mitigating patient mortality and reducing morbidity. Although it is generally assumed that nausea and vomiting, ileus, and generalized abdominal pain signify bowel injury, the most common postoperative presentation of bowel injury is severe pain at a single trocar site, abdominal distension, diarrhea, and leukopenia, sometimes followed by acute cardiopulmonary collapse secondary to sepsis that often occurs within 96 hours of surgery [37]. Once recognized, bowel injury should be addressed promptly.

Potential other complications of partial cystectomy and bladder diverticulectomy include common postoperative complications such as infection, voiding dysfunc-tion occurring as a result of the newly configured bladder, postoperative adhesions, and bleeding. Another potential complication is urine leakage from the cystorrha-phy site [3]. The occurrence of urine leakage can also be mitigated by intraopera-tively testing for a watertight repair by filling the bladder with 150–200 cc of normal saline and addressing any leakage if identified. The use of an intra-abdominal drain aids in the diagnosis of a urine leak or postoperative bleeding.

Intraoperative bleeding from the bladder wall can usually be identified and addressed with electrocautery or placement of additional sutures, as cystorrhaphy routinely controls the majority of bleeding. Postoperative bleeding may require intervention if bleeding is brisk or does not resolve with conservative management. To reduce the risk of infection, sterile urine should be confirmed preoperatively and near the planned date of surgery. Appropriate infection prophylaxis should be fol-lowed per the infection control guidelines.

Conclusion

In appropriately selected patients, partial cystectomy is a viable option for the man-agement of urothelial carcinoma when considering bladder preservation therapy. When partial cystectomy is performed for oncological control, concomitant pelvic lymphadenectomy should be considered for staging purposes. Multifocal disease is a contraindication to performing partial cystectomy and must be excluded prior. In select settings, bladder diverticulectomy can also be performed for oncological con-trol of a bladder tumor within the diverticulum. Bladder diverticulectomy can also be performed for benign indications such as a large symptomatic diverticulum that does not appropriately drain with resultant lithiasis, recurrent infections, or ureteral reflux or obstruction. In this setting, the etiology of the bladder diverticulum should be addressed prior to surgery. Both partial cystectomy and bladder diverticulectomy can be performed safely using laparoscopic and robotic approaches. A variety of techniques can be employed for identification of the bladder diverticulum to be excised. The surgeon should attempt to minimize the risk of complications such as infection, urine leak, and bleeding with proper antibiotic prophylaxis, patient selection and optimization, and meticulous surgical technique. Vascular and bowel injuries should be identified as soon as possible and addressed promptly. As with any minimally invasive surgery, meticulous technique and delicate handling of the tissues should be employed to maximize the success of the procedure.

References

 1. Rovner ES. Campbell-Walsh urology. 9th ed. Philadelphia: Saunders Elsevier; 2007.
 2. Thorner DA, Blaivas JG, Tsui JF, Kashan MY, Weinberger JM, Weiss JP. Outcomes of reduction cystoplasty in men with impaired detrusor contractility. Urology. 2014;83(4):882–6.
 3. Rha KH, Lorenzo EI, Oh CK. Smith's textbook of endourology. 3rd ed. West Sussex: Blackwell; 2012.
 4. Chang SS, Bochner BH, Chou R, Dreicer R, Kamat AM, Lerner SP, et al. Treatment of non-metastatic muscle-invasive bladder cancer: AUA/ASCO/ASTRO/SUO guideline. J Urol. 2017;198(3):552–9.
 5. Milowsky MI, Rumble RB, Booth CM, Gilligan T, Eapen LJ, Hauke RJ, et al. Guideline on muscle-invasive and metastatic bladder cancer (European Association of Urology Guideline): American Society of Clinical Oncology Clinical Practice Guideline Endorsement. J Clin Oncol. 2016;34(16):1945–52.
 6. Knoedler J, Frank I. Organ-sparing surgery in urology: partial cystectomy. Curr Opin Urol. 2015;25(2):111–5.
 7. Knoedler JJ, Boorjian SA, Kim SP, Weight CJ, Thapa P, Tarrell RF, et al. Does partial cystectomy compromise oncologic outcomes for patients with bladder cancer compared to radical cystectomy? A matched case-control analysis. J Urol. 2012;188(4):1115–9.
 8. Larcher A, Sun M, Schiffmann J, Tian Z, Shariat SF, McCormack M, et al. Differential effect on survival of pelvic lymph node dissection at radical cystectomy for muscle invasive bladder cancer. Eur J Surg Oncol. 2015;41(3):353–60.
 9. Abdollah F, Sun M, Schmitges J, Djahangirian O, Tian Z, Jeldres C, et al. Stage-specific impact of pelvic lymph node dissection on survival in patients with non-metastatic bladder cancer treated with radical cystectomy. BJU Int. 2012;109(8):1147–54.
10. Burnett AL, Epstein JI, Marshall FF. Adenocarcinoma of urinary bladder: classification and management. Urology. 1991;37(4):315–21.
11. James K, Vasdev N, Mohan SG, Lane T, Adshead JM. Robotic partial cystectomy for primary urachal adenocarcinoma of the urinary bladder. Curr Urol. 2015;8(4):183–8.
12. Williams CR, Chavda K. En bloc robot-assisted laparoscopic partial cystectomy, urachal resection, and pelvic lymphadenectomy for urachal adenocarcinoma. Rev Urol. 2015;17(1):46–9.
13. Wadhwa P, Kolla SB, Hemal AK. Laparoscopic en bloc partial cystectomy with bilateral pelvic lymphadenectomy for urachal adenocarcinoma. Urology. 2006;67(4):837–43.
14. Cui HW, Turney BW, Griffiths J. The preoperative assessment and optimization of patients undergoing major urological surgery. Curr Urol Rep. 2017;18(7):54.
15. Fleisher LA, Fleischmann KE, Auerbach AD, Barnason SA, Beckman JA, Bozkurt B, et al. 2014 ACC/AHA guideline on perioperative cardiovascular evaluation and management of patients undergoing noncardiac surgery: a report of the American College of Cardiology/American Heart Association Task Force on practice guidelines. J Am Coll Cardiol. 2014;64(22):e77–137.
16. Abreu AL, Chopra S, Dharmaraja A, Djaladat H, Aron M, Ukimura O, et al. Robot-assisted bladder diverticulectomy. J Endourol. 2014;28(10):1159–64.
17. Tareen BU, Mufarrij PW, Godoy G, Stifelman MD. Robot-assisted laparoscopic partial cystectomy and diverticulectomy: initial experience of four cases. J Endourol. 2008;22(7):1497–500.
18. Kural AR, Atug F, Akpinar H, Tufek I. Robot-assisted laparoscopic bladder diverticulectomy combined with photoselective vaporization of prostate: a case report and review of literature. J Endourol. 2009;23(8):1281–5.

19. Ganesamoni R, Ganpule AP, Desai MR. Robot-assisted laparoscopic bladder diverticulectomy in a seven-year-old child: case report and points of technique. Indian J Urol. 2012;28(4):434–6.
20. Moore CR, Shirodkar SP, Avallone MA, Castle SM, Gorin MA, Gorbatiy V, et al. Intravesical methylene blue facilitates precise identification of the diverticular neck during robot-assisted laparoscopic bladder diverticulectomy. J Laparoendosc Adv Surg Tech A. 2012;22(5):492–5.
21. Myer EG, Wagner JR. Robotic assisted laparoscopic bladder diverticulectomy. J Urol. 2007;178(6):2406–10; discussion 10
22. Eyraud R, Laydner H, Autorino R, Panumatrassamee K, Haber GP, Stein RJ. Robot-assisted laparoscopic bladder diverticulectomy. Curr Urol Rep. 2013;14(1):46–51.
23. Elands S, Vasdev N, Tay A, Adshead JM. Robot-assisted laparoscopic bladder diverticulectomy and ureteral re-implantation for a diverticulum containing high grade transitional cell carcinoma. Curr Urol. 2015;8(2):104–8.
24. Holzbeierlein JM, Lopez-Corona E, Bochner BH, Herr HW, Donat SM, Russo P, et al. Partial cystectomy: a contemporary review of the Memorial Sloan-Kettering Cancer Center experience and recommendations for patient selection. J Urol. 2004;172(3):878–81.
25. Kassouf W, Swanson D, Kamat AM, Leibovici D, Siefker-Radtke A, Munsell MF, et al. Partial cystectomy for muscle invasive urothelial carcinoma of the bladder: a contemporary review of the MD Anderson Cancer Center experience. J Urol. 2006;175(6):2058–62.
26. Smaldone MC, Jacobs BL, Smaldone AM, Hrebinko RL Jr. Long-term results of selective partial cystectomy for invasive urothelial bladder carcinoma. Urology. 2008;72(3):613–6.
27. Capitanio U, Isbarn H, Shariat SF, Jeldres C, Zini L, Saad F, et al. Partial cystectomy does not undermine cancer control in appropriately selected patients with urothelial carcinoma of the bladder: a population-based matched analysist. Urology. 2009;74(4):858–64.
28. Leveridge MJ, Siemens DR, Izard JP, Wei X, Booth CM. Partial cystectomy for urothelial carcinoma of the bladder: practice patterns and outcomes in the general population. Can Urol Assoc J. 2017;11(12):412–8.
29. Finelli A, Gill IS, Desai MM, Moinzadeh A, Magi-Galluzzi C, Kaouk JH. Laparoscopic extended pelvic lymphadenectomy for bladder cancer: technique and initial outcomes. J Urol. 2004;172(5 Pt 1):1809–12.
30. Yuan JB, Zu XB, Miao JG, Wang J, Chen MF, Qi L. Laparoscopic pelvic lymph node dissection system based on preoperative primary tumour stage (T stage) by computed tomography in urothelial bladder cancer: results of a single-institution prospective study. BJU Int. 2013;112(2):E87–91.
31. Singh I. Robot-assisted pelvic lymphadenectomy for bladder cancer – where have we reached by 2009. Urology. 2010;75(6):1269–74.
32. Kaouk JH, Goel RK, White MA, White WM, Autorino R, Haber GP, et al. Laparoendoscopic single-site radical cystectomy and pelvic lymph node dissection: initial experience and 2-year follow-up. Urology. 2010;76(4):857–61.
33. Bazzi WM, Kopp RP, Donahue TF, Bernstein M, Russo P, Bochner BH, et al. Partial cystectomy after neoadjuvant chemotherapy: memorial Sloan Kettering Cancer Center Contemporary Experience. Int Sch Res Notices. 2014;2014:702653.
34. Ma B, Li H, Zhang C, Yang K, Qiao B, Zhang Z, et al. Lymphovascular invasion, ureteral reimplantation and prior history of urothelial carcinoma are associated with poor prognosis after partial cystectomy for muscle-invasive bladder cancer with negative pelvic lymph nodes. Eur J Surg Oncol. 2013;39(10):1150–6.
35. Chandler JG, Corson SL, Way LW. Three spectra of laparoscopic entry access injuries. J Am Coll Surg. 2001;192(4):478–90; discussion 90-1
36. Woodson B, Lee BR. Laparoscopic and robotic access. In: Best SL, Nakada SY, editors. Minimally invasive urology. New York: Springer Science+Business Media; 2015. p. 1–10.
37. Bishoff JT, Allaf ME, Kirkels W, Moore RG, Kavoussi LR, Schroder F. Laparoscopic bowel injury: incidence and clinical presentation. J Urol. 1999;161(3):887–90.

Pediatric Bladder Augmentation and Urinary Diversion

19

Rana Kumar and Mohan S. Gundeti

Abbreviations

CIC	Clean intermittent catheterization
MAPV	Mitrofanoff appendicovesicostomy
RALI	Robotic-assisted laparoscopic augmentation ileocystoplasty
RALIMA	Robotic-assisted laparoscopic augmentation ileocystoplasty and Mitrofanoff appendicovesicostomy
RALMA	Robotic-assisted laparoscopic Mitrofanoff appendicovesicostomy
VP shunt	Ventriculoperitoneal shunt

Introduction

Pediatric bladder augmentation/ileocystoplasty and urinary diversion procedures, while infrequently performed, are an invaluable part of the complete surgical armamentarium for the management of impaired bladder function in patients with neurogenic bladder and non-neurogenic neurogenic bladder (NNNB) and less commonly with bladder exstrophy complex, posterior urethral valves (PUV), and prune belly syndrome (PBS) [1]. Traditionally, it is accomplished with an open surgical approach which is considered

Supplementary Information The online version of this chapter (https://doi.org/10.1007/978-3-030-50196-9_19) contains supplementary material, which is available to authorized users.

R. Kumar (✉)
Department of Urology, University of Chicago, Chicago, IL, USA

M. S. Gundeti
Department of Surgery, Chicago Medicine, Chicago, IL, USA
e-mail: mgundeti@surgery.bsd.uchicago.edu

© Springer Nature Switzerland AG 2022
M. D. Stifelman et al. (eds.), *Techniques of Robotic Urinary Tract Reconstruction*, https://doi.org/10.1007/978-3-030-50196-9_19

215

the benchmark against which all future surgical technical innovations, including laparoscopic and robot-assisted laparoscopic surgery, should be compared.

With an established long-term safety and efficacy record in adult patients, the use of robot-assisted laparoscopic surgery has gradually expanded to the pediatric population with favorable long-term safety and efficacy outcomes for upper tract reconstructive procedures [2, 3]. With increasing comfort and good safety and efficacy outcomes, more and more complex pediatric urological procedures such as ureteric reimplantation [4], Mitrofanoff appendicovesicostomy (MAPV) [5], bladder augmentation [6], and bladder neck reconstruction [7] are now being done completely robotically with comparable safety and efficacy outcomes.

In this chapter, our point of focus will be on robot-assisted laparoscopic augmentation ileocystoplasty and Mitrofanoff appendicovesicostomy (RALIMA), where we discuss in detail its indications, preparations, surgical techniques, outcomes, complications and their management, as well as future directions.

Preoperative Indications

Pediatric bladder augmentation is a complex lower urinary tract reconstruction procedure that is performed in patients with impaired bladder function to protect children from progressive renal damage and to achieve good social continence. Impaired bladder function implies reduced capacity of the bladder and/or poor compliance with high pressure voiding. It is commonly encountered in children with neurogenic bladder secondary to congenital neural tube defects such as spina bifida, myelomeningocele, and tethered spinal cord syndrome or, less commonly, a sequel to traumatic spinal cord injury, transverse myelitis, or anorectal malformations. Other important etiologies of bladder dysfunction in children can be non-neurogenic neurogenic bladder, posterior urethral valves, prune belly syndrome (PBS), and bladder exstrophy complex. Other etiologies include tuberculosis or schistosomiasis of the bladder with severe contracture of the urinary bladder [8].

The first-line management of neurogenic or idiopathic bladder dysfunction is clean intermittent catheterization (CIC), anticholinergic medication (orally or intravesically), and certain lifestyle and behavioral modifications [8]. The option of bladder augmentation is usually offered to patients who have failed this first-line management. Bladder augmentation offers the advantage of increased capacity with improved compliance and better protection of the upper tracts and can also lead to better continence [8]. It should be noted that successful performance of clean intermittent catheterization is a mandatory requirement before bladder augmentation.

A Mitrofanoff appendicovesicostomy (MAPV) is often an adjunct procedure with bladder augmentation. This is offered to patients in whom CIC is either difficult or impossible via the urethra. These include patients with extreme discomfort in performing CIC, as well as patients with difficult CIC due to noncompliance, urethral trauma, urethral stricture disease, female sex and morbid obesity with difficult access to the urethra, and disability secondary to quadriplegia [9].

Patient selection is of prime importance before considering a child for bladder augmentation and continent urinary diversion. The parents and caregivers must undergo elaborate preoperative counseling before the procedure. Prior history of short or irradiated bowel and inflammatory bowel disease such as Crohn's disease are absolute contraindications to bladder augmentation [10]. A Mitrofanoff procedure cannot be contemplated in patients with previous appendectomy, but small bowel segments can be used instead using the Yang-Monti procedure. However, this requires a bowel anastomosis and can be associated with slightly higher complication rates [11]. Traditionally, chronic kidney disease with severe renal functional impairment has been a relative contraindication for bladder augmentation, but a recent study found that bladder augmentation did not appear to hasten the progression to end-stage kidney disease in patients with severe renal insufficiency and neuropathic bladder [12].

Multiple prior abdominal surgeries and certain body habitus such as severe kyphoscoliosis with extensive bowel adhesions or difficulty in achieving pneumoperitoneum may pose additional challenge in performance of these procedures robotically and may necessitate conversion to an open procedure.

Technical Considerations

The surgical technique described here as well as in the video has been published previously by the chapter's senior author [6, 13, 15].

Preparation

Patients are not given any preoperative antibiotic or mechanical bowel preparation as per the approach of Gundeti et al. [14]. Preoperatively, all patients receive a weight-based dose of cefazolin, gentamicin, and metronidazole 1 hour before the procedure. In cases with ventriculoperitoneal (VP) shunt in situ, the antibiotic regimen is broadened to include vancomycin. We prefer heparin (LMW) 1 hour before surgery for patients who are wheelchair bound for deep vein thrombosis prophylaxis.

Patient Positioning, Port Placement, VP Shunt Management, and Robot Docking

The patient is placed in low lithotomy and slight Trendelenburg position (10°–20°) with the arms tucked at the side (Fig. 19.1). Appropriate foam padding of the arms, legs, torso, and face is done to prevent any compression injury. The patient is prepped and draped with a Foley catheter placed in sterile field to permit access by the assistant during the procedure. The initial 12 mm trocar is placed through the umbilicus using the Hassan technique, keeping in mind to maintain a minimal distance of about 10–12 cm between this port site and the pubic symphysis. If needed,

Fig. 19.1 Patient positioning

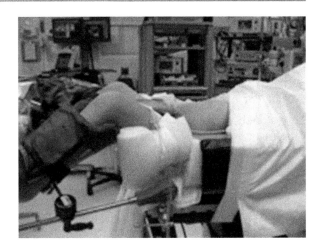

Fig. 19.2 Patient position and port placement. 12 mm camera port, 8 mm secondary robotic arm ports, 5 mm and 10–12 mm assistant port

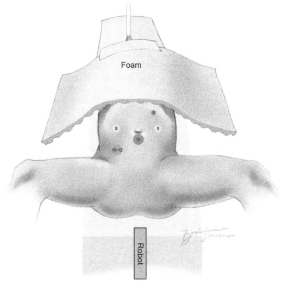

RALIMA UOC Technique–M. Gundeti et-al

a supraumbilical port placement can be done instead. Once pneumoperitoneum is safely achieved, two 8 mm robotic ports are then placed 7 cm lateral to midline at the level of the umbilicus under direct vision. Additionally, 12 mm (on the left side) and 5 mm (on the right side) robotic ports are placed 7 cm lateral to the previously placed side ports, to introduce sutures easily into the working area and to assist with retraction (Fig. 19.2). The umbilical port incision is typically used for stoma maturation at the end of the procedure. A diagnostic peritoneoscopy is performed to assess for the amount of adhesions, as well as identification and calibration of the appendix in terms of length and lumen diameter, and to assess the bladder. In general, the appendix should be at least 5–6 cm in length and also allow the passage of a 10F or 12F catheter. If a VP shunt is present, it is placed in an Endopouch specimen retrieval bag (Ethicon, Somerville, NJ, USA) and placed in the subhepatic space to avoid its contamination with bowel contents [15]. The robot is then docked from the caudal end between the legs.

ILEAL Loop Isolation and Bowel Anastomosis

A 20 cm loop of the ileum is identified 15–20 cm proximal to the ileocecal junction using a premeasured silk tie. The segment is then marked at both ends and kept under traction using two stay sutures with Keith needles that are passed through the abdominal wall (Fig. 19.3a). The adequacy of its mesenteric length to reach the pelvis without much tension is then verified before creating the mesenteric windows. The ileal segment is then incised using monopolar scissors (Fig. 19.3c). The seromuscular ileoileal anastomosis is then performed in an end-to-end manner using a running 4-0 or 5-0 polydioxanone (PDS) suture (Fig. 19.3b). The mesenteric windows are similarly closed.

Appendiceal Isolation and Harvest

A traction suture is placed at the tip to aid complete visualization of the appendix and its mesentery. Mesenteric windows to mobilize the appendix are then made, taking care to preserve its blood supply (Fig. 19.4a). A 4-0 polyglactin purse-string suture is then placed at its base, and the appendix is separated from the cecum. The purse-string suture is tied to close the cecal opening in one layer. Often we prefer to take part of the cecum to prevent future stomal stenosis.

Detrusorotomy and Appendicovesicostomy

Keeping the mesenteric orientation in mind, the appendix is implanted into the posterior bladder wall. The bladder is partially distended with sterile saline. A 4 cm detrusorotomy is made on the right posterior wall of the bladder. Bladder retraction using stay sutures to the dome of the bladder, passed transabdominally using Keith needle, as described previously, simplifies this step. The tip of the appendix is now excised and spatulated approximately 1 cm to allow intubation with an 8 French feeding tube. The initial anastomotic suture (using 5-0 PDS II suture) is placed at

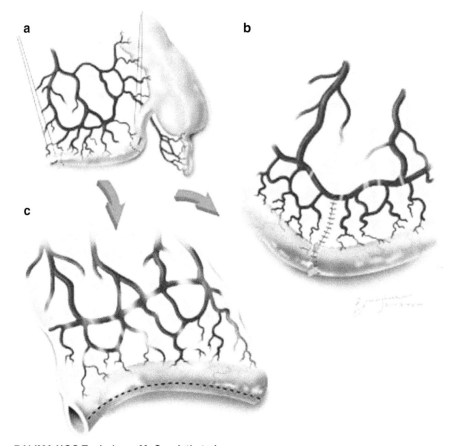

RALIMA UOC Technique–M. Gundeti et-al

Fig. 19.3 (**a**). Traction suture on the ileum. (**b**). Ileoileal anastomosis and closure of mesenteric defect. **c**. Isolation of 20 cm ileal loop

the apical tip of the appendix to the caudal apex of the detrusorotomy incision. Subsequently, a 1 cm incision is made over the bladder mucosa, and the appendico-vesical anastomosis is performed over the 8 French feeding tube in a continuous fashion, using a similar suture. The detrusor muscle is then imbricated over the appendix, using 4-0 polyglactin sutures, to function as an anti-refluxing continence mechanism (Fig. 19.4b). Recently, this technique has been modified to perform the posterior wall anastomosis in the coronal plane following detrusorotomy with an intravesical approach to reduce the operating time.

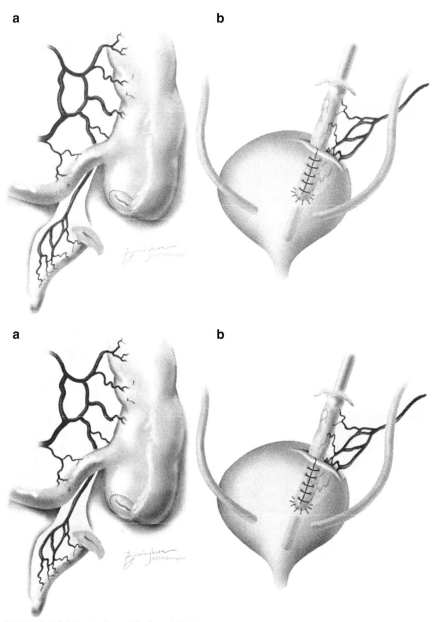

RALIMA UOC Technique–M. Gundeti et-al

Fig. 19.4 (**a**). Appendix isolation and closure of appendicocecal junction. (**b**). Appendicovesicostomy and detrusor imbrication of the posterior bladder wall

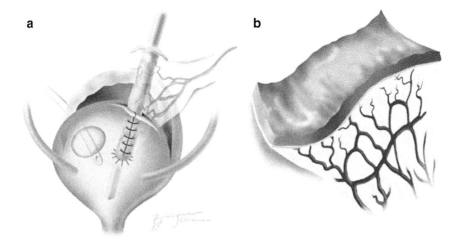

RALIMA UOC Technique–M. Gundeti et-al

Fig. 19.5 (**a**). Detubularization of the ileum on anti-mesenteric border. (**b**). Cystotomy in coronal plane from right ureteral orifice to left ureteral orifice

The orientation of the mesentery will decide the stoma location at the umbilicus or right iliac fossa, and accordingly, the detrusor tunnel is made oblique or straight.

Cystotomy and Ileovesical Anastomosis

A coronal cystotomy is performed starting from the right to the left side, with the ureteric catheter in situ aiding its identification, creating a bivalve bladder (Fig. 19.5). For the intravesical approach MAPV, at this stage, tunneling and anastomosis are performed. The isolated ileal segment is now incised along its anti-mesenteric side (Fig. 19.5). Initial corner sutures are placed on the posterior edge of the ileal segment to the respective apices of the bladder wall to aid the anastomosis. Using a running 2-0 coated Vicryl suture, the posterior edge of the bowel is now sutured to the posterior wall of the bladder. Similarly, the anterior anastomosis is accomplished taking care to avoid torsion of the bowel mesentery (Fig. 19.6). An 18 French suprapubic catheter is brought through the left lower quadrant abdominal wall and inserted into the neo-bladder before completion of the anastomosis and is fixed using a purse-string suture. The bladder is then filled with saline to confirm the anastomotic integrity. We prefer to place two suprapubic catheters for optimal drainage.

Fig. 19.6 Completion of
ileocystoplasty and
appendicovesicostomy

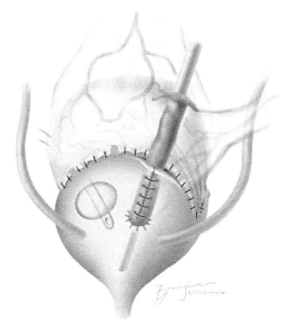

RALIMA UOC Technique–M. Gundeti et-al

The proximal end of the appendix is now exteriorized through the umbilical port site or the right lower quadrant port. This end of the appendix is now spatulated and then anastomosed to the skin using a V flap or a VQZ flap [16], which provides the advantage of cutaneous coverage of the intestinal mucosa.

If there is a need for antegrade colonic enema (ACE) and depending on the appendix length, split technique MAPV and ACE or cecal flap ACE is performed.

The augmented bladder is drained with an 18 French Foley suprapubic catheter (until starting clean intermittent catheterization usually after 4 weeks), a 16 French Foley urethral catheter (for 7–10 days), and an 8 French feeding tube through the appendicovesicostomy. A pelvic drain is also placed toward the end of the procedure.

Postoperative Care and Follow-Up

Patients are administered intravenous ketorolac for the initial 48 hours along with acetaminophen for pain management. Ibuprofen is given as needed after the last dose of ketorolac. A regular diet is instituted immediately after both MAPV and bladder augmentation. Patients with baseline constipation are started on their home bowel regimen. The abdominal drain is usually removed on postoperative day 3 after documentation of minimal drainage. The Foley catheter (per urethra) is removed on day 5. The discharge criteria include tolerating a diet well, being pain free, and achieving comfort with the drainage tubes. This usually takes 5–7 days.

The MAPV and suprapubic catheters are maintained for 4 weeks. With increasing experience, we no longer perform a routine postoperative cystography to test the integrity of the augmented bladder. Patients are taught clean intermittent catheterization (CIC) through the MAPV at the 4 week mark, while maintaining the suprapubic catheter as a safety valve for 1 more week or until the family is comfortable with CIC. We advise CIC to be done with a 10 French catheter every 4 hours.

Upper tract evaluation using renal ultrasound is routinely performed postoperatively. Long-term follow-up of the augmentation is needed to prevent future complications.

Outcomes and Complications

The existing data on outcomes and complications of RALIMA are based on small case series reported from highly specialized centers performing these procedures. In the absence of any prospectively designed randomized controlled trial, it would be impossible to directly compare this data to the standard open approach. However, the preliminary results from these centers do support the notion that these complex urinary tract reconstructive procedures can be accomplished robotically both safely and efficaciously, [5, 6, 9, 13, 17–19] with early results comparable to open series reported in the literature [20–23].

In one of the largest published series of RALIMA, the authors have shared their experience of 15 patients who underwent robotic-assisted laparoscopic augmentation ileocystoplasty (RALI), of whom 11 had a concomitant MAPV with a median follow-up of 43 months [18]. The median operative time was significantly longer in the RALI group (623 vs 287 min; p = 0.01). However, the median length of stay (LOS) was shorter in the RALI group (6 vs 8 days; p = 0.01). There were no statistical difference between the groups in terms of postoperative percentage increase in bladder capacity, estimated blood loss, return to regular diet, narcotic usage, and complication rates [18]. In this study, however, the patients in RALI group were significantly heavier, older, and with less patients who had prior abdominal surgery.

In one of the largest reported series of RALMA, the authors have shared their experience of 18 patients with a mean follow-up of 24.2 months [24]. The overall long-term continence rate as reported by the authors was 94.4%.

The complications of RALIMA reported in the literature are bladder stone formation (20%), stoma revision surgery (20%), stomal incontinence (6.7%), and parastomal hernia revision (6.7%) [18]. Other important long-term complications after bladder augmentation with a follow-up of 3 years, as reported in the open series, were re-augmentation (5.2%), bladder perforation (3.5%), and bowel fistula (2%) [23]. In the RALI group with a mean follow-up of 43 months, the authors have not observed any of these major complications such as re-augmentation. Other complications of ileocystoplasty include urinary tract infections, metabolic derangements, or renal deterioration.

Surgical Tips

The complex nature of surgery as well as unique challenges encountered in many of these patients with neurogenic bladder merits discussion of tips and tricks to troubleshoot these problems.

In our experience, many of these patients have associated obesity, kyphoscoliosis, and presence of ventriculoperitoneal (VP) shunts. The presence of these can portend unique challenges to the successful performance of the surgery. We discuss ways to troubleshoot these problems.

Patients with VP Shunt

Patients with preexisting VP shunt are administered additional vancomycin coverage over and above the usual antibiotic regimen (cefazolin + gentamicin + metronidazole) 1 hour before the procedure. Presence of a VP shunt in the abdomen can lead to a great amount of adhesions. In our experience, the adhesions shift the appendix from its usual location to a subhepatic location. We always prefer performing a diagnostic laparoscopy to confirm its location, perform adhesiolysis, and if possible, place the appendix in a more accessible location. To reduce the risk of bacterial contamination of the VP shunt, we routinely place the distal end of the shunt into a 5 mm Endopouch bag (Ethicon, Endosurgery), cinch it around the tube, and place in the subhepatic space. We also reduce the pneumoperitoneum to less than or equal to 12 mmHg to minimize pressure-induced changes to the shunt.

Patients with Obesity

Patients with a high body mass index (BMI) present a unique set of technical challenges. One needs to be highly proficient in managing simpler cases with minimal obesity before advancing to more difficult cases. Bariatric ports and instruments should be available on standby for these technically challenging cases. Another technical challenge noted in these patients is a fatty mesentery and short ileal mesenteric vessels. Fatty mesentery can be managed with incision of the bowel on the anti-mesenteric side, and then taking down of the mesentery for better visualization of the vessels. Use of contrast and Firefly, if available, may be considered. Short ileal mesenteric vessels may be managed by reducing the Trendelenburg position which may bring the bowel loop into the pelvis.

Patients with Kyphoscoliosis

Patient with severe kyphoscoliosis is a strict contraindication for robotic surgery due to profound difficulties with positioning and achieving pneumoperitoneum. Patients with spina bifida and associated kyphoscoliosis may have shorter pubo-umbilical lengths. However, in patients with kyphoscoliosis allowing adequate positioning, shifting the camera port proximally toward the xiphoid and sternum may be helpful. Also, placement of a fourth robotic port may help with traction.

Current Controversies

Median operative time in the RALIMA and RALMA group as reported by the authors is 623 and 323 minutes, respectively, which is significantly higher than the open group [18, 24]. In another series, Nguyen reported a mean operative time of 5.4 hours in the RALMA group, versus 4.5 hours in the open group [19]. However, they reported a mean operative time of 3.7 hours in their last three cases, possibly explained by expected longer times when early on the learning curve. In the future, with increasing experience, further reductions in the mean operative time can be expected.

Another important controversial issue related to RALMA is the location of the MAPV channel on the bladder wall. Traditionally, the MAPV channel is placed in the posterior bladder wall. Published literature on open MAPV series have reported on increased incidence of bladder stone formation and urinary tract infection in the anteriorly placed conduit. However, published series of RALMA, reporting the use of either anterior or posterior [19] or anterior only MAPV conduit [18], did not identify bladder stone formation as a complication.

One of the most important concerns with regard to widespread adoption of robotic technology is the cost issue. At present, the cost of robotic surgery is definitely high when compared to conventional laparoscopic or standard open approaches, but with the presence of multiple robotic options in the commercial market with consequent heightened competitiveness and with technology development resulting in availability of reusable instruments, differences in cost may be further shortened. From the view point of the patients, the advantage of minimally invasive surgery including less postoperative pain medication usage, early convalescence, and better cosmesis may drive future medical decision-making.

Future Directions

The role of robotic surgery is now well established in the management of adult urological disease. Its adoption in the pediatric population is gradually on the rise. Today pediatric urologists and surgeons in tertiary-level settings are getting more and more comfortable performing common surgeries such as pyeloplasty and ureteric reimplantation. However, only a few advanced centers have been performing complex urological procedures such as MAPV or augmentation cystoplasty robotically.

For widespread dissemination of the technology, it is important to start a robotic curriculum to train residents and fellows on these techniques. They should be facilitated with appropriate credentialing before embarking onto more complex procedures such as RALMA and RALIMA.

There is a need for development of pediatric-specific robotic components, keeping in mind the inherent issues in this patient population such as small body habitus with limited working spaces. Development of miniaturized instruments is expected to further advance adoption of the technology in the future.

With surgeons controlling the robot from a console, the time may come for remote procedure where the surgical procedure can be performed by the surgeon sitting at another location. Telesurgery, as it is known technically, may aid in disseminating the advantages of robotic surgery to different parts of the world, including developing economies currently unable to support the current high costs. Although it may appear simple, it will be a daunting task to overcome the social, political, and economic hurdles associated with it.

The use of bowel segments for augmentation of the bladder is the Achilles' heel of the surgery, contributing to some of the short- and long-term complications associated with the procedure. Atala and colleagues, utilizing the concept of tissue engineering, described their initial experience of using engineered bladder tissue created from collagen-based scaffolds with implanted autologous cells and wrapped by omentum, with promising early results [25]. However, subsequent phase II studies describing its use in children and adolescent with spina bifida reported no improvement in bladder capacity or compliance [26]. Further research in the field of regenerative medicine is warranted to find a more ideal and durable tissue alternative for the bladder.

Conclusion

Pediatric surgeons and urologists are now becoming increasingly comfortable performing complex surgical procedures such as RALIMA. Results from early case series endorse the feasibility of doing the procedure robotically and have shown its safety and efficacy. The potential benefits with robotic surgery are decreased postoperative pain medication usage, reduced length of stay, and better cosmesis. The short-term outcomes and complications data is comparable to that achieved with open surgery. However, it is important to understand that it reflects the results of the procedure performed at advanced centers with the availability of highly skilled robotic surgeons. Also, these benefits must be weighed against the steep learning curve, higher operative times, and cost.

References

1. Lazarus J. Intravesical oxybutynin in the pediatric neurogenic bladder. Nat Rev Urol. 2009;6(12):671–4.
2. Minnillo BJ, Cruz JA, Sayao RH, Passerotti CC, Houck CS, Meier PM, et al. Long-term experience and outcomes of robotic assisted laparoscopic pyeloplasty in children and young adults. J Urol. 2011;185:1455–60.
3. Cundy TP, Harling L, Hughes-Hallett A, Mayer EK, Najmaldin AS, Athanasiou T, et al. Meta-analysis of robot-assisted vs conventional laparoscopic and open pyeloplasty in children. BJU Int. 2014;114(4):582–94.

4. Gundeti MS, Kojima Y, Haga N, Kiriluk K. Robotic-assisted laparoscopic reconstructive surgery in the lower urinary tract. Curr Urol Rep. 2013;14(4):333–41.
5. Pedraza R, Weiser A, Franco I. Laparoscopic appendicovesicostomy (Mitrofanoff procedure) in a child using the da Vinci robotic system. J Urol. 2004;171(4):1652–3.
6. Gundeti MS, Eng MK, Reynolds WS, Zagaja GP. Pediatric robotic-assisted laparoscopic augmentation ileocystoplasty and Mitrofanoff appendicovesicostomy: complete intracorporeal – initial case report. Urology. 2008;72(5):1144–7.
7. Bagrodia A, Gargollo P. Robot-assisted bladder neck reconstruction, bladder neck sling, and appendicovesicostomy in children: description of technique and initial results. J Endourol. 2011;25(8):1299–305.
8. Biers SM, Venn SN, Greenwell TJ. The past, present and future of augmentation cystoplasty. BJU Int. 2012;109(9):1280–93.
9. Cohen AJ, Pariser JJ, Anderson BB, Pearce SM, Gundeti MS. The robotic appendicovesicostomy and bladder augmentation: the next frontier in robotics, are we there? Urol Clin North Am. 2015;42(1):121–30.
10. Khoury JM, Webster GD. Evaluation of augmentation cystoplasty for severe neuropathic bladder using the hostility score. Dev Med Child Neurol. 1992;34(5):441–7.
11. Piaggio L, Myers S, Figueroa TE, Barthold JS, González R. Influence of type of conduit and site of implantation on the outcome of continent catheterizable channels. J Pediatr Urol. 2007;3(3):230–4.
12. Ivančić V, Defoor W, Jackson E, Alam S, Minevich E, Reddy P, Sheldon C. Progression of renal insufficiency in children and adolescents with neuropathic bladder is not accelerated by lower urinary tract reconstruction. J Urol. 2010;184(4 Suppl):1768–74.
13. Gundeti MS, Acharya SS, Zagaja GP. The University of Chicago technique of complete intracorporeal pediatric robotic-assisted laparoscopic augmentation ileocystoplasty and Mitrofanoff appendicovesicostomy. J Robot Surg. 2009;3(2):89–93.
14. Gundeti MS, Godbole PP, Wilcox DT. Is bowel preparation required before cystoplasty in children? J Urol. 2006;176:1574–6.
15. Marchetti P, Razmaria A, Zagaja GP, Gundeti MS. Management of the ventriculo-peritoneal shunt in pediatric patients during robot-assisted laparoscopic urologic procedures. J Endourol. 2011;25(2):225–9.
16. Landau EH, Gofrit ON, Cipele H, et al. Superiority of the VQZ over the tubularized skin flap and the umbilicus for continent abdominal stoma in children. J Urol. 2008;180:1761–6.
17. Gundeti MS, Acharya SS, Zagaja GP, Shalhav AL. Paediatric robotic-assisted laparoscopic augmentation ileocystoplasty and Mitrofanoff appendicovesicostomy (RALIMA): feasibility of and initial experience with the University of Chicago technique. BJU Int. 2011;107(6):962–9.
18. Murthy P, Cohn JA, Selig RB, Gundeti MS. Robot-assisted laparoscopic augmentation ileocystoplasty and Mitrofanoffappendicovesicostomy in children: updated interim results. Eur Urol. 2015;68:1069–75.
19. Nguyen HT, Passerotti CC, Penna FJ, Retik AB, Peters CA. Robotic assisted laparoscopic Mitrofanoff appendicovesicostomy: preliminary experience in a pediatric population. J Urol. 2009;182:1528–34.
20. Harris CF, Cooper CS, Hutcheson JC, Snyder HM 3rd. Appendicovesicostomy: the mitrofanoff procedure-a 15-year perspective. J Urol. 2000;163:1922–6.
21. Thomas JC, Dietrich MS, Trusler L, DeMarco RT, Pope JC 4th, Brock JW 3rd, Adams MC. Continent catheterizable channels and the timing of their complications. J Urol. 2006;176:1816–20.
22. Flood HD, Malhotra SJ, O'Connell HE, Ritchey MJ, Bloom DA, McGuire EJ. Long-term results and complications using augmentation cystoplasty in reconstructive urology. Neurourol Urodyn. 1995;14(4):297–309.
23. Schlomer BJ, Copp HL. Cumulative incidence of outcomes and urologic procedures after augmentation cystoplasty. J Pediatr Urol. 2014;113:468–75.

24. Famakinwa OJ, Rosen AM, Gundeti MS. Robot-assisted laparoscopic Mitrofanoff appendicovesicostomy technique and outcomes of extravesical and intravesical approaches. Eur Urol. 2013;64:831–6.
25. Atala A, Bauer SB, Soker S, Yoo JJ, Retik AB. Tissue-engineered autologous bladders for patients needing cystoplasty. Lancet. 2006;367:1241–6.
26. Joseph DB, Borer JG, De Filippo RE, Hodges SJ, McLorie GA. Autologous cell seeded biodegradable scaffold for augmentation cystoplasty: phase II study in children and adolescents with spina bifida. J Urol. 2014;191(5):1389–95.

Robot-Assisted Bladder Surgery for Nonmalignant Conditions in the Pediatric Patient (Bladder Diverticulectomy, Urachal Cyst Excision, and Cystolithotomy)

20

Jonathan A. Gerber and Chester J. Koh

Background and Epidemiology

Bladder diverticula, urachal anomalies, and bladder stones in children are individually rare occurrences. Bladder diverticula have been reported to occur in 1.7% of children with most being asymptomatic [1, 2]. Urachal anomalies have been estimated to occur in roughly 1% of the general pediatric population [3]. Of these 1%, roughly 8% will require extirpative surgery [3]. Bladder stones are more likely to occur in pediatric patients with prior bladder augmentation due to altered bladder dynamics, poor compliance with mucous irrigation, and metabolic changes associated with intestinal augmentation. When bladder stones occur, extraction is required to reduce the risk of infection, obstruction, and bladder perforation. This chapter reviews surgical techniques for the minimally invasive treatment of these conditions.

Bladder Diverticulum

Bladder diverticula may be asymptomatic and thus not require any intervention. However, symptomatic diverticula require surgical excision. Symptomatic

Supplementary Information The online version of this chapter (https://doi.org/10.1007/978-3-030-50196-9_20) contains supplementary material, which is available to authorized users.

J. A. Gerber
Division of Pediatric Urology, Department of Surgery, Texas Children's Hospital, Houston, TX, USA

Scott Department of Urology, Baylor College of Medicine, Houston, TX, USA

C. J. Koh (✉)
Division of Pediatric Urology, Texas Children's Hospital - Baylor College of Medicine, Houston, TX, USA
e-mail: ckoh@bcm.edu

© Springer Nature Switzerland AG 2022
M. D. Stifelman et al. (eds.), *Techniques of Robotic Urinary Tract Reconstruction*, https://doi.org/10.1007/978-3-030-50196-9_20

diverticula most often present as recurrent urinary tract infections (UTI) due to urinary stasis within the adynamic diverticulum. In rare instances, very large diverticula may prolapse and cause obstruction of the urethra which can subsequently result in bladder perforation. Traditionally, the management of symptomatic diverticula is with open surgical excision. Over the last 30 years, however, laparoscopic surgery has come to the forefront of the surgical world due to its ability to provide a more cosmetically pleasing result and shorter postoperative hospital stay compared to open surgery. More recently, traditional laparoscopy has been replaced by the use of the da Vinci robot surgical system (Intuitive Surgical, Sunnyvale, California). The wide acceptance of these technologies has spread into the realm of pediatric surgery as well, with a larger number and variety of procedures being performed robotically. Many case reports and one small series of 14 patients who underwent robot-assisted laparoscopic bladder diverticulectomy have been published in the pediatric literature [4–6].

Port Placement and Instrumentation

In general, the robot-assisted laparoscopic approach to all pelvic and bladder surgeries will require similar port placement with only minor adjustments as needed for each particular case. In all cases, a cystoscopy is recommended to aid in the recognition of divergent anatomy and proximity of pathology to the ureteral orifices and to allow placement of a ureteral stent to help identify the ureters during dissection and excision. A Foley catheter should then be placed on the sterile field to allow complete drainage of the bladder during port placement so as to avoid injury to the bladder. The presence of a Foley will also allow the bedside assistant to distend the bladder, once indicated, for identification of the diverticulum for excision.

In our experience, most bladder surgeries will involve a standard setup with placement of an 8.5 mm (12 mm optional) camera port at the umbilicus and two 5 mm (8 mm optional) instrument ports on each side of the camera port, lateral to the rectus muscles, at the level of the umbilicus (Fig. 20.1). An assistant port is optional and can be placed superiorly, between one instrument port and the camera port.

Our preferred method of obtaining pneumoperitoneum is via the open Hasson technique or with the aid of a Veress needle at the umbilicus. The 8.5 or 12 mm camera port is then placed, with port size based on patient size and surgeon preference. A zero degree camera is inserted via the camera port to assess for any damage caused by the Veress needle or camera port insertions. Next, the two 5 mm (or 8 mm) instrument ports are placed at the midaxillary lines, lateral to the rectus muscles, at the same level as the camera port, under direct vision. At this point, approximately 30° Trendelenburg position should be obtained to allow for cephalad displacement of the intestines out of the pelvis. After successful port placement and adjustment into Trendelenburg position, the robot should be docked from the foot position. If the patient's height precludes docking at the feet, then the robot can be brought in from the side of the legs. Our preferred instruments are the DeBakey grasper in the left hand and the monopolar hook or scissors in the right hand.

Surgical Approach

The bladder is then distended with saline via the Foley catheter to allow visualization of the bladder and diverticulum. Some surgeons, as noted in studies on adult patients, advocate utilizing a cystoscope in order to illuminate and better identify the diverticulum from within the bladder [7]. Once the diverticulum is identified, an opening in the peritoneum is made at the level of the diverticulum, and dissection is carried down to the neck of the diverticulum (Fig. 20.2). If the edge of the neck of the diverticulum is an adequate distance from the ureteral orifice, the diverticulum

Fig. 20.1 Standard port placement for pelvic surgery

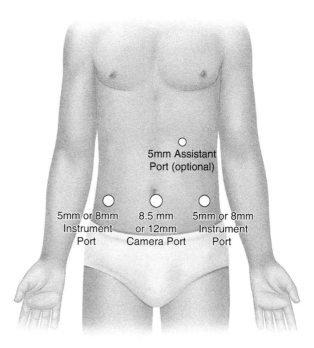

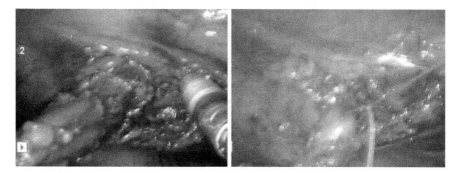

Figs. 20.2 and 20.3 Identification of the neck of the diverticulum and placement of a purse-string stitch at the neck of the diverticulum

may be excised circumferentially. Placement of a purse-string stitch at the level of the neck of the diverticulum is an option at this point, prior to excision of the diverticulum (Fig. 20.3). Dissection and excision are done with both blunt and sharp dissection as well as electrocautery. Once the diverticulum is excised, the cystotomy is closed in two layers starting with the mucosal layer. A 4-0 absorbable suture is used for both the mucosal and muscle layers. If a purse-string stitch was used, the mucosal layer should be closed adequately; therefore only closure of the detrusor layer is required.

When the diverticulum is near the ureteral orifice and there is concern about its proximity, it is recommended to place a ureteral catheter. When vesicoureteral reflux (VUR) is present in association with a diverticulum, then an extravesical ureteroneocystostomy can be performed concomitantly.

Once the cystotomy is closed, we ensure that it is watertight by filling the bladder with saline to visualize any leakage. If a leak is noted, a simple figure-of-eight stitch with the same 4-0 absorbable suture will usually suffice. The Foley catheter is then replaced and should remain in place for at least 1 day, although longer durations are optional. A Jackson-Pratt (JP) drain can be placed at the surgeon's discretion.

Urachal Anomalies

Urachal anomalies are most often discovered incidentally at the time of abdominal imaging obtained for other reasons [3]. Roughly 8% of incidentally discovered urachal anomalies will subsequently undergo surgery for a multitude of reasons—UTIs, abdominal pain, and/or persistent umbilical drainage [3]. The standard of care for symptomatic urachal anomalies remains extirpative therapy with surgical excision. Most often, excision is performed in an open fashion; however many urologists both in the adult and pediatric realm have demonstrated equivalent success with laparoscopic and robot-assisted laparoscopic approaches compared to the open approach [8–10].

Port Placement and Instrumentation

At the outset of the procedure, we first perform a cystoscopy and possible cystography to aid in the identification of a possible connection between the bladder and the urachal remnant. A Foley catheter is then placed on the sterile field to drain the bladder completely. Similar to our approach to bladder diverticulum as described previously, the patient is placed in the supine position, all pressure points are padded, and pneumoperitoneum is obtained via the open Hasson technique or with the aid of a Veress needle. In contrast to our port placement during bladder diverticulectomy, the camera port is placed in a more cephalad position to provide better visualization of the more cephalad urachal structure. An 8.5 or 12 mm camera port is placed in the midline roughly midway between the umbilicus and xyphoid process. Instrument ports (5 or 8 mm, depending on availability and surgeon preference) are placed at the midaxillary lines bilaterally at, or just slightly cephalad to, the level of the umbilicus (Fig. 20.4). An assistant port is optional and may be placed in the

Fig. 20.4 Port placement for urachal anomaly excision

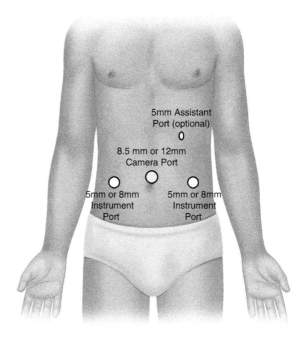

upper abdominal quadrant on either side, depending on the location of the bedside assistant.

The patient is then placed into 30° Trendelenburg to displace the intestines cephalad and out of the pelvis. The robot is then brought in over the feet and docked. We advocate using a DeBakey grasper in the left hand and either a hook (5 mm) or monopolar-connected scissors (8 mm only) in the right hand for dissection purposes. The camera is a zero degree lens.

Surgical Approach

Initial dissection focuses on lysis of omental adhesions which often are present and adherent to the urachal remnant. Identification of the bilateral obliterated umbilical arteries (medial umbilical ligaments) is required to aid in the definition of the relevant anatomy (Fig. 20.5). Next, cauterization and division of one or both obliterated umbilical arteries are advised in order to gain access to the anterior bladder wall. The superior aspect of the urachus is then freed from the abdominal wall and used as a handle to aid in the dissection of the remainder of the urachus from the abdominal wall to the level of the bladder dome. Dissection is extended until adequate visualization of the anterior bladder wall caudal to the urachus is obtained. At this point, a hitch stitch placed into the anterior bladder wall is useful to maintain visualization during and after excision of the urachus with a bladder cuff. Next, the urachus is excised using a combination of sharp and electrocautery dissection with a small bladder cuff included with the urachal specimen (Fig. 20.6). The bladder

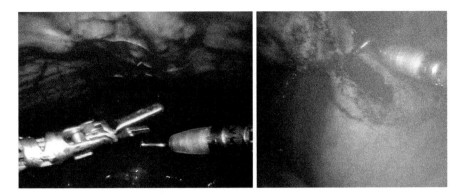

Figs. 20.5 and 20.6 Identification of medial umbilical ligaments and excision of bladder cuff attached to urachal remnant

defect is closed in two layers using 4-0 absorbable suture in a running fashion. Leak testing is performed with instillation of saline via the Foley catheter. The specimen is then placed into a laparoscopic pouch and removed under direct visualization via one of the port sites.

Bladder Stones

Patients with bladder stones comprise a significant portion of adult urology practices. For pediatric urologists, bladder stones are seen at a much lower rate and almost exclusively occur in children with a history of bladder augmentation. Studies have shown the incidence of bladder stones in children with prior bladder augmentation at 10–11% [11, 12]. Upon discovery of bladder stones, surgical removal is warranted. Historically, cystolithotomy has been done in an open fashion with excellent results. With the trend toward minimally invasive approaches, laparoscopic and robot-assisted laparoscopic approaches to bladder stones have become more prevalent.

Port Placement and Instrumentation

As seen in Fig. 20.1, the port placement for robotic cystolithotomy is identical to that of bladder diverticulectomy. The camera port is placed at the umbilicus (if no appendicovesicostomy (APV) at the umbilicus) or 5 cm superior to the umbilicus if an APV is present. Two working instrument ports are placed at the level of the umbilicus just lateral to the rectus muscles, and an optional assistant port is placed superiorly between a working instrument port and the camera port, on either side. Thirty degrees Trendelenburg positioning is instituted to displace the intestines, and the abdominal anatomy is inspected. Special attention is necessary at this step as many patients with bladder augmentation had concomitant placement of an APV which requires careful consideration of anatomy in order to avoid disruption of a sometimes tenuous appendiceal mesentery and blood supply. Intestinal adhesions are taken down only in the areas where there is impediment of safe access to the bladder or for improved working space for the robotic instruments. The bladder is filled with saline via the Foley catheter to aid in the identification of the anatomy. Two hitch stitch sutures of 2-0 PDS are placed through the anterior surface of the bladder near the dome. These sutures aid in retraction upon entry into the bladder. After placement of the hitch stitches, the bladder is opened vertically between the sutures. Entry into the bladder should be done with electrocautery to avoid excessive blood loss. Occasionally, prior augmentation precludes entry into the native bladder, and entry into the augmented portion of the bladder is required. The approach is the same in either instance. Special attention is needed if there is an APV or the ureters were previously reimplanted in order to avoid damage to these vital structures. Once the cystotomy is made, the bladder stones should be readily visible. A specimen removal bag is then placed via the assistant port, and the bladder stones are removed from the bladder and placed into the specimen bag. Once all stones have been removed, bladder closure is performed in two layers with 4-0 absorbable suture. The hitch stitches should be loosened incrementally during the cystorrhaphy to reduce tension on the suture line. Once the cystorrhaphy is completed, the hitch stitches should be removed. Leak test is performed by filling the bladder with saline and looking for evidence of leakage. A JP drain may be placed at the surgeon's discretion.

Next, the robot is undocked, the patient is replaced into the supine position, and the specimen bag is removed via the umbilical camera port incision. The fascia is closed followed by closure of the skin in the usual fashion. Due to the history of bladder augmentation, the Foley can remain in place for an extended period (3–5 days) to avoid bladder leakage. A cystogram may be performed postoperatively according to surgeon preference.

Conclusion

Benign bladder conditions, such as bladder diverticula, urachal anomalies, and bladder stones, are rare in children. Robot-assisted laparoscopic techniques offer a minimally invasive treatment option as an alternative to open surgery.

References

1. Psutka SP, Cendron M. Bladder diverticula in children. J Pediatr Urol. 2013;9(2):129–38. https://doi.org/10.1016/j.jpurol.2012.02.013.
2. Blane CE, Zerin JM, Bloom DA. Bladder diverticula in children. Radiology. 1994;190(3):695–7. https://doi.org/10.1148/radiology.190.3.8115613.
3. Gleason JM, Bowlin PR, Bagli DJ, Lorenzo AJ, Hassouna T, Koyle MA, Farhat WA. A comprehensive review of pediatric urachal anomalies and predictive analysis for adult urachal adenocarcinoma. J Urol. 2015;193(2):632–6. https://doi.org/10.1016/j.juro.2014.09.004.

4. Noh PH, Bansal D. Pediatric robotic assisted laparoscopy for paraureteral bladder diverticulum excision with ureteral reimplantation. J Pediatr Urol. 2013;9(1):e28–30. https://doi.org/10.1016/j.jpurol.2012.06.011.

5. Christman MS, Casale P. Robot-assisted bladder diverticulectomy in the pediatric population. J Endourol. 2012;26(10):1296–300. https://doi.org/10.1089/end.2012.0051.

6. Meeks JJ, Hagerty JA, Lindgren BW. Pediatric robotic-assisted laparoscopic Diverticulectomy. Urology. 2009;73(2):299–301. https://doi.org/10.1016/j.urology.2008.06.068.

7. Macejko AM, Viprakasit DP, Nadler RB. Cystoscope- and robot-assisted bladder diverticulectomy. J Endourol. 2008;22(10):2389–92. https://doi.org/10.1089/end.2008.0385.

8. Yamzon J, Kokorowski P, Filippo RED, Chang AY, Hardy BE, Koh CJ. Pediatric robot-assisted laparoscopic excision of urachal cyst and bladder cuff. J Endourol. 2008;22(10):2385–8. https://doi.org/10.1089/end.2008.0338.

9. Lee H-E, Jeong CW, Ku JH. Robot-assisted laparoscopic management of urachal cysts in adults. J Robot Surg. 2010;4(2):133–5. https://doi.org/10.1007/s11701-010-0190-2.

10. Madeb R, Knopf JK, Nicholson C, Donahue LA, Adcock B, Dever D, et al. The use of robotically assisted surgery for treating urachal anomalies. BJU Int. 2006;98(4):838–42. https://doi.org/10.1111/j.1464-410x.2006.06430.x.

11. Kronner KM, Casale AJ, Cain MP, Zerin MJ, Keating MA, Rink RC. Bladder calculi in the pediatric augmented bladder. J Urol. 1998;160(3 Pt 2):1096–8; discussion 1103

12. DeFoor W, Minevich E, Reddy P, Sekhon D, Polsky E, Wacksman J, Sheldon C. Bladder calculi after augmentation cystoplasty: risk factors and prevention strategies. J Urol. 2004;172(5) Pt 1:1964–6.

Part VII

Urinary Diversion: Introduction

Lee Zhao

This section covers robotic urinary diversions. The visualization and dexterity of robotics allows one to adhere to the principles of delicate tissue handling, edge to edge approximation, and watertight anastomosis. All these advantages should lead to potential benefits for better ureterointestinal and vesicourethral anastomosis. Another benefit is the ease of revision surgery. While the primary goal of surgery is to reduce complications, the need for revision surgery in some patients is inevitable. Decreased bowel handling from robotic surgery leads to fewer adhesions, meaning that access to the peritoneum is easier, which reduces a barrier to revision surgery.

Surgical Complications After Robot-Assisted Radical Cystectomy

21

Ahmed S. Elsayed, Naif A. Aldhaam, Richard Sarle,
Ahmed A. Hussein, and Khurshid A. Guru

Introduction

Robot-assisted radical cystectomy (RARC) has been shown to provide equivalent oncologic outcomes when compared to open radical cystectomy (ORC) [1, 2]. Regardless of the approach, radical cystectomy remains a morbid procedure with high complication rate (24–64%) [3, 4]. While nonstandardization of reporting complications may have contributed to the high rate of complications, efforts have been made to incorporate care pathways to improve quality of care. RARC is a technically demanding procedure, especially with intracorporeal urinary diversion [5, 6], with an acceptable level of proficiency that can be achieved by the 30th case [7]. Currently, robot-assisted repair for most surgical complications related to RARC is feasible but limited to high-volume and experienced surgeons. Other complications such as gas embolism, stress ulcer, deep vein thrombosis, pulmonary embolism, urinary tract infections, vesicoureteral reflux, vitamin B12 deficiency, and skin maceration are out of the scope of this chapter. This chapter addresses preventive measures and tips of robot-assisted surgical repair for complications that usually require surgical intervention.

Supplementary Information The online version of this chapter (https://doi.org/10.1007/978-3-030-50196-9_21) contains supplementary material, which is available to authorized users.

A. S. Elsayed · N. A. Aldhaam · A. A. Hussein · K. A. Guru (✉)
Department of Urology, Roswell Park Comprehensive Cancer Center, Buffalo, NY, USA
e-mail: Ahmed.Elsayed@roswellpark.org; Naif.Aldhaam@roswellpark.org; Ahmed.aly@roswellpark.org; Khurshid.Guru@roswellpark.org

R. Sarle
Michigan State University, Lansing, MI, USA

Sparrow Hospital, Lansing, MI, USA

© Springer Nature Switzerland AG 2022
M. D. Stifelman et al. (eds.), *Techniques of Robotic Urinary Tract Reconstruction*, https://doi.org/10.1007/978-3-030-50196-9_21

Intraoperative Complications

Rectal Injury

The incidence of rectal injury during RARC is 0.2–1.5% [4]. Rectal injury is more common in male patients with a previously irradiated pelvis and in high-stage bladder cancer (T3b-T4). It occurs due to either direct injury or indirect transmitted thermal energy.

How to Prevent Rectal Injury During RARC?
It is best avoided by meticulous dissection with forward sweeping of the posterior bladder wall and prostate away from the rectum, with athermal dissection while developing the anterior rectal space. The plane between posterior and anterior layers of Denonvilliers' fascia is preferred to the dissection, rather than the perirectal fat.

Diagnosis
Immediate diagnosis intraoperatively is vital. Appearance of bowel or fecal contents in the pelvic cavity, positive rectal test (performed by irrigating the pelvis with saline and observed for the presence of air bubbles upon slow introduction of air through the rectal tube), or visualization of blood on examining finger during digital rectal examination.

Management

Intraoperative Identification
Immediate repair is the hallmark for management. The repair depends on the type of injury (thermal vs sharp cut), size, and degree of spillage of fecal matter. For small injuries (<2 cm) with minimal spillage, repair of the rectal wall is performed with two-layer closure after refreshing the edges and copious irrigation (Fig. 21.1). The first layer is full thickness, interrupted in a watertight fashion with absorbable sutures (2/0 Vicryl). The second layer includes the perirectal fat and serosal layer of the rectum for reinforcement in continuous manner with absorbable sutures (Video 21.1). The repair is preferably covered with an omental flap (Video 21.2). For larger (>2 cm) or massive thermal injuries (especially monopolar) or gross spillage, it is preferred to perform a diverting colostomy.

Late Identification
The patient usually presents with fever, nausea, vomiting, signs of peritonitis, and leukopenia or leukocytosis (with left shift) on complete blood picture. Computed tomography (CT) scan with oral and rectal contrast is the mainstay for diagnosis. If rectal injury is confirmed, an immediate exploratory laparotomy should be performed to achieve three goals: generous irrigation of the abdomen with saline, repair

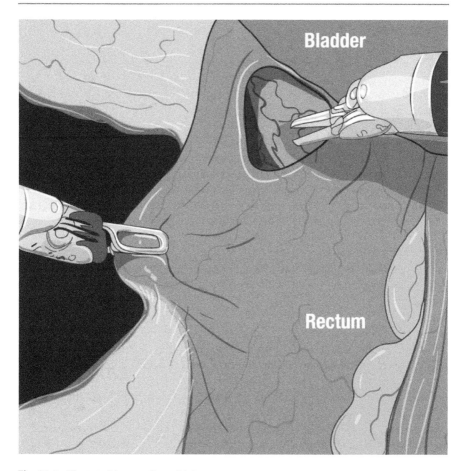

Fig. 21.1 Illustrated image of rectal injury

of the rectal injury if possible, and a diverting colostomy and GI surgery consultation if needed.

Postoperative Care

Nothing per oral (NPO) intake for at least 2 days postoperatively with a nasogastric tube for 1–2 days. Patients are instructed to ambulate as soon as they are able to. Once the patient is clinically stable with active bowel sounds, the NGT is clamped, and a clear fluid diet is started. Once tolerated, diet can be further advanced gradually. Once the patient tolerates full diet and passes stool, the intra-abdominal drain can be removed, and the patient is discharged. For patients with diversion colostomy, closure of the colostomy may be performed 6 weeks later after ensuring rectal integrity.

Bowel Injury

Bowel injury can happen during the Veress needle insertion, trocar placement, direct injury with robotic instruments, or thermal injury. Reports from large multi-institutional studies of laparoscopic (Lap) and robot-assisted urologic procedures reported an incidence of approximately 1.3 per 1000 cases [3].

How to Prevent Bowel Injury During RARC?
Insulation and integrity of lap/robotic instruments in use should be confirmed. It is critical to introduce and keep the instruments under vision all the time. Assistants should be careful when advancing instruments into the surgical field without direct visualization. Patients with previous abdominal surgeries and/or radiation may have intra-abdominal adhesions and are more susceptible to injuries during adhesiolysis [8].

Diagnosis
Immediate diagnosis intraoperatively is of paramount importance. Injury may vary from superficial serosal to full-thickness tears or thermal injuries.

Management
Bowel injuries vary according to the type of bowel injured (small vs large bowel). The management of both will follow the same principles, but for large bowel injuries, the surgeon should have a low threshold for a diverting colostomy in case of significant fecal spillage. The bowel loops are inspected carefully looking for any bowel content spillage or serosal tear. If the injury is small and less than 30% of bowel circumference, it can be repaired with two layers of interrupted sutures (serosa should be sutured). For large or full-thickness bowel wall injuries, resection and primary anastomosis are preferred. The continuity of the bowel can be restored intracorporeally with the aid of a suprapubic port to ease bowel reanastomosis. A 60-mm Endo GIA stapler is inserted through the short 12 mm suprapubic port. Two sequential side to side anastomoses are performed after both ends of the bowel are aligned along their anti-mesenteric borders (Fig. 21.2). The open ends of the two anastomosed intestinal segments are stapled by firing an Endo GIA stapler horizontally via the assistant's port. The mesentery window is closed using a 3-0 silk suture to avoid internal hernia.

Postoperative Care
It is advisable to keep the nasogastric tube for 1–2 days. Once the patient is clinically stable with active bowel sounds, the NGT is clamped, and clear fluid diet can be started. Diet should be advanced as tolerated and the NGT is removed.

Vascular Injury

Vascular injury is less than 5% following RARC [9]. The most common site of bleeding is avulsion of small tributaries of the common iliac vein during extended pelvic

Fig. 21.2 Illustrated image showing side to side bowel anastomosis

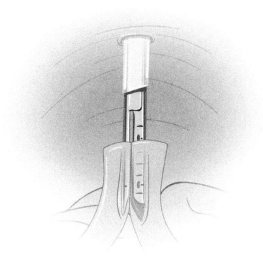

lymph node dissection [10]. Vascular injury can be divided into abdominal wall related (inferior epigastric vessels) and those the pelvis or the retroperitoneum.

Iliac Vessels

This can occur during a bulky pelvic lymph node dissection, using thermal dissection around the vein, extensive traction, or poor handling of the vessels.

How to Prevent Iliac Vessel Injury During RARC?

Sound knowledge of the pelvic vascular anatomy is a key (Fig. 21.3). Blunt dissection should be carried out along the vessels with direct visualization of the vessels. If thermal instruments are used, care should be taken to avoid contact with vessels.

Diagnosis

Any vascular injury needs to be repaired immediately.

Management

The first step is applying adequate compression to control the bleeding and then raising the pneumoperitoneum to 20 mm Hg. 4-0 or 5-0 Prolene sutures are used to repair the defect in a continuous fashion. There is a low threshold to convert to open and to consult vascular surgery if needed (Video 21.3).

Fig. 21.3 Illustrated
pelvic vascular anatomy

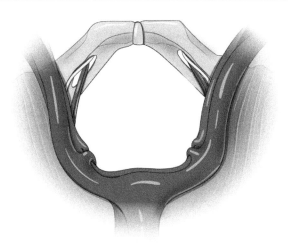

Postoperative Care

Anticoagulants may be needed during the postoperative course based on the extent
of the injury and the vascular surgery recommendations. Ipsilateral lower limb viability needs to be monitored.

Obturator Nerve Injury

The obturator nerve is encountered during the pelvic lymph node dissection. Injury
might occur while performing a bulky lymphadenectomy.

How to Prevent Obturator Nerve Injury During RARC?

During pelvic lymph node dissection, sound knowledge of the pelvic anatomy is
important (Fig. 21.4). We adopted the zonal dissection technique of the pelvic
lymph nodes. Lymph nodes lateral and proximal to the common iliac vessels are
dissected first followed by the triangle of Marseille and then connected anteriorly
with the area near the obturator nerve. This technique allows better visualization of
the obturator nerve [11].

Diagnosis

The best time to repair the injury is intraoperatively. Postoperative presentation of nerve
injuries are confirmed by electrophysiological and neurosonographic studies [12].

Management

If the obturator nerve is completely transected (neurotmesis) and identified intraoperatively [13], this injury should be repaired immediately through an epineural
end-to-end repair microscopically by the neurosurgical team using 9-0 or 10-0

Fig. 21.4 Illustrated image of the obturator nerve

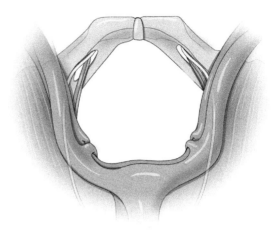

nylon sutures [12]. If identified later (clinical presentation of neuropraxia or axonotmesis), management may differ due to the presence of an accessory obturator nerve in 25% of the patients. Therefore, the patient's presentation determines further management [13].

Postoperative Care
Physiotherapy will be needed with almost full recovery ranging between 6 weeks and 6 months according to the type of the injury and timing of the repair for neurotmesis cases [14].

Acute Postoperative Complications

Bowel-Related Complications

Bowel Obstruction
Bowel obstruction after RARC is common and usually involves the small intestine. Reoperation due to small bowel-related complications after RARC occurs in 12% of cases [15]. In cases of mechanical bowel obstruction due to internal hernia, ischemia, or twisted bowel segment, most of the cases require surgical management after resuscitation of the patient.

How to Prevent Bowel Obstruction After RARC?
During RARC, the mesenteric defect after restoration of bowel continuity should be sutured and closed; avoid unnecessary manipulation and handling of the bowel, and use adhesive barriers if possible to reduce adhesions in the future. Bowel loops should be carefully inspected for any color changes. If noticed, warm packs should be applied, while observing for color changes and peristalsis. If this persists,

resection and primary anastomosis should be done. Indocyanine green (ICG) can be administered intravenously (10 mg) with the Firefly® fluorescence to assess blood perfusion to the bowel ends before anastomosis.

Diagnosis

The patient usually presents with nausea, vomiting, and abdominal distension. The diagnosis is initially suspected by an erect abdominal X-ray. CT scan of the abdomen/pelvis with oral and IV contrast and identification of a transition point or absence of contrast material in the rectum may be visulaized (Fig. 21.5).

Paralytic Ileus

Intracorporeal urinary diversion may decrease third space loss and decrease the incidence of ileus [16]. The treatment is usually conservative (drip and suck) with replacing of electrolytes, NPO, insertion of nasogastric tube, and intravenous fluids.

How to Prevent Ileus After RARC?

Early patient ambulation, avoidance of opioids, and the use of prokinetic drugs will help prevent paralytic ileus [17].

Diagnosis

The patient usually presents with nausea, vomiting, and abdominal distension. The diagnosis is initially suspected by an erect abdominal X-ray. The best way to confirm bowel obstruction is with a CT scan of the abdomen/pelvis with oral and IV contrast.

Fig. 21.5 CT abdomen/pelvis showing dilate bowel loops most likely due to bowel obstruction

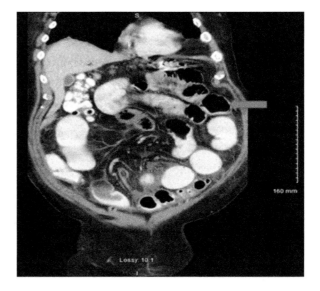

Management

Conservative management includes stabilization of the general condition, NGT placement, urethral catheter, correction of electrolyte imbalances, and maintaining patient's hydration. Prokinetic agents such as alvimopan and metoclopramide can help the recovery of bowel function. Judicious use of opioids as they may slow down bowel movement. Using acetaminophen and nonsteroidal anti-inflammatory drugs has been incorporated as part of enhanced recovery after surgery (ERAS) pathway to limit the effect of opioids on bowel recovery. Naldemedine is a new mu opioid agonist that has shown promising results [18].

If conservative measures fail or the clinical condition worsens (worsening pain, vomiting, fever, worsening distension, leukocytosis), surgical exploration is warranted. Open laparotomy is recommended; however, robot-assisted approach depends on the experience of the surgeon. For patients with signs of peritonitis, hemodynamic instability, or severely dilated bowel loops with small room for pneumoperitoneum, the open approach is preferred. For robot-assisted approach, use either Veress needle or open (Hasson) technique for pneumoperitoneum. The Veress needle can be inserted at a higher position or in the left upper quadrant (Palmer's point) to avoid possibly adherent bowel loops [19, 20]. Laparoscopic adhesiolysis may be needed to facilitate insertion of other robotic ports. Extensive adhesiolysis may be required which may affect bowel integrity. Bowel loops should be carefully inspected for any color changes. If noticed, warm packs should be applied, while observing for color changes and peristalsis. If this persists, resection and primary anastomosis should be done. Indocyanine green (ICG) can be administered intravenously (10 mg) with the Firefly® fluorescence to assess blood perfusion to the bowel ends before anastomosis.

If the cause of the obstruction is internal hernia, try to retrieve the herniated bowel segment through internal defect, and then assess viability; if viable close the internal defect with interrupted nonabsorbable sutures. Regardless of the cause, an intra-abdominal drain and nasogastric tube should be left in place.

Postoperative Care

The patient should be monitored clinically for nausea or vomiting, passing flatus, or stool and drain output. The NGT is removed on day 2 postoperatively. Once the patient is clinically stable with active bowel sounds, the NGT is clamped, and a clear fluid diet is started. If the patient is tolerating clear fluids, the NGT is removed. Then the diet should be advanced as tolerated.

Bowel Anastomosis Leakage

Urinary diversion is a fundamental step of RARC. The most commonly used intestinal segment during the diversion is the ileum. Gastrointestinal complications are the commonest post-RARC. The rate of anastomosis leak post-radical cystectomy ranges from 0.3% to 8.7% [21]. Predictors for bowel leak from the GI literature on a multivariate regression analysis included male gender, Charlson comorbidity index of three or more, intraoperative adverse events, and longer operative times [22].

How to Prevent Bowel Leakage After RARC?

There should be a sound surgical technique, maintenance of good nutritional status, and adherence to the enhanced recovery after surgery (ERAS) protocol. The bowel should be handled gently during surgery, ensuring adequate blood supply to the bowel ends, refreshing the the edges, and ensuring a watertight anastomosis. A stapler or hand-sewn anastomosis is equally effective [23].

Diagnosis

Postoperative bowel leakage may present acutely as peritonitis or a more insidious onset. Patients with peritonitis will complain of an agonizing abdominal pain, fever, abdominal tenderness, and rebound tenderness along with signs of sepsis. Insidious onset may be due to a contained bowel leakage. Insidious presentation will include low-grade fever, prolonged ileus, or diet intolerance. Clinical assessment can be confirmed with a CT abdomen and pelvis with both oral and IV contrast (Fig. 21.6).

Management

Management of this complication includes urgent patient's resuscitation and transfer to the OR. Urgent laparotomy is the choice through a midline incision. Formal exploration of the bowel is warranted with identification of the leaking anastomosis. A search for other bowel injury may be the cause and missed intra-operatively. After generous peritoneal irrigation, resection of the leaking anastomosis and refreshing of the intestinal edges are performed. Depending on intraoperative findings, bowel anastomosis or proximal diversion is performed. The abdomen is closed with two wide bore drains. In cases of early discovery of bowel leak, a robot-assisted approach may be feasible but limited to high-volume centers with expert robotic surgeons [15].

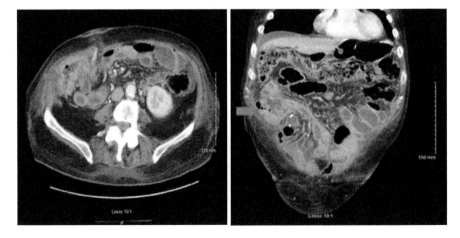

Fig. 21.6 CT abdomen/pelvis showing bowel anastomosis leak

Postoperative Care

The patient is kept NPO for at least 2 days postoperative with intra-abdominal drain and NGT for 1–2 days. The patient is instructed to ambulate as soon as possible. Once the patient is clinically stable with active bowel sounds, the NGT is clamped, and clear fluid diet is started. If the patient is tolerating clear fluids, the NGT is removed. Then the diet should be advanced as tolerated.

Urinary Leakage and Acute Urinary Tract Obstruction

Urinary leakage rate is 6% after RARC [15]. Usually, it happens due to edema or because of a technical error at the site of ureteroileal anastomosis. Slippage of the ureteric stents or clogging of the draining catheter with mucus in cases of orthotopic urinary diversion can also cause a urine leak. Acute urinary tract obstruction is usually related to poor surgical techniques such as incorporating the anterior and posterior wall of the ureter during ureteroileal anastomosis or because of the presence of ureteral edema from excessive handling.

How to Prevent Urine Leakage After RARC?

It is critical to adhere to the principles of anastomosis such as minimal handling of the ureters and the ileum, ensuring adequate blood supply to the ureteric ends, generous spatulation of the ureters, ensuring a watertight anastomosis, trans-anastomotic stenting, and good drainage. There is no difference in the leakage rates between the Bricker and Wallace techniques for ureteroileal anastomosis [24]. Indocyanine green (ICG) can be administered intravenously (10 mg) with the Firefly® fluorescence to assess blood perfusion to the bowel and ureters before anastomosis.

Diagnosis

Postoperative urine leakage is asymptomatic most of the time and usually present as an increased drain output. Diagnosis is confirmed by measuring creatinine level from the drain and CT urography or pouchogram.

Management

Management includes ensuring proper function of the draining catheter in orthotopic diversions and irrigation of the neobladder to avoid blockage by a mucus plug. A "wait and see" approach may be first adopted until the edema of the site of anastomosis resolves. If failed, urinary diversion with nephrostomy tube or antegrade stenting may be performed.

Postoperative Care

The drain output is monitored. If the drain output is insignificant for 48 hours, it is removed, and the patient is discharged with nephrostomy tubes in place. Late consequences of urine leak may include ureteroileal anastomosis stricture (discussed later in this chapter).

Conduit/Orthotopic Diversion Necrosis

Diversion necrosis is a rare but morbid complication (0–0.7%) [21]. It occurs due to compromised vascular supply to the isolated intestinal segment. This may be due to the twisting of the mesentery or overstretching of the mesentery of the conduit.

How to Prevent Diversion Necrosis After RARC?

During RARC ensure adequacy of the blood supply and integrity of the mesentery of the created pouch. Intravenous ICG and Firefly® technology can be used to ensure the adequacy of the blood supply.

Diagnosis

Diagnosis of necrosis is made clinically (Fig. 21.7). Clinically, the color of the stoma will darken, and the stoma may retract (≥0.5 cm) from the skin edge. Pricking of the stoma will not reveal bleeding. Scoping the conduit will reveal necrosis of the conduit from inside as well. The patient may become septic if diagnosis is delayed. For orthotopic diversions, color cannot be used for assessment. However, urinary fistulae may develop or the patient might present with sepsis.

Management

Urgent patient resuscitation and transfer to the OR. Urgent laparotomy is the choice through a midline incision. Formal exploration of the bowel is warranted with isolation of the necrotic segment. A new bowel segment is selected, and a surface

Fig. 21.7 Illustrated image showing conduit necrosis

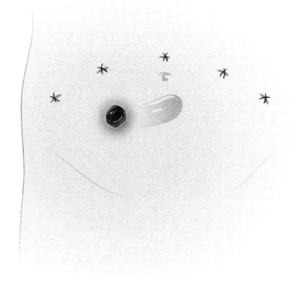

diversion is performed (either ileal conduit or uretero-cutaneous). The abdomen is closed over two wide bore drains.

Postoperative Care

The patient is kept NPO for at least 2 days postoperatively with an intra-abdominal drain, NGT for 1–2 days, and instructions to mobilize as soon as possible. Once the patient is clinically stable with active bowel sounds, the NGT is clamped. Clear fluid can be instated, and diet is advanced as tolerated.

Lymphocele

Lymphocele is the most common complication after pelvic lymphadenectomy. It occurs in 5% of the patients after open pelvic lymph node dissection [25].

How to Prevent Lymphocele After RARC?

A previous study showed that on multivariate analysis symptomatic lymphocele formation is associated with the number of lymph nodes dissected and the use of prophylactic low molecular weight heparin [26]. Another study has shown that the operating surgeon influences the rate of lymphocele formation [27]. Adequate clipping of all lymphatic vessels helps prevent lymphocele formation.

Diagnosis

The majority of the patients are asymptomatic, and lymphoceles are detected incidentally on follow-up images. Pelvic-abdominal ultrasound is the initial diagnostic tool and confirmation is achieved by CT abdomen/pelvis. Lymphoceles may get infected and cause fever and abdominal pain or compress the surroundings if large enough, for example, compression of pelvic veins causing lower extremity swelling [26].

Management

Asymptomatic small-volume lymphocele requires no treatment. Percutaneous drainage of the lymphocele is the treatment of choice if it is infected or if large enough to cause symptoms. For recurrent lymphoceles, laparoscopic marsupialization is preferred [27].

Late Postoperative Complications

Ureterointestinal Stricture

The cause of ureterointestinal stricture is either benign (ischemia) or malignant (primary or recurrence). Benign causes usually develop gradually over 1–2 years after RARC. Malignant causes are often symptomatic and progressive. Upper urinary tract recurrences are the most common late recurrences after cystectomy [28].

Ureteroileal strictures are more common on the left side (45% of all strictures) which may be attributed to higher dissection to facilitate crossing of the left ureter beneath the sigmoid mesentery [29]. Bilateral strictures occurred in 25%.

Hussein et al. reported the rate of 12% for surgical interventions for ureteroileal strictures after RARC [15]. Ureterointestinal stricture after RARC is associated with high body mass index (BMI), poor renal function preoperative, intracorporeal urinary diversion, urinary tract infections, and urine leak [29].

How to Prevent Occurrence of Stricture After RARC?

Minimal and meticulous ureteric handling, ensuring good blood supply (preserve adequate adventitia) for the distal ureteric stumps (can be confirmed with ICG and Firefly® technology fluorescence), generous spatulation, ensuring good drainage, excision of pathological segment, and stented anastomosis are excellent ways to avoid this complication. We prefer to retroperitonealize the ileal conduit to contain any leakage. There is no reported difference in stricture rates between the Wallace or Bricker techniques [24]. The use of tunneling anti-reflux mechanism (especially in the colon) was associated with higher risk of stricture.

Diagnosis

The patient might present with loin pain, recurrent urinary tract infections, or rising creatinine. The diagnosis of stricture is confirmed with CT urography, MAG3 renal scan, nephrostogram (if a nephrostomy tube was placed) (Fig. 21.8), or MRU.

Management

The first step is drainage of the dilated system with percutaneous nephrostomy tube to avoid consequences of obstruction such as infection or renal parenchymal loss. After drainage, the second step is to confirm the cause of the stricture (benign vs malignant). Endoscopic management should be tried first with dilatation and stenting, which will be enough in1/3 of cases [15]. Surgical revisions by open or robot-assisted approach give more durable results.

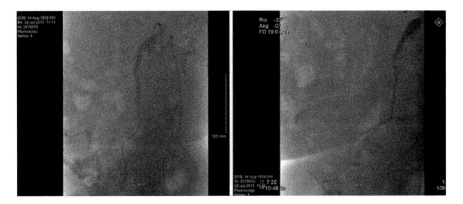

Fig. 21.8 Nephrostogram showing left ureteroileal stricture

Robotic revision of ureteroileal stricture is feasible with comparable results to open repair [15]. Laparoscopic adhesiolysis is usually required. Ureter is identified away from the site of stricture. This could be facilitated by injecting methylene blue through the nephrostomy tube. Dissection continues until the stenosed segment. The ureter is divided just proximal to the stricture, and the distal edge is sent to pathology. Generous spatulation is done. If there is tension, ureter should be dissected proximally to gain more length; if not successful, try to mobilize the conduit or neobladder toward the tethered ureter and fix it to the posterior wall of the peritoneum.

Bricker or Wallace (if bilateral) techniques may be employed. In the Bricker technique, each ureter is generously spatulated and anastomosed separately with the conduit or the neobladder without tension on the ureter. Before completion of the anastomosis, a single J stent is inserted in each ureter and fixed to the conduit with chromic catgut suture. In the Wallace technique, both ureters are held beside each other after spatulation with the fourth arm, and then the posterior wall of both ureters is anastomosed (Fig. 21.9) in a continuous manner with 4-0 Vicryl. Each side of

Fig. 21.9 Illustrated image for Wallace plate

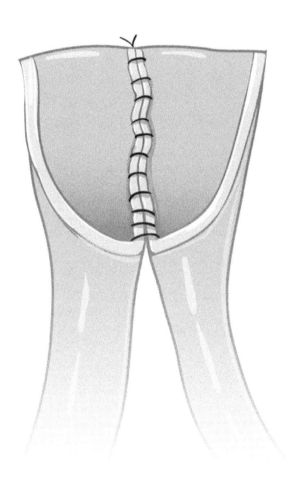

the ureter is sutured with the bowel in a continuous or interrupted manner until both sides meet anteriorly where both sutures are finally tied. While running the side sutures, insert bilateral single J stents through Foley's catheter, and fix them to the conduit or neobladder with chromic catgut suture (Video 21.4). Retroperitonealization of the anastomosis (covering the anastomosis with a peritoneal flap) is recommended to contain any leak. Intra-abdominal drain and Foley's catheter inside the pouch are placed.

Longer stricture segments with defects >3 cm may require an additional isoperistaltic ileal segment interposition to bridge the gap for ileal conduit urinary diversions. For continent urinary diversions, a longitudinal anterior wall segment of the pouch can be fashioned as a Boari flap to bridge the gap, provided the pouch size allows. Otherwise, a 10-cm isoperistaltic ileal segment interposition can be used [30]. Also buccal mucosal graft ureteroplasty was recently reported for long segment ureteric strictures [31, 32].

Postoperative Care

The percutaneous nephrostomy may be removed intraoperatively or the next day. Follow-up will be after 2 weeks with history, physical examination, renal function test, and urine analysis. The author prefers to clamp the nephrostomy tube and remove the stent after 2 weeks. If the patient is asymptomatic (no evidence of UTI or flank pain) and follow-up imaging shows no obstruction, we remove the nephrostomy tube. A pelvic-abdominal ultrasound is recommended 2–4 weeks after removal of the ureteric catheters to ensure patency of the uretero-enteric anastomosis. Then follow up after 3 months with an ultrasound of the kidneys or MAG 3 renal scan, and then follow-up is spaced every 6 months for at least 2 years with images and renal function tests.

Urethral-Enteric Anastomosis Stricture

The data about urethral-enteric anastomosis stricture after RARC in the literature is very limited. From open surgery, the incidence of benign stricture at anastomosis site is 1.2% [4]. The stricture usually develops due to tension at the anastomotic site.

How to Prevent Urethral-Enteric Stricture After RARC?

Techniques to prevent strictures include preservation of maximal urethral length, reduction of pneumoperitoneum, and incision of the mesentery to gain more length [33].

Diagnosis

Patients usually present with recurrent UTI, difficult self-intermittent catheterization, or overflow incontinence. The best way to confirm the diagnosis is cystoscopy combined with an ascending urethrogram. Rectal (in males) and vaginal exam (in females) should be done simultaneously to rule out tumor recurrence.

Management

Endoscopic approach should be tried first especially for thin and short strictures with visual internal urethrotomy; if the stricture recurs, surgical revision should be implemented for definitive treatment. The repair is accomplished by resection of the stenosed segment, trimming of the urethral edges, and reanastomosis with a new enterotomy site. Revision of the whole pouch may be an option or even a conduit diversion may be performed.

Fistula Formation

The incidence of reoperation for fistula repair is 3% in first 2 years after RARC [15]. Management strategies and outcomes are poorly defined in the literature due to its rarity. The fistula tract might form between the bowel and pouch (bowel-pouch fistula), pouch with skin (pouch-cutaneous), pouch with vagina (vaginal-pouch), or pouch with rectum (rectum-pouch).

How to Prevent Fistula Formation After RARC?

Strategies to prevent a fistula include ensuring adequate perioperative nutrition by either oral or parenteral route, adhering to the anastomotic principles in bowels or urinary tract reconstruction, minimizing surgical trauma to the bowels or ureters, trying to cover the anastomosis with omental flap, and treating any leak or infection promptly. For organ confined tumors in sexually active females, organ-sparing cystectomy may be an option with lower fistulae rates.

Diagnosis

Symptoms consistent with possible fistula formation are pneumaturia, incidental radiographic findings of air in the urinary system, recurrent UTIs, or passage of feculent debris via the wound, urine, or the vagina [32]. Diagnostic modalities for diagnosis are pouchogram (Fig. 21.10), CT pouchogram, CT scan urography, or MRU. Some surgeons prefer to perform cystoscopy/looposcopy which may show the fistulous tract or an area of inflammation at the site of the fistulae. At the time of repair, a guide wire or ureteral catheter may be placed to facilitate identification of the fistulae at the time of repair.

Management

Fistula management starts with conservative treatment such as diversion of urine with urethral or nephrostomy catheters, a low residual diet, and/or hyperalimentation. If the conservative measures failed, then surgical repair through either open or robot-assisted approach is performed.

Robot-assisted enteric-pouch fistula repair is feasible and depends on the experience of the surgeon. Hussein et al. report, after 406 RARCs performed, 11 patients that developed fistulous complications. Five of them underwent robot-assisted repair, and the rest underwent open repair with no difference in long-term outcomes [15]. Robot-assisted repair starts with adhesiolysis until identification of the

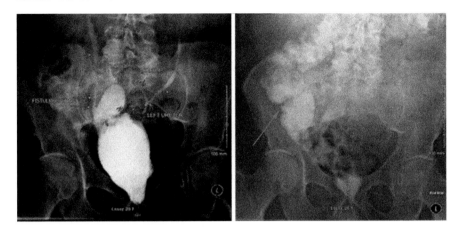

Fig. 21.10 Pouchogram showing enteric-pouch fistula

fistulous site. It then resected. If the ureter is involved or near the fistula site, then reimplantation of the ureter is highly recommended. Closure of the two sides of the fistulous tract with absorbable suture and omental, peritoneal, or adipose tissue interposition is performed (Video 21.5).

In cases of bowel-pouch and rectum-pouch fistulae, the bowel segment involved is usually resected if necessary. A diverting colostomy may also be considered, especially with rectal involvement. For vaginal-pouch fistulae, after dissection of the anterior vaginal wall from the pouch, the anterior vagina is closed in two layers, and an omental (peritoneal) flap may be interposed between the pouch and the vagina.

The integrity of the pouch is checked by filling the pouch with 150 cc of methylene blue. A drain and Foley's catheter are placed.

Postoperative Care

The percutaneous nephrostomy tube is clamped after surgery. Keep the catheter for 10–14 days, and then remove it if pouchogram/loopogram confirms no extravasation. If the ureter is reimplanted with a single J stent, leave the stents for at least 4 weeks, and then remove it with the flexible cystoscopy. Repeat CT scan or MRU after 3 months to confirm absence of fistuale.

Stomal Complications

Parastomal Hernia

Parastomal hernia (PSH) is defined as the protrusion of abdominal contents through the stomal defect in the abdominal wall. It is the most common stomal complication [34]. Hussein et al. reported a 20% incidence of PSH post-RARC [35], and the Indiana group reported 29% after open surgery [36]. The mechanism of PSH occurrence is due to either poor surgical technique or patient-related factors.

Moreno-Matias classification is used to differentiate PSH into three types: (1) the hernia sac contained prolapsed bowel forming the stoma; (2) the sac contained abdominal fat or omentum; (3) the sac contained herniated loops of bowel other than that forming the stoma [37].

How to Prevent the Risk of PSH After RARC?

Narrow the fascial defect, avoid resection of the fat, use fatty fascial anchoring sutures (debatable), and improve the nutritional status of the patient [35]. Prolonged pneumoperitoneum may increase the risk of PSH. De-insufflation of the abdomen is necessary before preparing the conduit site to avoid shift of the conduit site away from the rectus muscle. Surgeons have suggested the use of a prophylactic mesh at the time of RARC to avoid subsequent PSH.

Diagnosis

Most of the patients with PSH are asymptomatic; only 30% of the patients with PSH post-RARC present with symptoms [35]. PSH presentation may be acute (bowel obstruction, strangulation, or urinary obstruction) or chronic (problems with fitting the stomal appliance, urine leakage, skin maceration, recurrent partial bowel obstruction, and/or abdominal pain). The best way for diagnosis is CT scan of the abdomen with oral and IV contrast (Fig. 21.11).

Management

The mainstay of treatment is patient education about the symptoms and signs of bowel obstruction. For symptomatic patients, conservative management using the hernia belt is initial treatment, and only 15% of the patients require surgical intervention [35]. Management of obstructed PSH includes resuscitation of the patient

Fig. 21.11 CT scan showing grade 3 parastomal hernia

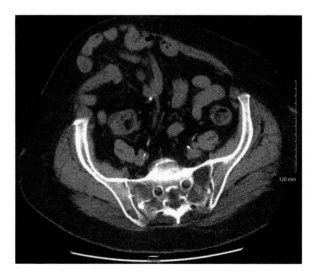

and exploratory laparotomy with reduction of the herniated loops. Followed by assessment of the loops, unviable loops are resected and reanastomosed. The stomal defect is repaired primarily.

Chronic symptomatic patients can be managed by robot-assisted approach, with reduction of the herniated contents and primary repair of the defect using a mesh. An intraperitoneal onlay mesh is wrapped around the stoma and fixed to the abdominal wall using interrupted Vicryl sutures. The mesh needs to extend 5–10 cm beyond the defect [38, 39]. We prefer using a mesh rather than primary repair, due to the high failure rate of the primary repair (46–100%) [40]. In rare occasions the conduit may be moved to a new site [41]. Stoma relocation to the other side may be an option for large defects with weak abdominal muscles [42].

Postoperative Care
For postoperative management monitor the patient clinically for nausea, vomiting, passing flatus, or stool and drain output.

Stomal Prolapse
Stomal prolapse is defined as increase in the size and/or length of the stoma after maturation [43]. There is a limited data on stomal prolapse. Patients may present with poorly fitting appliances, ulceration, dryness, and bleeding of the stoma. The hypothesis behind stomal prolapse is thought to be due to a wide fascial opening. Management is indicated for persistent symptoms or signs of vascular compromise. Care must be taken for a concurrent PSH. The literature suggests releasing of the prolapsed stoma from the abdominal wall, resecting redundant bowel, and reconstructing the stoma. Relocation may be done for larger fascial defects not amenable for repair [44].

Stomal Stenosis
Stomal stenosis is defined as failure to pass the small finger or a 6 Fr Hegar dilator through the stomal opening [44]. This may occur due to bowel ischemia or narrowing of the skin and/or fascial opening. Median time for occurrence of stomal stenosis is 9 years with an incidence of 2.1% [45]. A loopogram study may be performed to confirm the diagnosis. Management includes intermittent catheterization, regular dilatation, or surgical revision. Surgical revision is done by releasing the stoma from the abdominal wall, refreshing the bowel edges and the skin, and followed by reconstructing the stoma.

Neobladder Rupture

It is a rare complication. Regular examination for post-voiding residual urine along with the need for clean intermittent catheterization (CIC) is essential. Patient compliance is a key factor, and lifelong commitment from the patient to CIC if indicated is warranted if continent urinary diversion is performed [46, 47].

How to Prevent Neobladder Rupture?

Patient education is of key importance. Avoidance of over distention of the pouch and abdominal trauma can prevent neobladder ruptures [47].

Diagnosis

The patient usually presents with an acute abdomen. Proper history taking and examination are needed to reach the correct diagnosis. A pouchogram showing contrast leakage confirms the diagnosis.

Management

Patient stabilization and placement of a 22 Fr hematuria catheter are the first steps. Conservative management has been reported for small tears in stable patients. A large caliber catheter is inserted and left to drain the pouch for 3–4 weeks, and then a repeat pouchogram is performed [48]. Laparotomy, peritoneal irrigation, repair of the perforation in two layers using 2/0 Vicryl sutures, and closure of the abdomen over two peritoneal drains [47]. The drains are removed after return of the bowel function and minimum drainage. A pouchogram is performed after 3 weeks and the catheter is removed if there is no leakage.

Urinary Incontinence

Continence rates after RARC vary widely. Daytime continence rates range from 68% to 100%, and nighttime continence rates vary from 57% to 85% [49–51].

How to Prevent Urinary Incontinence After Neobladders?

Ensuring adequate urethral function and continence of the patient prior to surgery is a key for patient selection and realistic expectation of outcomes after surgery. Forming a reservoir with an adequate volume, low pressure, and globular shape is a key. Avoid opening the endopelvic fascia, and nerve preservation when oncologically feasible will help with continence.

Diagnosis

Patient reported outcomes using the urinary function questionnaires at follow-up visits. Secondary causes of incontinence such as urinary tract infections and inflammation of the pouch should be excluded through a urine analysis, culture, and sensitivity. Total versus overflow incontinence should be differentiated by a post-voiding residual urine measurement, and sometimes a urodynamic study is needed.

Management

Exclude infection and pouchitis. For overflow incontinence timed voiding along with CIC is enforced to the patient. Regular assessment is needed by pelvic ultrasound for post-voiding residual urine. For total incontinence patient education and pelvic floor exercises are key. Continence may take up to 6 months until the neobladder reaches its full size. The use of male slings or artificial urinary sphincter may be needed [50, 51]. The use of other methods of diversion such as ileal conduits have been reported as a final resort [52].

Conclusion

Complications are common after radical cystectomy whatever the approach used. When conservative measures fail to manage complications after RARC, surgical revision is warranted with good outcomes. Robot-assisted revision of these complications is feasible and offers less morbidity for the patients if performed with enough experience and planned steps.

References

1. Nix J, Smith A, Kurpad R, Nielsen ME, Wallen EM, Pruthi RS. Prospective randomized controlled trial of robotic versus open radical cystectomy for bladder cancer: perioperative and pathologic results. Eur Urol. 2010;57(2):196–201.
2. Parekh DJ, Reis IM, Castle EP, Gonzalgo ML, Woods ME, Svatek RS, et al. Robot-assisted radical cystectomy versus open radical cystectomy in patients with bladder cancer (RAZOR): an open-label, randomised, phase 3, non-inferiority trial. Lancet. 2018;391(10139):2525–36.
3. Khan MS, Elhage O, Challacombe B, Rimington P, Murphy D, Dasgupta P. Analysis of early complications of robotic-assisted radical cystectomy using a standardized reporting system. Urology. 2011;77(2):357–62.
4. Niegisch G, Albers P, Rabenalt R. Perioperative complications and oncological safety of robot-assisted (RARC) vs. open radical cystectomy (ORC). In Urologic Oncology: Seminars and Original Investigations Elsevier. 2014;32(7):966–74.
5. Hussein AA, Dibaj S, Hinata N, Field E, O'Leary K, Kuvshinoff B, et al. Development and validation of a quality assurance score for robot-assisted radical cystectomy: a 10-year analysis. Urology. 2016;97:124–9.
6. Patel H, Cerantola Y, Valerio M, Persson B, Jichlinski P, Ljungqvist O. Enhanced recovery after surgery: are we ready, and can we afford not to implement these pathways for patients undergoing radical cystectomy. Eur Urol. 2014;65(2):263–6.
7. Wilson TG, Guru K, Rosen RC, Wiklund P, Annerstedt M, Bochner BH, et al. Best practices in robot-assisted radical cystectomy and urinary reconstruction: recommendations of the Pasadena consensus panel. Eur Urol. 2015;67(3):363–75.
8. Schrenk P, Woisetschläger R, Rieger R, Wayand W. Mechanism, management, and prevention of laparoscopic bowel injuries. Gastrointest Endosc. 1996;43(6):572–4.
9. Smith AB, Woods ME, Raynor MC, Nielsen ME, Wallen EM, Pruthi RS. Prevention and management of complications following robot-assisted radical cystectomy: lessons learned after> 250 consecutive cases. World J Urol. 2013;31(3):441–6.
10. Poch MA, Raza J, Nyquist J, Guru KA. Tips and tricks to robot-assisted radical cystectomy and intracorporeal diversion. Curr Opin Urol. 2013;23(1):65–71.
11. Hussein AA, Hinata N, Dibaj S, May PR, Kozlowski JD, Abol-Enein H, et al. Development, validation and clinical application of pelvic lymphadenectomy assessment and completion evaluation: intraoperative assessment of lymph node dissection after robot-assisted radical cystectomy for bladder cancer. BJU Int. 2017;119(6):879–84.
12. Antoniadis G, Kretschmer T, Pedro MT, König RW, Heinen CP, Richter H-P. Iatrogenic nerve injuries: prevalence, diagnosis and treatment. Dtsch Arztebl Int. 2014;111(16):273.

13. Vasilev SA. Obturator nerve injury: a review of management options. Gynecol Oncol. 1994;53(2):152–5.
14. Kretschmer T, Antoniadis G, Braun V, Rath SA, Richter HP. Evaluation of iatrogenic lesions in 722 surgically treated cases of peripheral nerve trauma. J Neurosurg. 2001;94(6):905–12.
15. Hussein AA, Hashmi Z, Dibaj S, Altartir T, Fiorica T, Wing J, et al. Reoperations following robot-assisted radical cystectomy: a decade of experience. J Urol. 2016;195(5):1368–76.
16. Hussein AA, May PR, Jing Z, Ahmed YE, Wijburg CJ, Canda AE, et al. Outcomes of Intracorporeal urinary diversion after robot-assisted radical cystectomy: results from the international robotic cystectomy consortium. J Urol. 2018;199(5):1302–11.
17. Giannarini G, Crestani A, Inferrera A, Rossanese M, Subba E, Novara G, et al. Impact of Enhanced Recovery After Surgery (ERAS) protocols versus standard of care on perioperative outcomes of radical cystectomy: a systematic review and meta-analysis of comparative studies. Minerva Urol Nefrol. 2019; https://doi.org/10.23736/S0393-2249.19.03376-9.
18. Esmadi M, Ahmad D, Hewlett A. Efficacy of naldemedine for the treatment of opioid-induced constipation: a meta-analysis. J Gastrointestin Liver Dis. 2019;28(1):41–6.
19. Jain N, Sareen S, Kanawa S, Jain V, Gupta S, Mann S. Jain point: a new safe portal for laparoscopic entry in previous surgery cases. J Hum Reprod Sci. 2016;9(1):9.
20. Chang F, Lee C, Soong Y. Use of palmer's point for insertion of the operative laparoscope in patients with severe pelvic adhesions: experience of seventeen cases. J Am Assoc Gynecol Laparosc. 1994;1(4, Part 2):S7.
21. Lawrentschuk N, Colombo R, Hakenberg OW, Lerner SP, Månsson W, Sagalowsky A, et al. Prevention and management of complications following radical cystectomy for bladder cancer. Eur Urol. 2010;57(6):983–1001.
22. Trencheva K, Morrissey KP, Wells M, Mancuso CA, Lee SW, Sonoda T, et al. Identifying important predictors for anastomotic leak after colon and rectal resection: prospective study on 616 patients. Ann Surg. 2013;257(1):108–13.
23. Witzke JD, Kraatz JJ, Morken JM, Ney AL, West MA, Van Camp JM, et al. Stapled versus hand sewn anastomoses in patients with small bowel injury: a changing perspective. J Trauma. 2000;49(4):660–5; discussion 5–6
24. Davis NF, Burke JP, McDermott T, Flynn R, Manecksha RP, Thornhill JA. Bricker versus Wallace anastomosis: a meta-analysis of ureteroenteric stricture rates after ileal conduit urinary diversion. Can Urol Assoc J. 2015;9(5–6):E284.
25. Sogani PC, Watson RC, Whitmore WF. Lymphocele after pelvic lymphadenectomy for urologic cancer. Urology. 1981;17(1):39–43.
26. Gotto GT, Yunis LH, Guillonneau B, Touijer K, Eastham JA, Scardino PT, et al. Predictors of symptomatic lymphocele after radical prostatectomy and bilateral pelvic lymph node dissection. Int J Urol. 2011;18(4):291–6.
27. Musch M, Klevecka V, Roggenbuck U, Kroepfl D. Complications of pelvic lymphadenectomy in 1,380 patients undergoing radical retropubic prostatectomy between 1993 and 2006. J Urol. 2008;179(3):923–9.
28. Schnoeller T, Finter F, Hautmann RE, Volkmer BG. Upper urinary tract recurrence after cystectomy for bladder cancer: who is at risk? J Urol. 2009;181(4S):632.
29. Ahmed YE, Hussein AA, May PR, Ahmad B, Ali T, Durrani A, et al. Natural history, predictors and management of ureteroenteric strictures after robot assisted radical cystectomy. J Urol. 2017;198(3):567–74.
30. Nassar OAH, Alsafa MES. Experience with ureteroenteric strictures after radical cystectomy and diversion: open surgical revision. Urology. 2011;78(2):459–65.
31. Arora S, Campbell L, Tourojman M, Pucheril D, Jones LR, Rogers C. Robotic buccal mucosal graft ureteroplasty for complex ureteral stricture. Urology. 2017;110:257–8.
32. Zhao LC, Weinberg AC, Lee Z, Ferretti MJ, Koo HP, Metro MJ, et al. Robotic ureteral reconstruction using buccal mucosa grafts: a multi-institutional experience. Eur Urol. 2018;73(3):419–26.

33. Almassi N, Zargar H, Ganesan V, Fergany A, Haber G-P. Management of challenging urethro-ileal anastomosis during robotic assisted radical cystectomy with intracorporeal neobladder formation. Eur Urol. 2016;69(4):704–9.
34. Kouba E, Sands M, Lentz A, Wallen E, Pruthi RS. Incidence and risk factors of stomal complications in patients undergoing cystectomy with ileal conduit urinary diversion for bladder cancer. J Urol. 2007;178(3):950–4.
35. Hussein AA, Ahmed YE, May P, Ali T, Ahmad B, Raheem S, et al. Natural history and predictors of parastomal hernia after robot-assisted radical cystectomy and ileal conduit urinary diversion. J Urol. 2018;199(3):766–73.
36. Liu NW, Hackney JT, Gellhaus PT, Monn MF, Masterson TA, Bihrle R, et al. Incidence and risk factors of parastomal hernia in patients undergoing radical cystectomy and ileal conduit diversion. J Urol. 2014;191(5):1313–8.
37. Moreno-Matias J, Serra-Aracil X, Darnell-Martin A, Bombardo-Junca J, Mora-Lopez L, Alcantara-Moral M, et al. The prevalence of parastomal hernia after formation of an end colostomy. A new clinico-radiological classification. Color Dis. 2009;11(2):173–7.
38. LeBlanc K, Bellanger D, Whitaker J, Hausmann M. Laparoscopic parastomal hernia repair. Hernia. 2005;9(2):140–4.
39. Mancini G, McClusky D, Khaitan L, Goldenberg E, Heniford B, Novitsky Y, et al. Laparoscopic parastomal hernia repair using a nonslit mesh technique. Surg Endosc. 2007;21(9):1487–91.
40. Donahue TF, Bochner BH, Sfakianos JP, Kent M, Bernstein M, Hilton WM, et al. Risk factors for the development of parastomal hernia after radical cystectomy. J Urol. 2014;191(6):1708–13.
41. Martin L, Foster G. Parastomal hernia. Ann R Coll Surg Engl. 1996;78(2):81.
42. Cheung M-T, Chia N-H, Chiu W-Y. Surgical treatment of parastomal hernia complicating sigmoid colostomies. Dis Colon Rectum. 2001;44(2):266–70.
43. Johnson P. Intestinal stoma prolapse and surgical treatments of this condition in children: a systematic review and a retrospective study. Surg Sci. 2016;7(09):400.
44. de Miguel VM, Escovar FJ, Calvo AP. Current status of the prevention and treatment of stoma complications. A narrative review. Cirugía Española (English Edition). 2014;92(3):149–56.
45. Shimko MS, Tollefson MK, Umbreit EC, Farmer SA, Blute ML, Frank I. Long-term complications of conduit urinary diversion. J Urol. 2011;185(2):562–7.
46. Haupt G, Pannek J, Knopf H-J, Schulze H, Senge T. Rupture of ileal neobladder due to urethral obstruction by mucous plug. J Urol. 1990;144(3):740–1.
47. Nippgen JBW, Hakenberg OW, Manseck A, Wirth MP. Spontaneous late rupture of orthotopic detubularized ileal neobladders: report of five cases. Urology. 2001;58(1):43–6.
48. Kristiansen P, Mansson W, Tyger J. Perforation of continent caecal reservoir for urine twice in one patient. Scand J Urol Nephrol. 1991;25(4):279–81.
49. Desai MM, Gill IS, de Castro Abreu AL, Hosseini A, Nyberg T, Adding C, et al. Robotic intracorporeal orthotopic neobladder during radical cystectomy in 132 patients. J Urol. 2014;192(6):1734–40.
50. Asimakopoulos AD, Campagna A, Gakis G, Corona Montes VE, Piechaud T, Hoepffner J-L, et al. Nerve sparing, robot-assisted radical cystectomy with intracorporeal bladder substitution in the male. J Urol. 2016;196(5):1549–57.
51. Tyritzis S, Collins J, Khazaeli D, Jonsson M, Adding C, Hosseini-Aliabad A, et al. 1035 The Karolinska experience in 67 robot-assisted radical cystectomies with totally intracorporeal formation of an ileal neobladder. Oncological and complication outcomes. Eur Urol Supp. 2013;12(1):e1035.
52. Hautmann RE, De Petriconi R, Gottfried H-W, Kleinschmidt K, Mattes R, Paiss T. The ileal neobladder: complications and functional results in 363 patients after 11 years of follow-up. J Urol. 1999;161(2):422–8.

Orthotopic Ileal Neobladder and Continent Catheterizable Urinary Diversion

Alvin C. Goh and Gregory Chesnut

Indications

The three main forms of urinary diversion following radical cystectomy are ileal conduit, continent cutaneous urinary diversion (CCUD), and ileal orthotopic neobladder (ileal ONB). This chapter focuses on CCUD and ONB, showing patient selection criteria, intraoperative and postoperative considerations, a detailed description of our technique for each diversion, and descriptions of complications and their management. Principles shared by both types of continent urinary diversions include low-pressure urine storage that provides socially acceptable continence and ease of emptying. Surgeons employing a minimally invasive approach should be familiar with all techniques of urinary diversion.

Intracorporeal ileal ONB, replicating the principles learned from decades of open surgery, offers the benefit of voiding per urethra and has been associated with improved quality of life and improved body image [1]. Though several neobladder configurations have been described, techniques which allow for a low-pressure, large capacity, highly compliant reservoir which allows voluntary emptying without residual urine are key to achieving desired functional outcomes [2].

The continent cutaneous urinary diversion (CCUD) utilizes detubularized bowel to create a reservoir that can be emptied using intermittent catheterization via a stoma, most commonly located at the umbilicus or right lower quadrant. Since the first description of a catheterizable cecal reservoir in 1908, various techniques have

Supplementary Information The online version of this chapter (https://doi.org/10.1007/978-3-030-50196-9_22) contains supplementary material, which is available to authorized users.

A. C. Goh (✉) · G. Chesnut
Urology Service, Department of Surgery, Memorial Sloan Kettering Cancer Center, New York, NY, USA
e-mail: goha@mskcc.org; chesnutg@mskcc.org

been developed using a variety of bowel segments and continence mechanisms to achieve a reservoir of adequate size and compliance with a stoma that is easily accessible and which is continent [3–5]. With continence rates of 90–98%, the continent cutaneous urinary diversion offers higher rates of continence than ONB in appropriately selected patients and results in comparable quality of life [6–9].

While its principal benefit is to offer a continent reservoir in patients unsuitable for neobladder creation, the CCUD remains an important technique for all surgeons performing urinary diversion. CCUD offers an alternative urinary reconstruction for patients who may not be a candidate for a neobladder for oncologic or functional reasons. As an increasing number of radical cystectomies (RC) are now performed using a minimally invasive robotic approach, the ability to perform CCUD in this setting is an important tool for the urologic surgeon. Since Goh's initial description of robotic intracorporeal continent urinary diversion in 2015, the minimally invasive approach to CCUD has been shown to be effective and reproducible [8, 9].

Development of Robotic Cystectomy (RARC)

First described in 2003, robot-assisted radical cystectomy (RARC) has become increasingly adopted in urologic practice [10]. While adoption of RARC varies geographically, implementation of RARC continues to steadily increase with time. The minimally invasive approach was used in 25.3% of patients in the National Cancer Database in 2013, an increase from 12.8% in 2010 [11]. Along with the increase in RARC, intracorporeal urinary diversion (ICUD) rates have increased. Among members of the International Robotic Cystectomy Consortium (IRCC), 51% of 2125 robotic cystectomies performed between 2005 and 2016 were completed with ICUD [12]. Within this consortium, rates of ICUD grew from 9% in 2005 to 97% in 2016 [12]. In community practice, lower rates of ICUD persist, with a multi-institutional series showing that only 3% of patients undergoing RARC had an ICUD in the United States as of 2009 [13]. Further, from a global perspective, continent urinary diversion remains underutilized, with only around 20–25% undergoing this form of diversion after RC [12, 14]. At the authors' institution, around half of all patients undergoing RC are able to receive a continent diversion. This rate is consistent irrespective of the surgical approach. Specifically, CCUD is utilized in a minority of cases; its use varies from 0% to 39% in institutional series [15]. In a recent review, CCUD implementation in high-volume centers represented 10.4% of diversions [16]. With recent randomized trials showing comparable complication rates and short-term oncologic outcomes between RARC and open RC (ORC), we expect the utilization of RARC to continue to increase [17–19]. With increased robotic experience and standardization of technique, the rate of ICUD use will likely rise accordingly.

Incorporation of Intracorporeal Urinary Diversion (ICUD)

The evolution of ICUD has followed a stepwise approach. Early descriptions focused on the development of techniques for ileal conduit. Subsequent efforts showed the feasibility of ileal ONB, replicating the techniques refined from open surgery [20–23]. Several series have documented the learning curve to minimally invasive cystectomy and intracorporeal diversion, with most surgeons initially adopting simpler incontinent diversions and then progressing to more complex continent diversions [22]. Desai et al. reported a standardization of steps of the procedure and ways to optimize efficiency [20]. Experience and volume appear to correspond with reduction in complications and operative time [12, 13, 24, 25].

Initial experience with extracorporeal Indiana pouch following RARC has been reported with functional outcomes and complication rates comparable to those undergoing ORC with Indiana pouch [9]. Most recently, our group and others have shown the feasibility and safety of robotic CCUD, using detubularized right colon as the reservoir and the ileocecal valve as the continence mechanism [26, 27, 21]. These initial series appear to show functional outcomes similar to the extracorporeal approach but with fewer gastrointestinal and infectious complication rates [27, 28]. Similarly, as individual and institutional experience with intracorporeal ONB has increased, functional outcomes comparable to open surgery have been demonstrated [21, 28].

A completely minimally invasive cystectomy and intracorporeal diversion may offer some advantages. Randomized trials show evidence of lower blood loss, decreased risk for blood transfusion, and fewer wound complications following RARC compared to ORC [21, 28–31]. With a small incision, there is less pain and potential for enhanced recovery. During ICUD, there is less insensible fluid loss and bowel manipulation, which may result in quicker return of bowel function. Differences in postoperative recovery are currently being investigated in a prospective randomized trial [29]. Further, there is some indication that patients with compromised cardiopulmonary function may better tolerate minimally invasive cystectomy with ICUD [30]. Although there are only small series to date involving intracorporeal CCUD, the benefits conferred by RARC and ICUD, from decreased bowel manipulation and less wound morbidity, are expected to be similar [21, 31].

In general, patients desiring a continent urinary diversion in the presence of adequate renal and hepatic function and absence of colonic pathology would be candidates for either ONB or CCUD. Several oncologic factors, including urethral disease or bladder neck involvement in females, may preclude the option of an orthotopic diversion, in which case CCUD may be favored. CCUD may also be considered in patients who have received prior pelvic radiation and those desiring to mitigate the risk of urinary incontinence. Adequate manual dexterity and compliance are additional prerequisites for CCUD. Appropriate patient counseling and selection will be discussed further in the following section.

Preoperative Considerations and Evaluation

All patients being evaluated for RC should be counseled on the different types of urinary diversion options and advised of the risks and benefits of each one [32]. Delineation of patient expectations and preferences will help guide discussions of diversion type, as each type impacts quality of life in different ways. Patients considering ONB must be motivated to complete a timed voiding regimen and possess the ability to perform clean intermittent catheterization (CIC) if needed. Patients should be informed of the difference in voiding technique and requirement for timed voiding associated with ONB creation. Patients should be advised of the potential for urinary incontinence, which can vary during the daytime and nighttime. While older age is not a contraindication for ONB reconstruction, patients with advanced age should be counseled that there is a higher risk for delayed recovery of urinary control and that they are at higher long-term risk for nocturnal incontinence [1].

Patients considering undergoing CCUD must understand the requirement for regular CIC and be motivated to empty their pouch 4–6 times daily as well as perform regular pouch irrigation, particularly early in the recovery process. Patients must be able to demonstrate both the mental acuity and manual dexterity to manage self-catheterization. Patients with progressive degenerative neurologic disease, cognitive impairment, or frailty should be counseled that CCUD may be less favorable, since it requires dexterity and attention beyond what may be available with family caregivers, visiting nurses, or long-term care facilities [33].

Patients with malignancy at the bladder neck or prostatic urethra should be counseled regarding the increased risk of local recurrence when considering urinary diversion type. ONB may not be feasible. In the event of a positive urethral margin, neobladder would be contraindicated [20]. The presence of extensive local disease and the need for adjuvant radiation therapy are additional considerations when evaluating patients for continent diversion. Patients who have received radiation for previous gynecologic or pelvic malignancy should be counseled that ONB may result in increased complications and poor urinary function due to poor tissue characteristics following radiation exposure [33, 34]. In a cohort of salvage cystoprostatectomy with ONB after radiation therapy for prostate or bladder cancer, Bochner et al. showed that complications requiring reoperation increased (reoperation rate of 17%) and incontinence rates were higher (66% daytime and 56% nighttime continence) after radiation exposure [35]. These patients may benefit from CCUD or ileal conduit. Similarly, men with urethral stricture disease should be evaluated for CCUD rather than ONB. Patients with preexisting urinary incontinence should be counseled that superior continence may be available with CCUD than with ONB [36].

Female cystectomy patients represent another group that may benefit from evaluation for CCUD. Female patients with invasive cancer at the bladder neck, those with invasion of the anterior vaginal wall, and those with positive urethral margins are not candidates for ONB and may be more suitable for CCUD [16]. With proper staging and counseling, most women are now candidates for ONB, though 30–40%

of patients may not be eligible due to tumor characteristics [16]. Urinary retention rates in women following ONB have been reported as high as 50% [34]. With vaginal-sparing approaches and pelvic floor reconstruction, urinary function can be improved following ONB [37]. We have observed around 6–12% retention rate with ONB at our institution [28, 38].

Assessing renal and hepatic function is mandatory prior to performing both ONB and CCUD diversion, due to metabolic abnormalities that arise from urine solute reabsorption in the intestinal tract. Reabsorption of ammonium and potassium in the colon and ileum can lead to hyperchloremic, hypokalemic metabolic acidosis [39]. Factors that contribute to metabolic acidosis include the surface area of the bowel used and the contact time of the bowel with urine [16]. Chronic metabolic acidosis can lead to renal hyperfiltration injury, development of renal fibrosis, progression of kidney disease, and bone demineralization [40]. Ideal candidates for CCUD have a maximum serum creatinine of 2.5 mg/dL and glomerular filtration rate of 40 mL/min or greater. Similarly, as adequate hepatic function is required to manage the reabsorption of ammonium across the bowel mucosa, hepatic insufficiency is a contraindication for continent diversion [32].

Detailed past medical and surgical histories should focus on any prior abdominal surgeries or radiation. Personal and family history of colon cancer should be assessed, as well as history of any inflammatory bowel disease. Colonoscopy should be performed prior to the use of the colon in CCUD to rule out malignancy or evidence of chronic inflammatory bowel disease [33].

Preoperative evaluation, counseling, and education by a dedicated enterostomal therapist are critical. First, the site of the catheterizable stoma should be evaluated and shown to be accessible in standing or sitting positions. Secondly, a potential site for ileal conduit should be marked in case this diversion type is required. Standardized educational materials in addition to oral and written discussion are important to help patients understand the detail of the urinary diversion and help set appropriate expectations.

Additional preoperative preparation involves active smoking cessation intervention and inclusion of 30 minutes of daily exercise prior to surgery. Patients undergoing a small bowel diversion (ileal conduit or ONB) do not receive a bowel preparation. As a matter of routine, we do not utilize an antibiotic bowel preparation regimen [41]. For CCUD, which involves the large bowel, patients receive a complete mechanical bowel preparation, including a clear liquid diet 2 days before surgery and magnesium citrate. As part of a standardized enhanced recovery clinical care pathway, patients also receive carbohydrate loading, selective opioid receptor blockade, and narcotic-sparing perioperative pain management.

Step-by-Step Technique: ONB

Our ONB technique uses a standardized six port configuration (Figs. 22.1a and 22.1b).

Fig. 22.1a da Vinci Xi
port configuration for
orthotopic neobladder

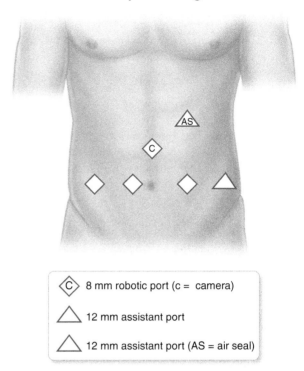

DaVinci Xi port configuration

⟨C⟩ 8 mm robotic port (c = camera)

△ 12 mm assistant port

△ 12 mm assistant port (AS = air seal)

Bowel Isolation and Reanastomosis

The white line of Toldt is opened lateral to the cecum to allow for mobilization of the small bowel to pelvis. Approximately 60 cm of the distal ileum is selected at a distance about 15 cm proximal to the ileocecal junction for the neobladder; 44 cm is used for the neobladder pouch and 10–15 cm for the afferent limb. An additional 5-cm discard segment is also measured proximally (Fig. 22.2). A pre-marked suture measuring 11 cm is inserted through the assistant port to facilitate measurements (video). Robotic tip-up fenestrated graspers are used for bowel manipulation. The distal ileum is manipulated to the pelvis, and a segment for urethroenteric anastomosis is chosen, which is at least 15 cm proximal to the ileocecal junction. The most mobile portion of the ileum that reaches the urethra without tension is selected. The anastomotic site is marked on the mesenteric and antimesenteric side. The antimesenteric side is marked with a barbed suture which will be used later to secure the bowel to Denonvilliers' fascia in order to take tension off the urethroenteric anastomosis. The undyed 11-cm pre-cut suture is used to measure the distance to the distal ileal transection (Fig. 22.3, video 00:47). This 11-cm segment of bowel will then be used to measure all remaining portions of the ileum; all bowel portions to be used on the neobladder are marked systematically with undyed sutures; bowel segments

Fig. 22.1b da Vinci Xi
port configuration
continent catheterizable
urinary diversion

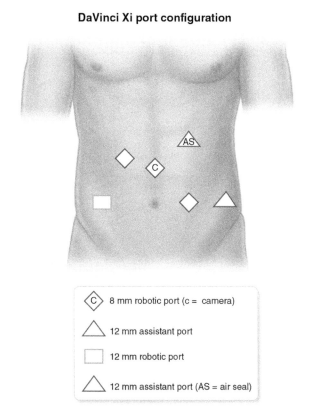

DaVinci Xi port configuration

not used in the diversion are marked with dyed sutures. The ileum is marked every 11 cm to a distance of 44 cm, which demarks the neobladder (Fig. 22.4, video 1:11). A 10–15-cm segment is measured proximally as the ileal chimney, and a 5-cm discard segment proximal to this is measured to ensure that the mesenteric window is off-tension and a deeper mesenteric division is not required. This also separates the suture lines of the neobladder and the staple line from the bowel anastomosis.

The distal ileal transection is performed with a 60-mm bowel load (3.5-mm thickness) stapler (Echelon Flex 60, Ethicon Inc., Cincinnati, OH). The initial load transects the small bowel and part of the adjacent mesentery (video 00:54). The mesenteric window can be deepened with an additional vascular load stapler (2.5-mm thickness) or a vessel sealer. Visualization of mesenteric blood vessels can be facilitated using near-infrared fluorescence with indigo cyanine green. The distal end of the transected bowel segment is marked with dyed 3-0 Vicryl suture, and 11-cm segments of neobladder are then marked on the antimesenteric border with 3-0 undyed Vicryl (Fig. 22.5). The proximal segment to be used for the afferent chimney is then measured from the 44-cm marked suture using a pre-marked Penrose drain and marked with another undyed Vicryl (Fig. 22.6, video 1:56). A 60-mm bowel load stapler is then used to divide the proximal ileum. A 5-cm discard

Fig. 22.2 Bowel segments used for ONB

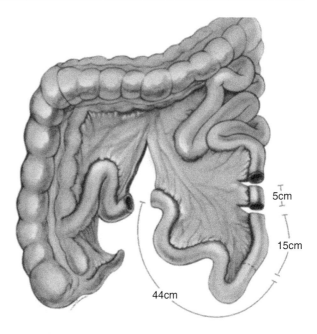

Fig. 22.3 Measuring neobladder from apex using pre-cut sutures

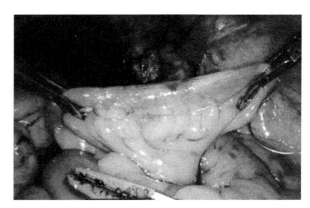

Fig. 22.4 Using the pre-measured 11-cm segment of the ileum to mark the 0-cm–44-cm segment of ileum for neobladder

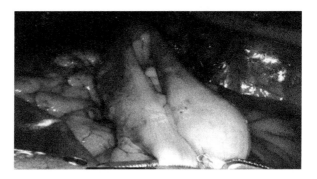

Fig. 22.5 11-cm segments of the neobladder are then marked on the antimesenteric border with 3-0 undyed Vicryl

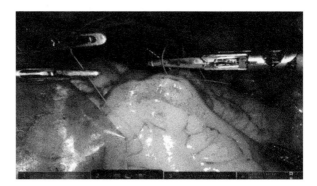

Fig. 22.6 Measuring the afferent limb and discard segment with a pre-marked Penrose drain

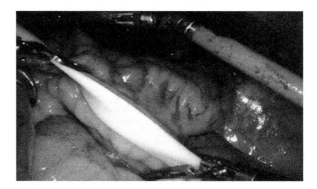

Fig. 22.7 Removal of discard segment

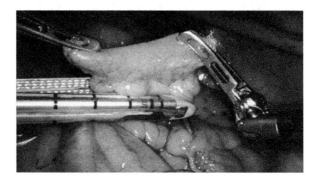

segment is measured and divided with sequential 60-mm bowel stapler loads (Fig. 22.7, video 2:22).

To restore bowel continuity, the antimesenteric corners of the proximal and distal stapled ileum to be anastomosed are cut, and a side-to-side ileoileal anastomosis is performed using a 60-mm bowel stapler placed from the left lateral port (Fig. 22.8). An additional bowel stapler load is deployed transversely to complete the anastomosis (Fig. 22.9). Interrupted sutures are used to reinforce the corner of the anastomosis (video 3:39).

Fig. 22.8 Side-to-side reanastomosis of the ileum using stapler from the patient's left side

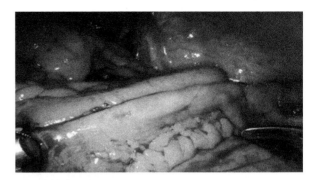

Fig. 22.9 Completing the entero-enteric anastomosis

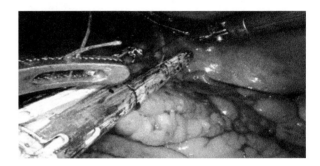

Configuration of Orthotopic Neobladder

The stapled end of the chimney is excised and closed with running 2-0 Vicryl barbed suture followed with a second imbricating layer. The fourth robotic arm is used to retract the bowel segment toward the pelvis, and 44 cm is detubularized with monopolar scissors, biasing the incision toward the mesenteric edge (video 3:50). A 24Fr chest tube is inserted into the ileum to facilitate detubularization (Fig. 22.10). Once fully detubularized, the posterior wall is aligned with several 2-0 Vicryl interrupted sutures (Fig. 22.11). The posterior wall is reapproximated with running 2-0 barbed sutures (Stratafix, Ethicon, Somerville, NJ, US, LLC).

After completing the posterior plate, the urethroileal anastomosis is performed. The posterior plate is rotated 90° counterclockwise, and caudal traction is applied to the 3-0 barbed suture (placed initially at 11 cm) to set up the anastomosis (video 5:19). This stay suture is then placed through Denonvilliers' fascia distally, adjacent to the rectourethralis muscle in order to provide for a tension-free anastomosis (Figs. 22.12 and 22.13).

Urethroileal Anastomosis and Neobladder Closure

A double-armed 3-0 Monocryl suture on an RB-1 needle is used to complete the urethroileal anastomosis in a running fashion, starting at the 6 o'clock position. The anastomosis is completed over a 22Fr Rusch catheter (Fig. 22.14, video 7:10). The neobladder is then cross-folded by placing a horizontal mattress suture dividing the

Fig. 22.10 Detubularization of ileal segment for
the neobladder

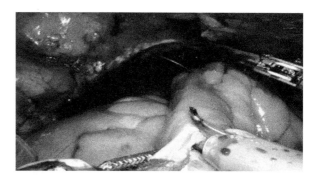

Fig. 22.11 Aligning the
posterior plate with
stay sutures

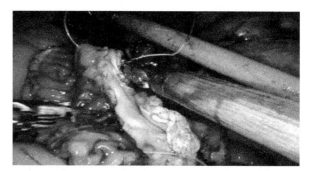

Fig. 22.12 Suturing the
dependent portion of the
neobladder to
Denonvilliers' fascia keeps
the urethroenteric
anastomosis off-tension

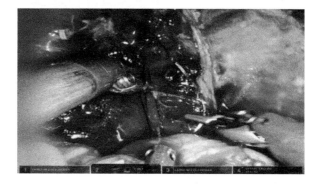

anterior suture line into two equal halves. The anterior wall closure is then started
with a 2-0 Stratafix Monocryl suture in a running fashion beginning at the urethroenteric anastomosis and working proximally. Several stay sutures may be placed to
ensure equal alignment for the anterior closure (video 10:30).

Ureteroileal Anastomoses

The ureters were previously clipped and transected during the cystectomy. The left
ureter is transposed under the sigmoid mesentery to the right side. The ureters are
aligned and partially transected and spatulated at the location of ureteroileal

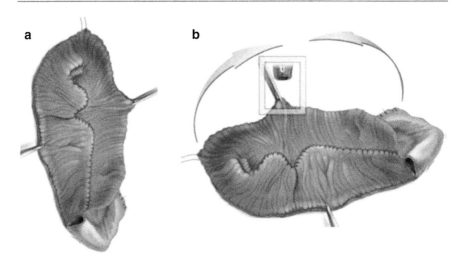

Fig. 22.13 (**a**) Posterior wall completed. (**b**) Alignment of urethroileal anastomosis by 90° counterclockwise rotation

Fig. 22.14 The urethroenteric anastomosis is completed over a 24Fr catheter using double-armed 3-0 Monocryl barbed suture

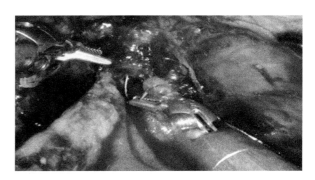

anastomosis. Indocyanine green is used to evaluate perfusion of the ureter, and each ureter is only handled at the tag or the distal ureteral segment, which will be discarded later (video 7:54). A small ileostomy is made, and each ureter is spatulated and anastomosed to the afferent limb using a running 4-0 Vicryl suture in a Bricker technique. After closing the posterior wall of the ureteroileal anastomosis, a 7Fr × 26 cm JJ ureteral stent is placed over a wire into the ureter percutaneously using a 2-mm port (Autosuture MiniPort 2 mm; Covidien, New Haven, CT). The excess ureter is then excised, and the ureteroileal anastomosis is completed (video 9:16).

Completion of Neobladder

The ureteral stents and Foley catheter are confirmed to be appropriately positioned within the neobladder. The remainder of the anterior bladder wall is closed with running 2-0 Stratafix Monocryl suture, and the neobladder is irrigated to confirm watertight integrity (video 12:14). A closed-suction drain is placed into the pelvis through a lateral port site. The specimen is then extracted through a low Pfannenstiel incision.

Step-by-Step Technique: CCUD

Our technique for intracorporeal CCUD (ICCUD) was developed to replicate well-established principles of the open surgical approach [42]. We have standardized the setup and steps of the procedure to improve efficiency and reproducibility. We have demonstrated feasibility with both platforms of the da Vinci® Si and Xi robot. The following section will provide a step-by-step description for robotic CCUD. *Table 22.1 shows supplies.*

Table 22.1 Recommended equipment

Robotic instruments	Fenestrated bipolar graspers
	Monopolar scissors
	Vessel sealer
	Tip-up fenestrated grasper
	Endowrist stapler (45-mm bowel load) for CCUD
	DeBakey forceps
	Potts scissors
	Large needle drivers
	Large clip (Weck) applier
Ports	8-mm robotic cannula
	12-mm robotic port (if using robotic stapler)
	12-mm assistant port
	12-mm assistant port (air seal)
	2-mm MiniPort; Covidien
Staplers	60-mm load (3.5 mm and 2.5 mm); Ethicon
Sutures	Pre-marked 2-0 Vicryl for intracorporeal measuring
	3-0 polyglactin SH
	2-0 silk SH
	4-0 polyglactin
	2-0 Stratafix Monocryl
	0-Vicryl on CT1
	0-Vicryl ties
Tubes	7Fr × 22 cm double-J ureteral stents
	22Fr Rusch hematuria catheter
	14Fr stomal catheter (capped)
	19Fr bulb-suction drain
Additional	Carter-Thomason
	10/12-mm endoscopic bag 10-mm endoscopic bag

Patient Positioning and Port Placement

Robotic cystectomy with extended pelvic lymph node dissection is performed with the patient in the dorsal lithotomy (Si) or supine (Xi) position in steep Trendelenburg configuration using previously reported standard six-port transperitoneal configuration [23].

Figure 22.1b illustrates port placement for extirpative component and intracorporeal CCUD component using the da Vinci Xi.

At the completion of the radical cystectomy, the patient is taken out of Trendelenburg and placed supine on the operating table with arms tucked and supported at the patient's sides. The patient is secured, and pressure points are padded to avoid pressure-related injury. The operating table is then tilted so the patient's right side is elevated in a modified lateral position. The robot is then docked and centered on the right side to facilitate bowel mobilization.

Mobilization and Segmentation of Bowel Segments

After identifying the ileocecal junction, the colon is mobilized from the cecum to the mid-transverse colon. Approximately 30 cm of ascending colon is selected for the pouch creation (video 00:45). The bowel is carefully manipulated using atraumatic tip-up graspers. Care is taken to clear the colon of mesocolic fat and adherent omentum to allow clear visualization of the colon and its mesentery to the transverse colon (video 1:05). A 10-cm segment of the terminal ileum is measured for the efferent catheterizable channel and stoma (video 1:25). Immediately proximal to this segment, a 12-cm segment of the ileum is measured to be used as an afferent chimney and to which the ureters will be anastomosed. Finally, a 5-cm segment proximal to this is measured to be excised and discarded to allow for separation between suture lines of the pouch and the bowel anastomosis (video 1:48).

A 60-mm bowel load (3.5-mm thickness) stapler (Echelon Flex 60, Ethicon Inc., Cincinnati, OH) is introduced via the 12-mm midline assistant port to divide the transverse colon and mesocolon using 2 or 3 staple loads between the hepatic flexure and middle colic artery. The left upper quadrant assistant port is used to introduce a 60-mm bowel load stapler (3.5-mm thickness) to transect the ileum (video 2:01). The antimesenteric sides of the proximal ileal segment and distal transverse colon segment are marked for orientation and manipulation (Fig. 22.15, video 2:06).

Restoration of Bowel Continuity

The terminal ileum and transverse colon are anastomosed in a side-to-side fashion to restore bowel continuity (video 3:15). A robotic 45-mm bowel load stapler is placed from the lateral robotic port on the patient's right side in order to facilitate the ileocolonic anastomosis (Fig. 22.16).

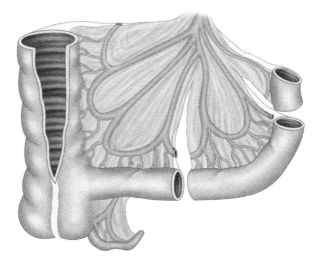

Fig. 22.15 A 30-cm segment of the colon is measured from the cecum to the transverse colon, and a 10-cm segment of terminal ileum is isolated for the efferent limb. A proximal 12-cm ileal segment is used to create the afferent ileal chimney, and a 5-cm proximal ileal segment is excised and discarded to separate the bowel anastomosis from the pouch

Fig. 22.16 Side-to-side ileocolonic anastomosis

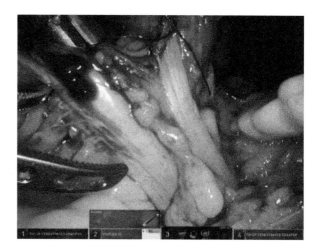

An additional bowel stapler load is deployed transversely to complete the anastomosis. Interrupted sutures are used to reinforce the corner of the bowel anastomosis.

Detubularization

The isolated colonic segment is then detubularized to begin pouch construction. The entire colonic segment is detubularized along the anterior tenia using monopolar

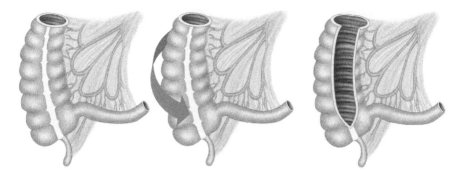

Fig. 22.17a A 30-cm segment of the colon is detubularized along the antimesenteric border to be used for the pouch

Fig. 22.17b Stay sutures at midpoint of detubularization will be used later for orientation during folding

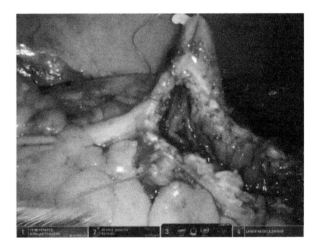

scissors (video 6:02). The contents of the colon are cleared during detubularization. Care is taken to avoid disrupting the ileocecal valve. Stay sutures are placed approximately 15 cm from the cecum on each side of the detubularized colon to mark the midpoint for folding the pouch. The stapled end of the efferent limb of the ileum is then excised and removed (Figs. 22.17a and 22.17b).

Tapering of the Efferent Limb

A 14Fr red rubber catheter is placed through the assistant port and inserted via the open ileal segment into the detubularized colon (video 6:15). This is secured with a purse-string suture at the end to be matured to the skin. The efferent limb is then tapered intracorporeally over the catheter using a bowel load stapler. Several staple loads are usually needed to traverse the length of the efferent limb (video 6:51). It is important to ensure the catheter passes easily and without kinking during tapering.

Fig. 22.18 The efferent limb is tapered over a 14Fr red rubber catheter intracorporeally

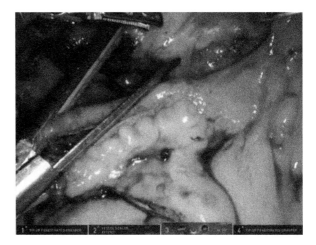

The ileocecal valve is reinforced for continence using interrupted 2-0 silk suture (Fig. 22.18, video 7:18).

Ureteroenteric Anastomosis

The ureters were previously tagged, clipped, and transected during the cystectomy. The tagged left ureter is then transposed under the sigmoid mesocolon to the right side. Traditionally, the ureters are anastomosed directly to the colon, though we have amended our technique to use an afferent ileal chimney. We describe both the traditional and new approaches. Sites for ureterocolonic anastomosis are identified on the posterior portion of the pouch to ensure creation of a tension-free anastomosis without angulation of the ureters after folding. A 1-cm colonic hiatus is created with monopolar scissors for each ureterocolonic anastomosis. The ureters are then passed from outside to inside of the colon and shortened to ensure redundant or poorly perfused ureter is excised. To assess the vascular perfusion of the distal ureter, indocyanine green (ICG) is injected intravenously (video 3:59). Poorly perfused distal ureteral tissue demonstrates less fluorescence when viewed under near-infrared light and is excised [43]. The rapid visualization of ICG approximately 1 minute after injection allows for quick assessment of ureteral perfusion [44] (Fig. 22.19).

The ureters are spatulated and anastomosed from inside the pouch. The distal ureter that will be discarded is used as a handle to manipulate the ureter for anastomosis. Individual Bricker anastomoses are performed using two running 4-0 polyglactin sutures with a PS-2 needle. The left arm utilizes robotic DeBakey forceps to allow for precise tissue manipulation. Full-thickness bites through the colon and ureter are taken. Once both ureterocolonic anastomoses are complete, a 7Fr × 26 cm double-J ureteral stent is placed into each ureter via a 2-mm port (Autosuture MiniPort 2 mm; Covidien, New Haven, CT).

Fig. 22.19 Indocyanine green shows distal ureteral vascularity, allowing poorly vascularized ureter to be excised and removed prior to ureterocolonic anastomosis

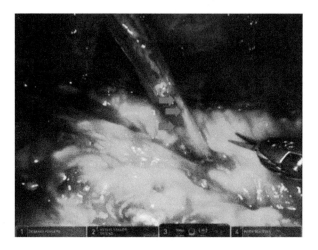

More recently, we updated our ureteroenteric anastomosis to incorporate an afferent ileal chimney. This approach replicates the standardized maneuvers of the intracorporeal ileal conduit and permits a ureteroileal anastomosis, in contrast to a ureterocolonic anastomosis. The ileal limb also reduces the length of the left ureter needed to reach the colonic diversion. After the segment to be used for ileal chimney has been isolated, the staple line is excised and the end closed in two layers with 2-0 Stratafix Monocryl (video 2:27). The sites for ureteroenteric anastomosis are identified and small ileostomies are made sharply. The vascularity of the ureters is assessed with ICG as described previously. The ureters are individually spatulated and the distal portion of the ureter is kept as a handle for positioning (video 3:56). The ureters are then anastomosed using Bricker anastomosis with two running 4-0 polyglactin sutures with PS-2 needle (video 4:32). Once half of the ureter is anastomosed to the chimney, a 7Fr single-J ureteral stent is placed into the ureter via a 2-mm port (Autosuture MiniPort 2 mm), and the second Monocryl suture is used to complete the running anastomosis (video 5:07).

Pouch Creation

With the ureterocolonic or ureteroileal anastomosis complete, the open colon segment is then folded and approximated using 2-0 polyglactin suture (Fig. 22.20). Several interrupted sutures are then placed to align the pouch for closure (video 8:11). The pouch is then closed in a running fashion using barbed absorbable sutures beginning medially and laterally (2-0 Stratafix Monocryl). The final configuration is displayed in Fig. 22.21. The proximal end of the ileal chimney is secured to the pouch with a running 2-0 Stratafix Monocryl suture as the pouch is being closed (video 8:27). An appendectomy is then completed (video 7:45). The single-J stents are passed through an opening in the pouch in preparation for externalization and are secured using a purse-string suture. A cecostomy tube (22Fr Rusch hematuria

Fig. 22.20 Folding
the pouch

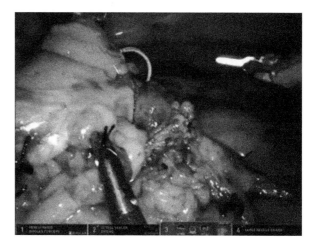

Fig. 22.21 Final
configuration of CCUD

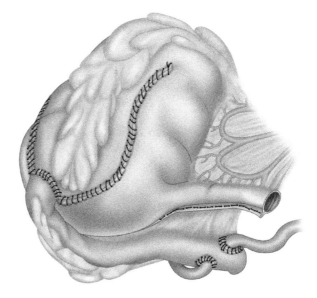

catheter) is then placed through the appendiceal opening and secured in place with
a purse-string suture. The pouch is then irrigated to confirm watertight integrity. The
abdomen is then irrigated and inspected. A 19 French drain is placed in the pelvis.

Stoma Creation

The robot is undocked and the specimen is extracted via a low transverse incision.
After removal of the specimen, the efferent limb is grasped and delivered through
the previously marked stoma site at the umbilicus or right lower quadrant using a
15-mm port. Excess ileum is excised and the catheterizable channel is spatulated.

Fig. 22.22 Post-operative visit

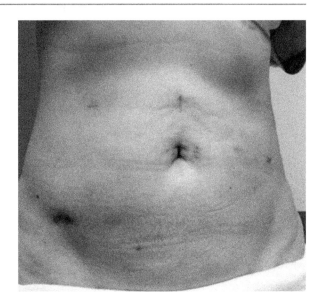

The stoma is matured to the skin using a V-shaped incision using interrupted 3-0 Vicryl suture. The stoma catheter is then placed in the channel and capped. Figure 22.22 shows a typical patient at their postoperative visit.

Intraoperative Considerations

Radical cystectomy with urinary diversion is a moderate-to-high risk major abdominal operation with the majority of patients being older and frequently with cardiopulmonary limitations. Standard general anesthetic considerations are applied, including noninvasive and invasive cardiac and pulmonary monitoring. Regional anesthetic block, such as transverse abdominis plane block, is routinely utilized for pain control management. Arterial line and large bore intravenous access are utilized. Central venous access is used at the discretion of the anesthesia department. Subcutaneous heparin and prophylactic antibiotics are administered prior to induction of anesthesia.

Respiratory response during the procedure is a critical consideration during RARC and ICUD. Attention should be paid to peak airway pressure, tidal volume, and end tidal CO_2 levels. Pulmonary response can be assessed at the start of the case by simulating the positioning. Adjustments to ventilator parameters and positioning can be made at this time. During the extirpative portion of the case, the patient is placed in steep Trendelenburg and then shifted to a modified lateral position for the intracorporeal CCUD. With continuous communication with the anesthesia provider, pneumoperitoneum pressures as well as the degree of Trendelenburg can be adjusted in accordance with pulmonary demands. The utilization of high-flow insufflation systems permits lower pneumoperitoneum pressure throughout the operation, which may be beneficial in patients with obstructive airway disease.

Multi-quadrant intra-abdominal access from the pelvis to the right upper abdomen permits extirpation and urinary reconstruction via a minimally invasive approach. One of the principal benefits of the intracorporeal approach is decreased bowel manipulation and exposure. Key components of the robotic bowel mobilization include mobilizing the colon from the cecum to the mid-transverse colon. The omentum and mesocolic fat are carefully cleared from the colon for transection. A small mesenteric window is made, taking care to preserve the mesenteric blood supply to the colon. The robotic stapler placed from the right side of the abdomen increases surgeon independence and provides a stable platform for the ileocolonic anastomosis. Articulation of the robotic stapler allows precise formation of the side-to-side anastomosis.

Near-infrared fluorescence imaging with indocyanine green (ICG) is also a useful tool during intracorporeal diversion. During bowel segmentation, it can be used to confirm vasculature anatomy and verify bowel perfusion after anastomosis. Further, ICG can be helpful to verify ureteral perfusion at the time of ureteral anastomosis. Redundant ureteral length can be discarded accordingly, and distal ureteral perfusion can be assessed at the anastomotic site. The utilization of fluorescent imaging to help reduce ureteral ischemia and subsequent ureteral stricture development is under active investigation.

As a component of enhanced recovery, fluids and blood products are carefully administered using a standardized goal-directed protocol. Stroke volume, stroke volume variation, and cardiac output are continuously monitored to aim for balanced fluid replacement. Care is taken to maximize homeostasis and minimize fluctuations in blood pressure and heart rate. Patient pressure points and extremity perfusion are checked throughout the procedure. Limiting of lithotomy position and repositioning every 4 hours are performed to reduce compartment syndrome risk.

Postoperative Care

After surgery, all patients follow a standardized enhanced recovery clinical pathway based on a 3–4-day hospital length of stay. Components of this pathway include early enteral feeding, aggressive mobilization, active prevention of nausea, and narcotic-sparing pain management. Multidisciplinary involvement of physical therapy, nursing, and case management is initiated immediately postoperatively.

Patients with ONB have only a 22Fr Rusch Foley catheter into the neobladder, and gentle irrigation of the neobladder begins in the recovery room. This catheter is routinely irrigated every 4–6 hours during postoperative hospital stay and at least twice daily at home after discharge. All CCUD patients have a suprapubic catheter (22Fr), which is secured off-tension and left to gravity drainage. This catheter is routinely irrigated with normal saline every 6 hours during the hospital course. Patients are instructed on catheter care and irrigation, which are continued twice daily at home until follow-up. The stoma catheter (14Fr) remains capped and secured during this period. The ureteral stents may be internalized within the pouch or externalized according to surgeon preference. A Jackson-Pratt (JP) drain is secured through a lateral port site and placed on bulb suction.

Postoperative day (POD) 0, patients are mobilized. Ambulation with assistance begins on POD 1. As patients receive a transversus abdominis plane (TAP) block preoperatively, intravenous (IV) patient-controlled analgesia (PCA) is generally not required. A narcotic-sparing pain management regimen is utilized, composed of scheduled acetaminophen, gabapentin, and nonsteroidal anti-inflammatory medication, renal function permitting. Oral and IV narcotic medication may be used as needed for breakthrough pain.

Diet is advanced from sips and ice chips on the day of surgery to full liquid diet on POD 1. If this is tolerated without abdominal distention or nausea, a regular diet is started on POD 2 or 3. Selective opioid receptor blockade with alvimopan is initiated preoperatively and continued until return of bowel function (ROBF) [45]. Gastrointestinal prophylaxis with a proton pump inhibitor and deep venous thrombosis (DVT) prophylaxis with low molecular weight heparin are instituted immediately postoperatively. DVT prophylaxis is continued for 28 days in the postoperative period [46].

Inpatient evaluation and education by wound ostomy nursing, physical therapy, occupational therapy, and respiratory therapy are critical components of the early postoperative rehabilitation program. Prior to discharge, the drain is removed after fluid creatinine is confirmed consistent with serum. The patient is discharged according to standard criteria, including afebrile status, stable labs, ability to ambulate with pain controlled, ability to tolerate a diet without nausea or distention, and appropriate outpatient support services established.

Patients are routinely contacted by nurses within 1–2 days following discharge. Immediate post-discharge follow-up occurs at 1 week. For ONB patients, the Foley catheter is removed around 3 weeks postoperatively. The ureteral stents are cystoscopically removed at the time of catheter removal. Figure 22.22 shows a postoperative result. For CCUD patients, a pouchogram is performed if indicated. The externalized stents are removed 1–2 weeks postoperatively. The stoma catheter is removed, while the suprapubic catheter is capped 2 weeks postoperatively. The patient then begins CIC at timed intervals along with daily pouch irrigation. A week later the suprapubic catheter is removed. Eventually, CIC intervals can be extended to every 4–6 hours as pouch capacity increases, usually by the third month.

Routine labs and cross-sectional imaging are performed at 3 months postoperatively. Patients are seen on a 3-month basis for the first year, and further surveillance imaging is tailored according to oncologic risk stratification.

Managing Complications and Next Steps

Radical cystectomy is a complex surgery associated with a significant risk for complications. Up to two-thirds of patients may experience a complication within the first 90 days after surgery [47]. Reports show that approximately 15–20% of complications may be high grade [48]. More than 60% of complications seen in this setting are related to the creation of the urinary diversion [47]. CCUD, whether performed using an open or intracorporeal approach, can be associated with increased short- and long-term complications compared to ileal conduit or ONB [6, 16, 48].

General Complications

Patients undergoing continent diversions remain susceptible to complications common to all patients undergoing RC with urinary diversion, in addition to CCUD-specific and ONB-specific complications. The most common complications in several series are gastrointestinal, infectious, and urinary [21, 48, 49]. Preoperative nutritional optimization and management of comorbid conditions are important in preparing RC patients for the surgical procedure and recovery [50, 51].

There is significant risk of perioperative venous thromboembolic events due to the presence of malignancy, major pelvic surgery, older age, and neoadjuvant chemotherapy [46]. For this reason, DVT prophylaxis with low molecular weight heparin is initiated preoperatively and continued for 28 days postoperatively.

Antibiotic prophylaxis with a second- or third-generation cephalosporin for the first 24 hours is provided, according to the American Urological Association's Best Practice Statement [52]. Antibiotic prophylaxis is also used prior to removing the cecostomy catheter and ureteral stents. Patients with CCUD will develop bacterial colonization, and further antibiotic treatment should be limited to those who are symptomatic [16].

Judicious perioperative fluid administration can limit bowel wall edema and aid in early functional recovery [53]. Postoperative enhanced recovery after surgery (ERAS) protocols which eliminate nasogastric tubes, limit opioid analgesia, encourage early ambulation, limit perioperative intravenous fluid hydration, and allow for early feeding can help reduce ileus as an early postoperative complication. Should ileus develop, supportive care with correction of electrolyte abnormalities, intravenous hydration, and bowel rest is recommended. In the event of emesis or persistent abdominal distention, early nasogastric decompression is recommended.

If ileus persists despite supportive care, abdominal imaging with computed tomography (CT) using oral contrast is indicated to rule out bowel obstruction. Serial abdominal examinations and blood work can identify signs of ischemia or perforation, which require abdominal exploration [54]. Bowel anastomotic leak is rare, seen in approximately 1% of patients [49]. Conservative management with bowel rest, antibiotics, and drain placement may be considered initially. Failure to progress with conservative measures may require exploration.

Pouch-Related Complications

Ureteroenteric stricture rates have been reported to be between 3% and 17% for intracorporeal ureteroenteric anastomoses [9, 21]. Ureterocolonic anastomotic stricture in CCUD was reported in 17% of 34 CCUDs performed extracorporeally after RARC, though this rate dropped to 9% after technical changes allowed confirmation of proper anastomosis orientation [9]. In a combined series of 17 patients undergoing totally intracorporeal CCUD, 2 patients were found to have anastomotic stricture, 1 of whom underwent operative reimplantation, while the other was managed with internal stenting [28]. Our use of afferent ileal chimney allows for a ureteroenteric anastomosis familiar to many urologists and may result in fewer anastomotic strictures.

To avoid injury to the ureter during mobilization, care should be taken to avoid over-dissection or skeletonization of the ureter. Atraumatic ureteral handling and preservation of periureteral adventitia are critical to avoid disruption of ureteral blood supply [55]. Stay sutures and discarding ureteral handles can be used to minimize ureteral handling and reduce the risk of injury. The authors routinely utilize fluorescence imaging to ensure robust ureteral perfusion and select the optimal site for anastomosis. Efforts are taken to create a straight ureteral path without redundancy or kinking to minimize the potential for ischemia or anastomotic leak [56].

Risk factors for benign ureteral anastomotic stricture include preoperative hydronephrosis, urine leak, perioperative urinary tract infection (UTI), prior abdominal surgery, and pelvic radiation. In the event of ureteroenteric anastomotic stricture, relief of obstruction with percutaneous nephrostomy tube and nephroureteral catheter placement should be first considered. Antegrade nephrostogram allows delineation of the stricture length and location. Endoscopic interrogation is needed to assess for malignant recurrence. Endoscopic management of the stricture may be considered for benign strictures, although the success of this approach has been reported to be only around 50%. In the authors' experience, robotic exploration and repair of benign ureteral strictures after open and robotic cystectomy can be feasible with a high degree of success. A minimally invasive approach allows for excision of the strictured segment with limited ureteral mobilization and verification of ureteral perfusion at the anastomotic site.

Urine leak from the suture line or ureteral anastomosis can occur in the early postoperative period. Urine leak can lead to chemical peritonitis and contribute to ileus. Resulting urinomas may become infected. Small leaks can be managed with decompression by cecostomy tube and closed suction (JP) drain. A leak should be suspected if JP drain output is elevated and is confirmed if the drain fluid creatinine is elevated above serum levels. Frequent gentle irrigation of the pouch can rid the pouch of mucous that may cause impaired drainage and contribute to early leak due to high intraluminal pouch pressure. In some cases, the JP drain can be withdrawn from closely overlying the pouch.

Fluoroscopic evaluation can show the site and extent of urine leak. Most urine leaks can be managed conservatively with tube drainage. If associated with leukocytosis or systemic symptoms, computed tomography is indicated to assess for fluid collection, which may require percutaneous drainage. Persistent urine leak may necessitate urinary diversion with nephrostomy tubes. Pouch revision is rarely needed and may be pursued in delayed fashion in the setting of controlled urinary fistula [57].

Difficulty Catheterizing/Stomal Stenosis

Patients are counseled to catheterize every 4–6 hours to avoid overdistention of the pouch. Difficulty catheterizing may be related to either stomal stenosis or efferent limb kinking. If the efferent limb is too long, the catheter may catch as it passes the fascia. For this reason, it is important to tailor the efferent limb to use a short segment and to test the ease of catheterization at the time of stoma maturation.

Patients should be educated that inability to catheterize necessitates urgent evaluation to avoid pouch rupture. If the pouch is overdistended, it may cause a kinking at the efferent limb that makes catheterization difficult. In the event of inability to catheterize via the stoma, a percutaneous drainage using an angiocatheter can be used for decompression. This can be performed at bedside under ultrasound guidance. Once the pouch is decompressed, a catheter can be placed. Endoscopic placement of a catheter over a wire may also be attempted in these situations. Leaving a catheter in place for several days can help avoid trauma to the tortuous efferent limb and aid healing. If difficulty catheterizing persists, efferent limb revision may be required.

Stomal stenosis can be avoided by spatulating the channel and incorporation of a well-vascularized skin flap. If the catheter cannot be placed due to stomal stenosis, gentle dilation with urethral sounds can be attempted. Stomal stenosis is more common in appendiceal channels and can be seen in 10–30% of cases [58]. For this reason, the authors favor the use of the ileum as the efferent limb. If dilation or incision of skin edge fails to alleviate the stenosis, revision with V-Y plasty or stomal revision may be required.

Recent studies showed urinary incontinence rates of 2–10% [4, 7] for CCUD. Among 17 patients recently undergoing intracorporeal CCUD, no incontinence was noted [23]. Adequate bowel length, detubularization, and folding all help to ensure low pressure within the pouch. Using an appropriate-length efferent limb segment can assist with continence; however, excessive length may lead to difficulty catheterizing due to mucosal folding and kinking [58].

As the colon can generate high-pressure contractions, urodynamics can be considered in patients who are experiencing stomal incontinence [3]. Pouch revision with an ileal patch can help alleviate incontinence in the case of high-pressure, low-volume pouch. Though some have attempted endoscopic injection of bulking agents, formal pouch revision with reinforcement of the ileocecal valve and efferent limb revision may be pursued less commonly [3, 59].

Incontinence following ONB can be expected to improve as the neobladder expands and with timed-voiding neobladder-training regimens. Daytime continence rates between 73% and 88% and nighttime continence rates of 55–58% have been reported in robotic intracorporeal ONB series, though standardized, validated assessments are needed for better characterization of continence in this population [28].

Pouch stones have been reported to impact up to 42% of CCUD patients [3]. This can be minimized by frequent complete catheterization and with manual irrigation using normal saline. Neobladder stone rates of 4–6% have been reported [60]. Endoscopic or percutaneous treatments are usually effective, though large stones may require open removal.

Efferent limb necrosis is a rare but potentially devastating complication of CCUD. This arises when vascular supply to the efferent limb is compromised. This can be avoided by taking care during bowel mobilization and through intraoperative observation of bowel perfusion. Some duskiness at the distal edge of the efferent limb can be serially monitored for resolution. If there is concern for more proximal necrosis, a flexible cystoscope can be used to directly visualize the efferent limb and pouch. Significant vascular compromise and limb necrosis require surgical revision.

Spontaneous perforation should be suspected in a patient presenting with acute abdominal pain and distention. This rare complication can occur due to poor compliance with catheterization or trauma and had an incidence of 1.6% in a large open Scandinavian series [61]. Some late perforations have no clear inciting event, though it may be more common among previously radiated patients [57]. Cystogram or CT cystogram can aid both in the diagnosis of perforation and in quick identification and surgical repair.

Metabolic Complications

Measures to prevent short- and long-term metabolic complications should be pursued in all patients with urinary diversions. The large bowel absorbs chloride, hydrogen, and ammonium, while excreting bicarbonate when in contact with urine, leading to hyperchloremic metabolic acidosis. Rates of metabolic acidosis range from 26% to 45% in CCUD patients and 6–13% in ONB patients [1, 62]. Prolonged urine-bowel contact time can increase these metabolic derangements. Routine electrolyte evaluation will allow for alkalinization if required. Dietary changes can help reduce acidosis. In severe cases, sodium bicarbonate or potassium citrate may be used for alkalinization. If there is significant renal dysfunction, nephrology referral is indicated. Routine comprehensive metabolic panel is checked every 3 months for the first 2 years and then on a 6-month basis.

In addition to renal deterioration, chronic acidosis can lead to bone demineralization and osteopenia [3]. Patients with preexisting renal insufficiency are at increased risk for this [62]. A SEER analysis of cystectomy patients recently found cystectomy patients to have a 21% greater risk of fracture (adjusted hazard ratio of 1.21) than those without cystectomy history [14]. Regular electrolyte evaluation with correction of acidosis, as well as calcium with vitamin D supplementation, may help prevent acidosis-related bone demineralization.

Patients undergoing ONB or CCUD with the use of the terminal ileum are at risk for vitamin B12 deficiency, as the terminal ileum is the site for B12 absorption. Depletion of B12 can take 3–4 years in the absence of absorption [63]. We routinely check B12 annually beginning after the first postoperative year and replenish as needed.

With bowel urinary diversion, chronic diarrhea may occur due to lower resorption of biliary salts. With the ileum or ileocecal valve harvested for the diversion, some unresorbed bile salts may enter the colon and lead to irritative diarrhea or steatorrhea due to fat malabsorption [62, 63]. A high-fiber diet and cholestyramine can be used to help mitigate persistent diarrhea [63].

Lifelong follow-up and health maintenance are required in all patients undergoing urinary diversion. Complication profiles change over time, and proactive vigilance is required for prevention and early detection.

Conclusion

Intracorporeal ONB or CCUD with RARC are important diversions for patients who desire urinary continence. The intracorporeal techniques demonstrated are feasible, safe, and reproducible. This minimally invasive approach aims to replicate the tenets established in open surgery. With incorporation of intracorporeal CCUD, the complete range of urinary diversions is available to all patients undergoing robotic cystectomy using techniques built on the principles of intracorporeal ileal conduit and neobladder. With experience, both intracorporeal ONB and CCUD can be performed with high continence rates and patient satisfaction.

References

1. Pearce SM, Daneshmand S. Continent cutaneous diversion. Urol Clin N Am. 2018;45:55–65.
2. Kock NG, Nilson AE, Nilsson LO, Norlen LJ, Philipson BM. Urinary diversion via a continent ileal reservoir: clinical results in 12 patients. J Urol. 1982;128:469–75.
3. Bricker EM. Symposium on clinical surgery; Bladder substitution after pelvic evisceration. Surg Clin N Am. 1950;3:1511.
4. Spencer ES, Lyons MD, Pruthi RS. Patient selection and counseling for urinary diversion. Urol Clin N Am. 2018;45:1–9.
5. Mansson A, Davidsson T, Hunt S, Mansson W. The quality of life in men after radical cystectomy with a continent cutaneous diversion or orthotopic bladder substitution: is there a difference? BJU Int. 2002;90:386–90.
6. Bihrle R. The Indiana pouch continent urinary reservoir. Urol Clin North Am. 1997;24(4):773–9.
7. Torrey RR, Chan KG, Yip W, Josephson DY, Lau CS, Ruel NH, Wilson TG. Functional outcomes and complications in patients with bladder cancer undergoing robotic-assisted radical cystectomy with extracorporeal Indiana pouch continent cutaneous diversion. Urology. 2012;79(5):1073–8.
8. Goh AC, Aghazadeh MA, Krasnow RE, Pastuszak AW, Stewart JN, Miles BJ. Robotic intracorporeal continent cutaneous diversion: primary description. J Endourol. 2015;29(11):1217–20.
9. Desai MM, Simone G, Abreu AL, Chopra S, Ferriero M, Guaglionone S, et al. Robotic intracorporeal continent cutaneous diversion. J Urol. 2017;198:436–44.
10. Pietzak EJ, Donahue TF, Bochner BH. Male neobladder. Urol Clin N Am. 2018;45:37–48.
11. Studer UE, Zingg EJ. Ileal orthotopic bladder substitutes: what we have learned from 12 years' experience with 200 patients. Urol Clin N Am. 1997;24(4):781–93.
12. Menon M, Hemal AK, Tewari A, Shrivastava A, Shoma AM, El-Tabey NA, et al. Nerve-sparing robot-assisted radical cystoprostatectomy and urinary diversion. BJU Int. 2003;92(3):232–6.
13. Hanna N, Leow J, Sun M, Friedlander D, Seisen T, et al. Comparative effectiveness of robot-assisted vs. open radical cystectomy. Urol Oncol. 2018;36:88.e1–9.
14. Hussein AA, May PR, Jing Z, Ahmed YE, Wijburg CJ, Canda AE, et al. Outcomes of intracorporeal urinary diversion after robot-assisted radical cystectomy: results from the international robotic cystectomy consortium. J Urol. 2017;199:1302–11.
15. Collins JW, Hosseini A, Sooriakumaran P, Nyberg T, Sanchez-Salas R, Adding C. Tips and tricks for intracorporeal robot-assisted urinary diversion. Curr Urol Rep. 2014;15:457–66.

16. Gupta A, Atoria CL, Ehdaie B, Shariat SF, Rabbani F, Herr HW, Bochner BH, Elkin EB. Risk of fracture after radical cystectomy and urinary diversion for bladder cancer. J Clin Oncol. 2014;32(29):3291–8.
17. Hautmann RE, Abol-Enein H, Lee CT, Mansson W, Mills RD, Penson DF. Urinary diversion: how experts divert. Urology. 2015;85(1):233–8.
18. Hautmann RE, Abol-Enein H, Davidsson T, Gudjonsson S, Hautmann SH, Holm HV, et al. ICUD-EAU international consultation on bladder cancer 2012: urinary diversion. Eur Urol. 2013;63:67–80.
19. Parekh DJ, Reis IM, Castle EP, Gonzalgo ML, Woods ME, Svatek RS, et al. Robot-assisted radical cystectomy versus open radical cystectomy in patients with bladder cancer (RAZOR): an open-label, randomized, phase 3, non-inferiority trial. Lancet. 2018;391:2525–36.
20. Bochner B, Dalbagni G, Sjoberg D, Silberstein J, Paz K, et al. Comparing open radical cystectomy and robot-assisted laparoscopic radical cystectomy: a randomized clinical trial. Eur Urol. 2015;67(6):1042–50.
21. Bochner B, Dalbagni G, Marzouk K, Sjoberg D, Lee J, et al. Randomized trial comparing open radical cystectomy and robot-assisted laparoscopic radical cystectomy: oncologic outcomes. Eur Urol. 2018;74(4):465–71.
22. Desai MM, de Abreu ALC, Goh AC, Fairey A, Berger A, Leslie S, et al. Robotic intracorporeal urinary diversion: technical details to improve time efficiency. J Endourol. 2014;28(11):1320–7.
23. Dason S, Goh AC. Contemporary techniques and outcomes of robotic cystectomy and intracorporeal diversions. Curr Opin Urol. 2018;28(2):115–22.
24. Wilson TG, Guru K, Rosen RC, Wiklund P, Annerstedt M, Bochner BH, et al. Best practices in robot-assisted radical cystectomy and urinary reconstruction: recommendations of the pasadena consensus panel. Eur Urol. 2015;67(3):363–75.
25. Goh AC, Gill IS, Lee DJ, Abreu ALC, Fairey AS, Leslie S, et al. Robotic intracorporeal orthotopic ileal neobladder: replicating open surgical principles. Eur Urol. 2012;62:891–901.
26. Hayn MH, Hussain A, Mansour AM, Andrews PE, Carpentier P, Castle E, et al. The learning curve of robot-assisted radical cystectomy: results from the international robotic cystectomy consortium. Eur Urol. 2010;58:197–202.
27. Moschini M, Simone G, Stenzl A, Gill I, Catto J. Critical review of outcomes from radical cystectomy: can complications from radical cystectomy be reduced by surgical volume and robotic surgery? Eur Urol Focus. 2016;2(1):19–29.
28. Dason S, Goh AC. Updates on intracorporeal urinary diversions. Curr Urol Rep. 2018;19:28–36.
29. Catto J, Khetrapal P, Ambler G, Sarpong R, Khan M, et al. Robot-assisted radical cystectomy with intracorporeal urinary diversion versus open radical cystectomy (iROC): protocol for a randomized controlled trial with internal feasibility study. BMJ Open. 2018;8:e020500. https://doi.org/10.1136/bmjopen-2017-020500.
30. Lamb B, Tan W, Eneje P, Bruce D, Jones A, et al. Benefits of robotic cystectomy with intracorporeal diversion for patients with low cardiorespiratory fitness: a prospective cohort study. Urol Oncol. 2016;34:417.e17–23.
31. Ahmed K, Khan SA, Hayn MH, Agarwal PK, Badani KK, Balbay MD, et al. Analysis of intracorporeal compared with extracorporeal urinary diversion after robot-assisted radical cystectomy: results from the international robotic cystectomy consortium. Eur Urol. 2014;65:340–7.
32. Daneshmand S, Bartsch G. Improving selection of appropriate urinary diversion following radical cystectomy for bladder cancer. Expert Rev Anticancer Ther. 2011;11(6):941–8.
33. DeCastro GJ, McKiernan JM, Benson MC. Ch 98: Cutaneous continent urinary diversion. In: WS MD, Wein AJ, Kavoussi LR, Partin AW, Peters CA, editors. Campbell-Walsh urology. 11th ed. Philadelphia: Elsevier; 2016. p. 2317.
34. Zlatev DV, Skinner EC. Orthotopic urinary diversion for women. Urol Clin N Am. 2018;45:49–54.
35. Bochner B, Figueroa A, Skinner E, Lieskovsky G, Petrovich Z, et al. Salvage radical cystoprostatectomy and orthotopic urinary diversion following radiation failure. J Urol. 1998;160(1):29–33.

36. Chopra S, Abreu ALC, Gill IS. Robotic urinary diversion: the range of options. Curr Opin Urol. 2016;26:107–13.
37. Littlejohn N, Cohn J, Kowalik C, Kaufman M, Dmochowski R, et al. Treatment of pelvic floor disorders following neobladder. Curr Urol Rep. 2017;18(1):5–10.
38. Shabsigh A, Korets R, Vora K, Brooks C, Cronin A, et al. Defining early morbidity of radical cystectomy for patients with bladder cancer using a standardized reporting methodology. Eur Urol. 2009;55(1):164–74.
39. Dahl DM. Ch 97: use of intestinal segments in urinary diversion. In: WS MD, Wein AJ, Kavoussi LR, Partin AW, Peters CA, editors. Campbell-Walsh urology. 11th ed. Philadelphia: Elsevier; 2016. p. 2310–1.
40. Tammaro G, Zacchia M, Zona E, Zacchia E, Capasso G. Acute and chronic effects of metabolic acidosis on renal function and structure. J Nephrol. 2018;31(4):551–9.
41. Maffezini M, Campodonico F, Canepa G, et al. Current perioperative management of radical cystectomy with intestinal urinary reconstruction for muscle-invasive bladder cancer and reduction of the incidence of postoperative ileus. Surg Oncol. 2008;17(1):41–8.
42. Rowland R. Continent cutaneous urinary diversion. Semin Urol Oncol. 1997;15(3):179–83.
43. Spinoglio G, Bertani E, Borin S, Piccioli A, Petz W. Green indocyanine fluorescence in robotic abdominal surgery. Updat Surg. 2018;70:375–9.
44. Tobis S, Knopf JK, Silvers CR, Marshall J, Cardin A, Wood RW, et al. Near infrared fluorescence imaging after intravenous indocyanine green: initial clinical experience with open partial nephrectomy for renal cortical tumors. Urology. 2012;79:958–64.
45. Tobis S, Heinlen JE, Ruel N, Lau C, Kawachi M, Wilson T, Chan K. Effect of alvimopan on return of bowel function after robot-assisted radical cystectomy. J Laparoendosc Adv Surg Tech A. 2014;24(10):693–7.
46. Schomburg J, Krishna S, Soubra A, Cotter K, Fan Y, Brown G, Konety B. Extended outpatient chemoprophylaxis reduces venous thromboembolism after radical cystectomy. Urol Oncol. 2018;36(2):77e9–77e13.
47. Anderson CB, McKiernan JM. Surgical complications of urinary diversion. Urol Clin N Am. 2018;45:79–90.
48. Namzy M, Yuh B, Kawachi M, et al. Early and late complications of robot-assisted radical cystectomy: a standardized analysis by urinary diversion type. J Urol. 2014;191(3):681–7.
49. Hautmann RE, Petriconi RC, Volkmer BG. Lessons learned from 1,000 neobladders: the 90-day complication rate. J Urol. 2010;184:990–4.
50. Johnson DC, Riggs SB, Nielson ME, Matthews JE, Woods ME, Wallen EM, Pruthi RS, Smith AB. Nutritional predictors of complications following radical cystectomy. World J Urol. 2015;33(8):1129–37.
51. Zhong J, Switchenko J, Jegadeesh NK, Cassidy RJ, Gillespie TW, Master V, et al. Comparison of outcomes in patients with muscle-invasive bladder cancer treated with radical cystectomy versus bladder preservation. Am J Clin Oncol. 2019;42(1):36–41.
52. Wolf JS, Bennett CJ, Dmochowski RR, Hollenbeck BK, Pearle MS, Schaeffer AJ, et al. Best practice policy statement on urologic surgery antimicrobial prophylaxis. American Urological Association Education and Research; 2008. 23p. http://www.auanet.org/guidelines/antimicrobial-prophylaxis-(2008-reviewed-and-validity-confirmed-2011-amended-2012). Accessed on 26 Feb 2020.
53. Lobo DN, Bostock KA, Neal KR, et al. Effect of salt and water balance on recovery of gastrointestinal function after elective colonic resection: a randomised controlled trial. Lancet. 2002;359:1812–8.
54. Mckiernan JM, Anderson CB. Ch 41: complications of radical cystectomy and urinary diversion. In: Complications of urologic surgery. Diagnosis, prevention, and management. 5th ed. New York: Elsevier; 2018. p. 437.
55. Fröber R. Surgical atlas: surgical anatomy of the ureter. BJU Int. 2007;100:949–65.
56. Richards KA, Cohn JA, Large MC, Bales GT, Smith ND, Steinberg GD. The effect of length of ureteral resection on benign ureterointestinal stricture rate in ileal conduit or ileal neobladder urinary diversion following radical cystectomy. Urol Oncol. 2015;33(2):65.e1–8.

57. Skinner EC, Zlatev D. Ch 46: complications of continent cutaneous diversion. In: Complications of urologic surgery. Diagnosis, prevention, and management. 5th ed. New York: Elsevier; 2018. p. 495.
58. Ardelt PU, Woodhouse CRJ, Riedmiller H, Gerharz EW. The efferent segment in continent cutaneous urinary diversion: a comprehensive review of the literature. BJU Int. 2012;109(2):288–97.
59. Kass-iliyya A, Rashid TG, Citron I, et al. Long-term efficacy of polydimethylsiloxane (Macroplastique) injection for Mitrofanoff leakage after continent urinary diversion surgery. BJU Int. 2015;115(3):461–5.
60. Simone G, Papalia R, Misuraca L, et al. Robotic intracorporeal padua ileal bladder: surgical technique, perioperative, oncologic and functional outcomes. Eur Urol. 2018;73:934–40.
61. Mansson W, Bakke A, Bergman B, et al. Perforation of continent urinary reservoirs. Scandinavian experience. Scand J Urol Nephrol. 1997;31(6):529–32.
62. Reddy M, Kader K. Follow-up management of cystectomy patients. Urol Clin N Am. 2018;45:241–7.
63. Roth JD, Koch MO. Metabolic and nutritional consequences of urinary diversion using intestinal segments to reconstruct the urinary tract. Urol Clin N Am. 2018;45:19–24.

Robotic-Assisted Ileal Conduit Urinary Diversion

Akbar N. Ashrafi, Luis G. Medina, and Monish Aron

Introduction

Bladder cancer is the 9th most commonly diagnosed malignancy worldwide with an incidence of 430,000 cases per year and is the 13th leading cause of cancer mortality annually [1]. Radical cystectomy (RC) with pelvic lymph node dissection and urinary diversion is the standard of care for localized muscle-invasive bladder cancer and is also recommended in non-muscle invasive bladder tumors at high risk of pathological progression [2, 3].

Robotic-assisted RC (RARC) has gained popularity in the last decade due to the potential benefits in improving blood loss, perioperative transfusion requirements, length of hospital stay, and postoperative convalescence without compromising oncological outcomes. In these patients, most surgeons adopted a hybrid approach with extracorporeal urinary diversion due to technical demands of a complete intracorporeal urinary diversion (ICUD). Intracorporeal RC with ileal conduit urinary diversion was first performed by Gill et al. using a purely laparoscopic technique in 2000 [4], followed by the first report using the robotic platform in 2003 [5]. Since the initial pioneering reports, the safety and feasibility of intracorporeal ileal conduit reconstruction have been demonstrated [6]. Increasing experience coupled with ongoing refinement of surgical technique has led to a significant increase in ICUDs following RARC in the last decade, which has primarily been driven by increased utilization of intracorporeal ileal conduit diversions [7].

Supplementary Information The online version of this chapter (https://doi.org/10.1007/978-3-030-50196-9_23) contains supplementary material, which is available to authorized users.

A. N. Ashrafi · L. G. Medina · M. Aron (✉)
USC Institute of Urology, Norris Comprehensive Cancer Center, Keck School of Medicine, University of Southern California, Los Angeles, CA, USA
e-mail: Akbar.Ashrafi@med.usc.edu; monish.aron@med.usc.edu

© Springer Nature Switzerland AG 2022
M. D. Stifelman et al. (eds.), *Techniques of Robotic Urinary Tract Reconstruction*, https://doi.org/10.1007/978-3-030-50196-9_23

In this chapter, we review the indications, preoperative preparation, step-by-step surgical technique, postoperative management, and potential complications of robotic-assisted ileal conduit urinary diversion.

Indications for Ileal Conduit Urinary Diversion

The choice of urinary diversion after RC is a shared decision-making process impacted by myriad patient, disease, and surgeon factors [8]. Patient factors include patient preference, comorbidities, baseline status, and perceived quality of life with each type of diversion. Disease characteristics include extent of bladder cancer and urethral margin status. Further, surgeon training, experience, and preference have a significant impact on the urinary diversion options presented to patients.

In the 2000s, the majority of urinary diversions were performed extracorporeally after RARC. More recently, over the last decade, there has been a trend toward increased utilization of ICUDs. A contemporary multi-institutional study of patients undergoing RARC demonstrated that, as of 2016, intracorporeal ileal conduit is the most popular method of urinary diversion (81% of all cases), followed by intracorporeal neobladder (17%) and extracorporeal diversions (2%) [7].

Patients with impaired hand function, neurologic conditions such as dementia or Parkinson's disease, intellectual impairment, urethral stricture disease, chronic inflammatory bowel disease, hepatic insufficiency, or renal impairment should be counseled for an ileal conduit as these are relative contraindications to a continent orthotopic or continent cutaneous urinary diversion. While there is no specific renal function cutoff, the ICUD-EAU International Consultation on Bladder Cancer recommended that patients with a glomerular filtration rate < 50 mL/min or a serum creatinine >150 μmol/L should be counseled against a continent diversion in favor of an ileal conduit [9].

Preoperative Considerations

Preoperative workup should include a complete medical and surgical history. In particular, the presence of prior neurologic, renal, or hepatic impairment, inflammatory bowel disease, prior abdominal surgery including small bowel resection, and previous pelvic irradiation should be assessed.

Laboratory testing should include baseline complete blood count, renal function, liver function, albumin, and preoperative type and screen. Nutrition consultation may be beneficial as poor nutritional status is associated with increased complications after RC and urinary diversion [10]. Exercise-based prehabilitation may improve muscle strength in patients undergoing RC [11], and preoperative carbohydrate loading has been associated with reduced length of stay in patients undergoing major abdominal surgery [12].

A complete metastatic workup with contrast-enhanced computerized tomography (CT) of the chest, abdomen, and pelvis is essential in patients undergoing RARC for bladder cancer. A delayed-phase CT urogram is recommended to exclude synchronous upper tract urothelial tumors. MRI may be performed for local pelvic staging particularly in patients with suspected extravesical disease. Brain MRI and whole-body bone scan are performed in symptomatic patients. While FDG-PET/CT is not routinely recommended, it may be considered if there is ongoing suspicion for metastases.

Patients undergoing robotic ileal conduit reconstruction should be counseled thoroughly on the risks, benefits, and potential complications and alternate treatment options for urinary diversion. A thorough preoperative anesthesiology assessment is mandatory. Cardiac workup, if required, typically comprises transthoracic echocardiography and a cardiac stress test. Lung function assessment is completed in patients with a history of smoking or pulmonary illness. Consideration of cardiac and pulmonary functions is particularly important given the need for prolonged steep Trendelenburg position during RARC and intracorporeal ileal conduit formation.

The stoma nurse plays an important role, and we prefer that the patients see the nurse early during the decision-making process on what type of urinary diversion to have. The nurse helps patients understand the body image changes associated with a stoma and teaches them how to care for the stoma and troubleshoot common stoma-related issues. The stoma site is marked on the patient's abdomen prior to surgery. Surgeons should be familiar with the main principles of siting the stoma, which are as follows [13]:

- The stoma site should be over the rectus abdominis muscle.
- The stoma should be over a flat section of the abdomen avoiding abdominal folds or creases.
- The stoma should avoid the belt line.
- The suitability of the stoma site should be confirmed with the patient in supine, sitting, and upright positions.

The patient is admitted on the day of surgery, and bowel preparation is omitted in patients undergoing RARC and ileal conduit urinary diversion. Bowel preparation may be considered if colonic conduit is a possibility or there is increased risk of bowel injury, for example, in patients with previous bowel resections or pelvic irradiation. Antiplatelet and anticoagulant medications are withheld prior to surgery according to hospital protocols. Broad-spectrum antibiotic prophylaxis with coverage of gram-positive, gram-negative, and anaerobic bacteria is recommended within 1 hour of surgery. Our preference is to administer intravenous cefoxitin. Fluconazole may also administered in diabetic or immunocompromised patients. A combination of mechanical and pharmacological thromboembolic prophylaxis and a single dose of alvimopan (a μ-receptor antagonist) is administered immediately prior to surgery.

Step-by-Step Technique

Patient Positioning and Port Placement

The patient is placed in the lithotomy position or supine position in male patients undergoing surgery with the Xi robot. Pneumoperitoneum is established using the Veress needle or Hasson technique according to surgeon preference. A six-port transperitoneal approach is used with a camera, three robotic, and two assistant

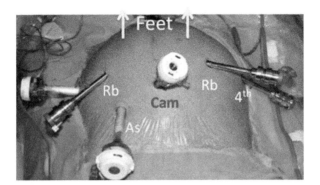

Fig. 23.1 Port configuration for the Si Surgical System. The Si robot is docked from between the patient's legs or the patient's right in females to allow access to the perineum. A six-port transperitoneal technique is used. The camera port is placed in midline 8 cm above the umbilicus. Four ports are placed in a horizontal line 2 fingerbreadths above the umbilicus including three robotic ports and a 15 mm assistant port on the patient's left. A 12 mm AirSeal port (ConMed, Utica, NY, USA) is placed in the left upper quadrant. (*As* assistant ports, *Cam* camera port, *Rb* robotic port, *4th* fourth arm)

ports. Port placement for the Si system is shown in Fig. 23.1. The camera port is placed 8 cm above the umbilicus, and four ports are placed in a horizontal line 2 fingerbreadths above the umbilicus. Two robotic ports are placed on the patient's right and one robotic port and a 15 mm assistant port on the patient's left. A 12 mm AirSeal port (ConMed, Utica, NY, USA) is placed in the left upper quadrant, triangulating between the camera port and left robotic port. The port configuration is similar to that used in robotic-assisted radical prostatectomy with a few important differences: all of the ports are placed in a more cephalad position to facilitate bowel handling and extended pelvic lymph node dissection, and two assistant ports are routinely used to facilitate the use of a laparoscopic bowel stapler during the procedure. Figure 23.2 depicts our preferred port placement for the Xi system if using the robotic stapler. For the Xi robot where a robotic stapler is preferred, two robotic ports are placed on the left including a hybrid port for the stapler at the left most lateral port at the level of the umbilicus, and the 15 mm assistant and AirSeal ports are placed on the right. Following port placement, the patient is placed in steep Trendelenburg. This position affords optimal working space in the pelvis due to cephalad displacement of the bowel. A 30-degree scope is used for the entire procedure. For the cystectomy, we use two Cadiere forceps, one monopolar scissor, and one robotic vessel sealer. For the diversion, we use the same instruments and add two large needle drivers.

Identification of the Ureters and Bowel Segment

By the time the ileal conduit diversion is commenced, both ureters have been clipped and divided and the left ureter transposed to the right posterior to the

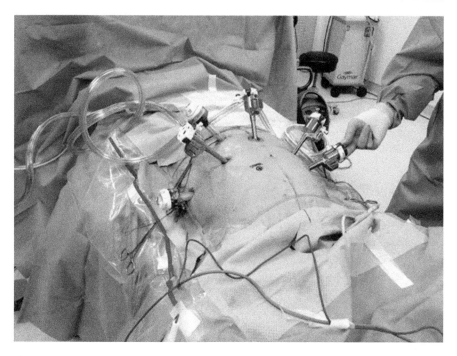

Fig. 23.2 Port configuration for the Xi Surgical System when using a robotic stapler. The Xi robot is side-docked from the patient's left. The camera port is placed in midline 8 cm above the umbilicus and three ports are placed in a horizontal line 2 fingerbreadths above the umbilicus a 12 mm hybrid robotic stapler port is placed at the left most lateral port at the level of the umbilicus, and the 15 mm assistant and 12 mm AirSeal ports are placed on the patient's right

sigmoid mesentery (Fig. 23.3a, b). The retromesenteric window is best created during lymph node dissection of the left common iliac and presacral nodes in cases of radical cystectomy. A Penrose drain may be looped around the sigmoid colon and used for retraction if required. We find that using fourth arm to deliver the left ureter through the retromesenteric window is easiest for this step. The ileocecal valve is identified, and 20 cm of the terminal ileum is measured from the ileocecal junction and preserved. This point marks the distal end of the bowel segment which will be used for the ileal conduit.

Isolation of the Bowel Segment

When using a handheld laparoscopic stapler, we prefer the Echelon Flex Powered Plus 60 mm stapler (Ethicon Inc., Somerville, NJ, USA) with a blue cartridge (3.5 mm staple height). When using the robotic stapler, we use the 45 mm blue cartridge for all bowel work.

The stapler is used to divide the small bowel 20 cm proximal to the ileocecal valve (Fig. 23.3c, d). This is followed by a further deepening of the mesenteric

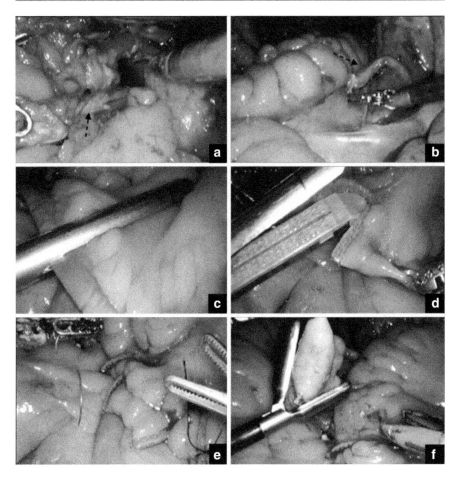

Fig. 23.3 **a** and **b**: Identification of the ureters; arrow points to the ureters. **c** and **d**: Isolation of the bowel segments. **e** and **f**: A 5 cm segment of the ileum may be discarded

division with a robotic vessel sealer if additional mobility is required. It is important to position the stapler perpendicular to the bowel segment and mesentery to minimize the risk of devascularization. The stapler is elevated to check that no bowel loops have been inadvertently caught underneath prior to firing the stapler. A 2-0 dyed Vicryl (Ethicon, Somerville, NJ, USA) stay suture is used to mark the distal bowel segment which will be used later for the side-to-side bowel anastomosis. The suture is placed on the mesenteric side of the bowel.

The segment of the small bowel used for the conduit is typically 15–20 cm long although occasionally the conduit needs to be longer than this to facilitate tension-free ureteroileal anastomosis. The fourth arm is used to elevate the distal end of the bowel segment to the anterior abdominal wall to ensure the conduit is of adequate length and can easily reach the prepared ureters before dividing the bowel. The proximal segment of the ileal conduit is then divided with the stapler, and depending on the mobility of the isolated segment, the vessel sealer can be used to deepen the mesenteric division. An undyed Vicryl suture is used to mark the proximal stump of the ileal conduit and is run in a horizontal mattress fashion to exclude the staple line from the conduit lumen. In our experience, this isolation of bowel is completed most efficiently using the stapler introduced through the left lateral port.

Bowel Anastomosis

In some cases, we discard a 5 cm segment of bowel proximal to the ileal conduit segment (Fig. 23.3e, f). The "discard segment" is isolated with the stapler and the mesentery is released using a vessel sealer immediately adjacent to the bowel so as to maintain good vascularity to the conduit and bowel anastomosis. The discard segment is removed through the 15 mm assistant port. This step can help ensure adequate separation and mobility of the ileal conduit from the bowel anastomosis that is to follow. Another dyed Vicryl stay suture is placed on the mesenteric border of the proximal bowel segment, which will aid in the identification and handling of the bowel segments used for the anastomosis.

The orientation of the bowel is checked by using the preplaced dyed Vicryl stay sutures ensuring it is not rotated. A side-to-side bowel anastomosis is then performed (Fig. 23.4a). It is important to ensure that the conduit is placed below the small bowel anastomosis. Two small enterotomies are made using electrocautery at the anti-mesenteric corners of the two bowel stumps marked by the dyed Vicryl stay sutures. A stapler is introduced from the left lateral port, and the two bowel segments are placed individually on to each blade of the stapler through their respective enterotomies. It is helpful to use the stay sutures to advance each bowel segment to the jaw of the stapler blades before closing the stapler. Care is taken to avoid inclusion of small bowel mesentery into the staple line before the stapler is fired. A second stapler load is introduced from the lateral port, passed simultaneously into the proximal and distal bowel segments, and stapled to ensure a widely patent side-to-side anastomosis. Finally, the stump of the side-to-side anastomosis is stapled off at the top, using a laparoscopic stapler from the medial assistant port or the robotic stapler from the left lateral hybrid port (Fig. 23.4b).

Ureteroileal Anastomosis

Our preference is to perform ureteroileal anastomosis using the Bricker technique. The ureters are checked to ensure there is no malrotation or kinking en route to the proximal end of the conduit and the most appropriate location for the ureteroileal anastomosis is determined. The ureters should be handled with great care using the clip or a stay suture to avoid crush injury and devascularization of the distal ureter. We typically perform the left ureteroileal anastomosis first, which usually lies closer to the ileal conduit stump and more medial compared to the right-sided anastomosis (Fig. 23.5). A small enterotomy is made at the appropriate location on

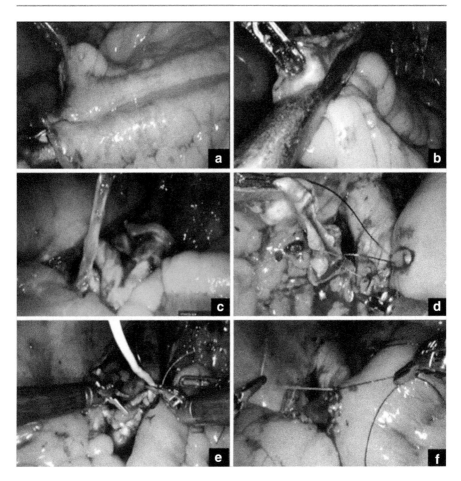

Fig. 23.4 **a**: Side-to-side anastomosis is performed for bowel reconstitution. **b**: Closure of the open end of the side-to-side anastomosis. **c**: Indocyanine green fluorescence imaging is used to ensure adequate vascularity of the ureters, ileal conduit, and bowel anastomosis. **d**: The ureter is spatulated, and the ureteroileal anastomosis is commenced at the apex of the spatulation. **e**: The ureter is catheterized with a double-J stent after the posterior wall of the ureteroileal anastomosis is completed. **f**: The ureteroileal anastomosis is completed

the conduit, close to the proximal end. Any distal ureteral segments with compromised vascularity or suspicion for malignancy are excised. The ureter is incised at an appropriate location taking care to maintain adequate length and vascularity. A distal ureteral "tail" is left attached and can be used as a handle during the ureteroileal anastomosis.

The ureters are spatulated, typically 1 cm, according to ureteral caliber. The ureteroileal anastomosis is completed using a 4-0 Vicryl suture in a continuous manner using a fine reverse cutting needle. The first suture is placed at the apex of the spatulation from outside to inside the ureter and then inside to outside the bowel (Fig. 23.4d). The posterior wall of the anastomosis is completed. A second suture is

Fig. 23.5 **6a**: Position of the left and right ureteroileal anastomosis. The left anastomosis is partially completed and the right side is marked with a red star

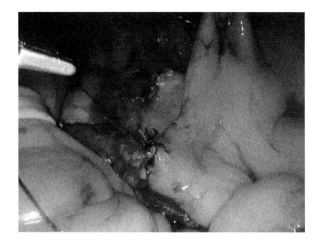

placed at the apex and the anterior wall of the anastomosis is commenced. At this point, the bedside assistant places a 2 mm MiniPort (Covidien, Mansfield, MA, USA) intra-abdominally under direct vision through a separate skin puncture in the right lower quadrant, and a 4.8F double-J ureteral stent is introduced (Fig. 23.4e). The stent is placed in the ureter and passed to the collecting system over a Glidewire using both the right and left robotic arms. The wire is removed, and the distal coil of the stent is placed within the conduit. The distal ureteral tail/handle is trimmed at this point, and the ureteroileal anastomosis is completed (Fig. 23.4f). This procedure is repeated for the right ureter.

The main objective of this step is to achieve a spatulated, tension-free, watertight, mucosa-to-mucosa anastomosis of healthy well-vascularized ureter to well-vascularized bowel. It is critical to observe these principles to minimize the risk of anastomotic leaks and ischemic anastomotic strictures. The fourth arm can be used during the anastomosis to gently retract the distal ureteral tail or position the proximal end of the conduit to aid suture placement. Note that our preference is to use double-J stents which simplifies stent placement, minimizes the risk of stent extrusion, and facilitates stoma bag changes during the early postoperative phase.

Stoma Creation

A locking Allis grasper is introduced from the left lateral port and used to grasp the distal end of the conduit, and a 19F Blake drain is placed in the pelvis, lateral to the conduit. The robot is undocked, and a circular skin incision is made over the stoma site, and a cylinder of tissue is removed from the skin down to the fascia. The fascia is opened in a linear fashion and four fascial sutures are placed using 2-0 Vicryl. The rectus muscle is bluntly separated, and the posterior sheath is divided to accommodate two fingers. The distal conduit is pushed toward the stoma site with the locking Allis and pulled through the abdominal wall using long Babcock forceps. This is achieved under direct vision using a handheld scope. The correct

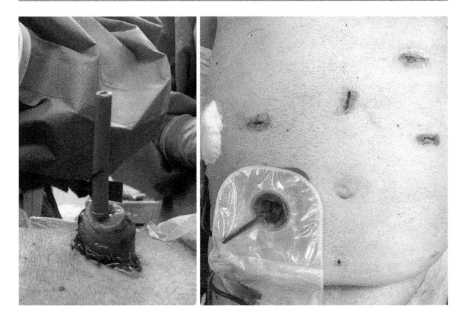

Fig. 23.6 a: 16F Red Rubber catheter within the ileal conduit secured with a nylon suture. **b**: Surgical wounds, stoma appliance, and Red Rubber catheter at the end of the procedure

orientation of the conduit is confirmed intra-abdominally. The abdomen is now desufflated and the specimen extracted through a Pfannenstiel or midline incision. The ileal conduit stoma is fashioned in the usual rosebud manner. The four fascial sutures are placed at the base of the conduit to anchor it. The caliber of the conduit is reviewed. Maturation and fixation of the conduit are completed using interrupted 3-0 Vicryl sutures ensuring the mucosa is everted. The aim is to fashion a stoma that is everted and sits proud on the abdomen to facilitate stoma bag attachment and prevent urinary leak and irritation to the skin. A Red Rubber catheter (BARD, Covington, GA, USA) is placed inside the conduit and is secured to the skin with a silk suture (Fig. 23.6a, b). The maneuver facilitates drainage of the conduit during the early postoperative period.

Adjunct Intraoperative Procedures

Indocyanine Green Fluorescence Angiography

Accurate assessment of ureteral vascularity using traditional white light is subjective and hence inherently prone to inaccuracy. Despite meticulous tissue handling, ureteral vascularity may be compromised even in experienced hands leading to ischemic ureteroileal strictures. Indocyanine green (ICG) is a nontoxic, fluorescent, exogenous tracer that is not visualized with white light but can be seen with near-infrared fluorescence (NIRF) and has emerged as a useful technique to assess tissue perfusion and vascularity [14]. The console surgeon can switch between white and near-infrared light facilitating real-time detection of ICG fluorescence and thus vascularity [15]. At our institution, we have been using ICG routinely during ICUD for several years [16]. ICG is prepared by mixing 25 mg ICG in 10 mL sterile water, and following isolation and preparation of the ileal conduit, 5 mL of ICG is injected intravenously. We then use NIRF to visually assess the vascularity of the ileal conduit and small bowel anastomosis and distal ureteral segments (Fig. 23.4c). Any poorly vascularized segments of ureter are excised. In our experience, the use of ICG leads to better assessment of ureteral and bowel vascularity compared to white light and better identification and subsequent excision of nonviable segments of the distal ureter prior to ureteroileal anastomosis. The introduction of ICG at our institution has allowed us to better identify long-segment devascularized distal ureters leading to an increase in the proportion of patients getting long-segment (>5 cm) ureteral resection compared to white light (18 vs 6%, $p < 0.05$) and has reduced our rate of ureteroileal anastomotic stricture from 10.6% to zero after a median follow-up of 12 months ($p = 0.02$) [17].

Intraoperative Frozen Section Analysis

In bladder cancer patients, the proximal ureteral segment may be sent for intraoperative frozen section to ensure a negative ureteral margin. If the ureteral margin is positive, some surgeons recommend further excision until a negative result is achieved. We do not advocate this approach due to known propensity for skip lesions in urothelial carcinoma. Approximately 13% of the patients will have ureteral involvement. While these patients may be at an increased risk of upper tract recurrence, microscopic ureteral margin involvement has not been shown to adversely impact anastomotic recurrence, cancer-specific survival, or overall survival [18, 19].

Adjunct Procedures to Ensure Tension-Free Ureteroileal Anastomosis

Occasionally, despite adequate assessment prior to isolation of the ileal segment, the ureter may not reach the ileal conduit, for example, if a large ischemic ureteral segment is removed. Some maneuvers can be used to achieve a tension-free anastomosis. First, it is important to check that both ureters have a smooth path to the conduit. If required, the ureters can be mobilized further proximally, and the sigmoid mesenteric window can be extended cranially so the left ureter takes a straighter, more direct path to the right side. In some cases, the proximal end of the conduit can be tunneled through the sigmoid mesentery window to reach the left ureter. Finally, a second segment of the small bowel can be used to reconnect to the previously harvested ileal segment, or a completely new ileal conduit can be made.

Postoperative Management

The use of enhanced recovery after surgery (ERAS) programs has gained wide-spread popularity after major abdominal surgery, and our institution has been a pioneer in developing ERAS pathways after RC and urinary diversion [20]. ERAS pathways include avoiding bowel preparation, standardized feeding schedules and avoiding opioid analgesia, and the use of prokinetics. Intraoperatively a targeted fluid resuscitation strategy is used, and any orogastric or nasogastric tubes are removed at the end of the procedure. The implementation of ERAS pathways has been shown to be associated with earlier recovery of bowel function and reduced blood loss, transfusions, and length of stay without compromising oncological outcomes [21–23].

Postoperatively, we start clear fluid oral intake as soon as the patient is alert, and oral intake is advanced to free fluids and a solid diet as tolerated. A strict fluid balance is maintained, and oral intake is supplemented with intravenous fluids to achieve a minimum urine output of >0.5 mL/kg/hour. Adequate pain control is essential to expediting recovery, and regular nonnarcotic analgesia is used such as acetaminophen and nonsteroidal anti-inflammatory medications. Alvimopan is continued postoperatively for a maximum of 7 days, which has been shown to significantly reduce the time to tolerating a solid diet and length of hospital stay. Chewing gum has been shown to reduce the time to flatus and bowel movement [24]. Early ambulation, breathing exercises, and incentive spirometry are implemented on postoperative day 1 with physiotherapy and nursing assistance. Incentive spirometry has been shown to improve lung function and may reduce postoperative pulmonary complications [25, 26]. The ileal conduit is assessed daily. Laboratory tests include complete blood count, a basic metabolic panel, and drain fluid creatinine. A midline venous catheter is inserted prior to discharge to facilitate home intravenous fluids on discharge. In our practice, patients are discharged with extended thromboembolic prophylaxis with low-molecular-weight heparin for 4 weeks after surgery, which has been shown to decrease the incidence of thromboembolism after major abdominal and pelvic oncological surgery.

The patient is typically discharged home on postoperative day 3–5 with oral sulfamethoxazole/trimethoprim for a week. Diabetic or immunocompromised patients also receive oral fluconazole for a week. Home nursing assistance is provided, and 1 L of intravenous fluids is administered every other day. The patient returns to the clinic at 1 week, 2 weeks, 1 month, 2 months, and 4 months. Our algorithm is to see the patient 1 week after surgery to discuss histopathology in patients who have had a cystectomy and remove the Red Rubber catheter. At 2 weeks, the pelvic drain is removed. The patient then returns at 4 weeks after completing their course of extended thromboembolic prophylaxis, and the double-J ureteral stents are removed. The patient returns at 2 months for clinical review and then at 4 months with surveillance CT imaging. A complete blood count and basic metabolic panel are completed prior to each visit (see Appendix).

Complications and Management

Gastrointestinal Complications

Gastrointestinal complications after intracorporeal urinary diversions is estimated to be 5–10% [27, 28]. Some reports suggest that gastrointestinal complications may be less common in patients with intracorporeal compared to extracorporeal urinary diversion [28]. In our experience, ileus remains the most common gastrointestinal complication though the use of alvimopan and ERAS protocols have helped improve recovery of bowel function. Parenteral nutrition is recommended if ileus persists more than 7 days. Bowel obstruction is rare after intracorporeal ileal conduit formation [29]. The management of bowel obstruction is usually conservative with nasogastric tube drainage and intravenous fluids, while persistent bowel obstruction warrants surgical exploration. Bowel leak from the bowel anastomosis is a rare but potentially fatal complication and requires expedient surgical exploration. Poor nutritional status, diabetes, abdominopelvic irradiation, and ischemia or tension at the bowel anastomosis are risk factors [30]. Ischemia and necrosis of the conduit are rare and require revision surgery. The incidence of bowel-related complications may be minimized by gentle handling using appropriate instruments such as the Cadiere forceps, maintaining the principles of anastomosis, assessment of bowel vascularity with ICG, and appropriate electrolyte replacement.

Stoma Complications

Stomal complications include stomal stenosis and parastomal hernias. Stomal stenosis may occur due to retraction of the stoma, chronic ischemia, or fascial narrowing and may require revision surgery. Parastomal hernias have been linked with patient factors such as increasing age, malnutrition, weak abdominal wall, obesity, history of radiation or increased intra-abdominal pressures from constipation, chronic coughing, or respiratory illnesses, while surgical risk factors include the omission of fascial anchoring sutures, inappropriate large fascial opening, and incorrect siting of the stoma. There is data from the colorectal literature that prophylactic placement of mesh at the time of stoma creation may reduce the rate of parastomal hernias. Urinary diversion poses additional risks due to the presence of both urinary and bowel anastomosis though retrospective data suggests that prophylactic mesh is safe and feasible in patients at high risk of parastomal hernias [31]. Surgical repair is recommended in patients with bothersome symptoms. Open surgical repair is challenging and is associated with high recurrence rates and often requires resiting the stoma to a new location which creates the potential for future hernias at both sites. Robotic repair of parastomal hernias using biological mesh has been described which simplifies the surgical technique, avoids excessive dissection, and avoids resiting the stoma site [32]. Robotic repair has been shown to be safe and feasible with minimal morbidity and good short-term outcomes [32].

Ureteroileal Anastomotic Complications

Ureteroileal anastomotic stricture can lead to pain, renal obstruction, infection, and renal failure. Meticulous handling, minimizing dissection of the ureters, placing the ureters in a retroperitoneal position, wide spatulation, and a tension-free anastomosis over a ureteral stent are key principles in minimizing risk of ureteroileal strictures. Nonetheless, anastomotic stricture rates as high as 12% have been reported after ICUD. The vast majority of strictures are thought to be of ischemic aetiology, and the use of ICG has improved our ability to assess distal ureteral vascularity and has reduced the stricture rates at our center [17]. As patients can often be asymptomatic, close follow-up is essential for early detection and prompt management of anastomotic strictures. Treatment includes endoscopic or percutaneous techniques and surgical revision which can be performed robotically [33]. Anastomotic urine leak is best managed by prolonged drainage with percutaneous nephrostomy tube and rarely requires revision surgery.

Disclosures Dr. Monish Aron is a consultant for Intuitive Surgical.

References

1. Antoni S, Ferlay J, Soerjomataram I, Znaor A, Jemal A, Bray F. Bladder cancer incidence and mortality: a global overview and recent trends. Eur Urol. 2017;71(1):96–108.
2. Alfred Witjes J, Lebret T, Comperat EM, Cowan NC, De Santis M, Bruins HM, et al. Updated 2016 EAU guidelines on muscle-invasive and metastatic bladder cancer. Eur Urol. 2017;71(3):462–75.
3. Babjuk M, Bohle A, Burger M, Capoun O, Cohen D, Comperat EM, et al. EAU Guidelines on Non-muscle-invasive urothelial carcinoma of the bladder: update 2016. Eur Urol. 2017;71(3):447–61.
4. Gill IS, Fergany A, Klein EA, Kaouk JH, Sung GT, Meraney AM, et al. Laparoscopic radical cystoprostatectomy with ileal conduit performed completely intracorporeally: the initial 2 cases. Urology. 2000;56(1):26–9; discussion 9–30.
5. Hubert J, Feuillu B, Beis JM, Coissard A, Mangin P, Andre JM. Laparoscopic robotic-assisted ileal conduit urinary diversion in a quadriplegic woman. Urology. 2003;62(6):1121.
6. Azzouni FS, Din R, Rehman S, Khan A, Shi Y, Stegemann A, et al. The First 100 Consecutive, Robot-assisted, Intracorporeal Ileal Conduits: Evolution of Technique and 90-day Outcomes. Eur Urol. 2013;63(4):637–43.
7. Hussein AA, May PR, Jing Z, Ahmed YE, Wijburg CJ, Canda AE, et al. Outcomes of Intracorporeal urinary diversion after robot-assisted radical cystectomy: results from the International Robotic Cystectomy Consortium. J Urol. 2018;199(5):1302–11.
8. Lee RK, Abol-Enein H, Artibani W, Bochner B, Dalbagni G, Daneshmand S, et al. Urinary diversion after radical cystectomy for bladder cancer: options, patient selection, and outcomes. BJU Int. 2013;113(1):11–23.
9. Hautmann RE, Abol-Enein H, Davidsson T, Gudjonsson S, Hautmann SH, Holm HV, et al. ICUD-EAU international consultation on bladder cancer 2012: urinary diversion. Eur Urol. 2013;63(1):67–80.
10. Allaire J, Leger C, Ben-Zvi T, Nguile-Makao M, Fradet Y, Lacombe L, et al. Prospective evaluation of nutritional factors to predict the risk of complications for patients undergoing radical cystectomy: a cohort study. Nutr Cancer. 2017;69(8):1196–204.

11. Jensen BT, Laustsen S, Jensen JB, Borre M, Petersen AK. Exercise-based pre-habilitation is feasible and effective in radical cystectomy pathways-secondary results from a randomized controlled trial. Support Care Cancer. 2016;24(8):3325–31.
12. Awad S, Varadhan KK, Ljungqvist O, Lobo DN. A meta-analysis of randomised controlled trials on preoperative oral carbohydrate treatment in elective surgery. Clin Nutr. 2013;32(1):34–44.
13. Salvadalena G, Hendren S, McKenna L, Muldoon R, Netsch D, Paquette I, et al. WOCN society and ASCRS position statement on preoperative stoma site marking for patients undergoing colostomy or ileostomy surgery. J Wound Ostomy Continence Nurs. 2015;42(3):249–52.
14. van den Berg NS, van Leeuwen FWB, van der Poel HG. Fluorescence guidance in urologic surgery. Curr Opin Urol. 2012;22(2):109–20.
15. Krane LS, Manny TB, Hemal AK. Is near infrared fluorescence imaging using indocyanine green dye useful in robotic partial nephrectomy: a prospective comparative study of 94 patients. Urology. 2012;80(1):110–8.
16. Melecchi Freitas D, Fay C, Ahmadi N, Abreu A, Shin T, Gill I, et al. V12–06 utilization of indocyanine green fluorescence angiography during intracorporeal uretero-ileal anastomosis following robotic Radical Cystectomy. J Urol. 2017;197(4):e1373.
17. Ahmadi N, Ashrafi, AN, Hartman N, et al.Use of indocyanine green to minimise ureteroenteric strictures after robotic radical cystectomy. BJU Int. 2019;124(2):302–307.
18. Raj GV, Tal R, Vickers A, Bochner BH, Serio A, Donat SM, et al. Significance of intraoperative ureteral evaluation at radical cystectomy for urothelial cancer. Cancer. 2006;107(9):2167–72.
19. Kim HS, Moon KC, Jeong CW, Kwak C, Kim HH, Ku JH. The clinical significance of intraoperative ureteral frozen section analysis at radical cystectomy for urothelial carcinoma of the bladder. World J Urol. 2015;33(3):359–65.
20. Djaladat H, Daneshmand S. Gastrointestinal complications in patients who undergo radical cystectomy with enhanced recovery protocol. Curr Urol Rep. 2016;17(7):50.
21. Daneshmand S, Ahmadi H, Schuckman AK, Mitra AP, Cai J, Miranda G, et al. Enhanced recovery protocol after radical cystectomy for bladder cancer. J Urol. 2014;192(1):50–5.
22. Pang KH, Groves R, Venugopal S, Noon AP, Catto JWF. Prospective implementation of enhanced recovery after surgery protocols to radical cystectomy. Eur Urol. 2017;73(3):363–71.
23. Koupparis A, Villeda-Sandoval C, Weale N, El-Mahdy M, Gillatt D, Rowe E. Robot-assisted radical cystectomy with intracorporeal urinary diversion: impact on an established enhanced recovery protocol. BJU Int. 2015;116(6):924–31.
24. Choi H, Kang SH, Yoon DK, Kang SG, Ko HY, Moon du G, et al. Chewing gum has a stimulatory effect on bowel motility in patients after open or robotic radical cystectomy for bladder cancer: a prospective randomized comparative study. Urology. 2011;77(4):884–90.
25. Overend TJ, Anderson CM, Lucy SD, Bhatia C, Jonsson BI, Timmermans C. The effect of incentive spirometry on postoperative pulmonary complications: a systematic review. Chest. 2001;120(3):971–8.
26. Othman E, Abaas S, Hassan H. Resisted breathing exercise versus incentive spirometer training on vital capacity in postoperative radical cystectomy cases: a pilot randomized controlled trial. Bull Fac Phys Ther. 2016;21(2):61–7.
27. Desai MM, de Abreu AL, Goh AC, Fairey A, Berger A, Leslie S, et al. Robotic intracorporeal urinary diversion: technical details to improve time efficiency. J Endourol. 2014;28(11):1320–7.
28. Ahmed K, Khan SA, Hayn MH, Agarwal PK, Badani KK, Balbay MD, et al. Analysis of intracorporeal compared with extracorporeal urinary diversion after robot-assisted radical cystectomy: results from the international robotic cystectomy consortium. Eur Urol. 2014;65(2):340–7.
29. Guru K, Seixas-Mikelus SA, Hussain A, Blumenfeld AJ, Nyquist J, Chandrasekhar R, et al. Robot-assisted intracorporeal ileal conduit: marionette technique and initial experience at Roswell Park Cancer Institute. Urology. 2010;76(4):866–71.
30. Donahue TBB. Complications of ileal conduit diversion. In: Daneshmand S, editor. Urinary diversion. 1st ed. Cham: Springer; 2017. p. 63–79.

31. Donahue TF, Cha EK, Bochner BH. Rationale and early experience with prophylactic place-
    ment of mesh to prevent parastomal hernia formation after ileal conduit urinary diversion and
    cystectomy for bladder cancer. Curr Urol Rep. 2016;17(2):9.
32. Mekhail P, Ashrafi A, Mekhail M, Hatcher D, Aron M. Robotic parastomal hernia repair with
    biologic mesh. Urology. 2017;110:262.
33. Hussein AA, Hashmi Z, Dibaj S, Altartir T, Fiorica T, Wing J, et al. Reoperations following
    robot-assisted radical cystectomy: a decade of experience. J Urol. 2016;195(5):1368–76.

Urinary Diversion: Robot-Assisted Laparoscopic Malone Antegrade Continence Enema (MACE) and Mitrofanoff Appendicovesicostomy (MAPV)

24

Aaron Wallace, Mayya Volodarskaya, Ciro Andolfi, and Mohan S. Gundeti

Indications

A Mitrofanoff appendicovesicostomy (MAPV), in which the appendix is used to create a continent catheterizable channel for urine, and a Malone antegrade continence enema (MACE) stoma, which utilizes the appendix and/or cecum to create a connection to the proximal colon for antegrade enema administration, can greatly improve the quality of life of patients suffering from bladder and bowel dysfunction. These issues may be secondary to neurogenic causes such as spina bifida, spinal cord injury, multiple sclerosis, transverse myelitis, tethered cord, sacral agenesis, cerebral palsy, or Arnold-Chiari malformation [1–3]. Bladder dysfunction may also be attributed to non-neurogenic etiologies including posterior urethral valve syndrome, urethral stricture, epispadias, and prune belly syndrome or idiopathic causes [4]. Patients with long-standing bladder dysfunction can progress to having diminished bladder capacity, reduced bladder compliance, and high-pressure voiding, which can impair not only renal function but also quality of life [1]. Patients with neurogenic bowel issues, which frequently coexist with neurogenic bladder

Supplementary Information The online version of this chapter (https://doi.org/10.1007/978-3-030-50196-9_24) contains supplementary material, which is available to authorized users.

A. Wallace (✉) · C. Andolfi · M. S. Gundeti
Department of Surgery, Chicago Medicine, Chicago, IL, USA
e-mail: aaron.wallace@uchospitals.edu; mgundeti@surgery.bsd.uchicago.edu

M. Volodarskaya
Department of Surgery, Rush University Medical Center, Chicago, IL, USA

© Springer Nature Switzerland AG 2022
M. D. Stifelman et al. (eds.), *Techniques of Robotic Urinary Tract Reconstruction*, https://doi.org/10.1007/978-3-030-50196-9_24

disease, often develop intractable constipation, fecal impaction, and fecal incontinence [2, 3]. In addition to the physical burden of these complications, urinary and fecal incontinence can lead to social isolation, making the achievement of social continence highly valuable.

Specifically, MAPV is indicated for patients with bladder-emptying difficulties when intermittent catheterization via the native urethra is not possible due to urethral sensitivity or anatomic issues such as urethral trauma, stricture, exstrophy-epispadias, or cloaca [1, 5]. Intermittent catheterization via the urethra may be particularly challenging for patients who are female or obese or who utilize a wheelchair, have limited dexterity, or suffer from lower extremity spasticity [6]. The same factors contribute to difficulty with administration of retrograde enemas, making the MACE also beneficial for such patients [7]. In addition to being indicated for neurogenic bowel issues, MACE is also indicated for patients with anorectal malformations [3]. Indications for isolated MAPV include prune belly syndrome and non-neurogenic bladder dysfunction [1, 8].

MAPV is absolutely contraindicated for patients who cannot perform catheterization and who have little or no access to caregivers capable of undertaking this task. It is also relatively contraindicated for patients with inflammatory bowel disease, short bowel, or a history of bowel radiation. MACE is contraindicated for patients in whom a left colon channel is preferred to the cecal site for enema delivery, and special consideration should be given to obese patients with a short appendix in whom maturation of the stoma may be difficult or delayed [3].

Although these procedures have been proven to be efficient and safe for patients via a conventional open surgical approach, robot-assisted laparoscopic (RAL) surgery may be the preferred option for many patients due to its minimally invasive nature. In general, RAL surgery has been shown to result in shorter hospital stays, less postoperative pain, and better cosmetic outcomes. Specific to the MAPV procedure, length of hospital stay and complication rates were comparable between the open and RAL approach [9]. Additionally, in a porcine model, RAL surgery was shown to cause fewer adhesions than an open approach, which may be beneficial for patients anticipating future additional abdominal surgery [10]. However, if a patient has previously had multiple abdominal surgeries, where significant intraperitoneal adhesions are expected, an open approach is recommended for the MAPV procedure. Additionally, contraindications to performing MAPV via RAL surgery include body habitus, such as for small children in whom intra-abdominal space may be limited, and patients with severe kyphoscoliosis or multiple previous abdominal surgeries which would prevent optimal patient positioning and port placement [1]. Additionally, patients with significantly impaired pulmonary or renal function may not be able to tolerate the pneumoperitoneum required for the procedure [9]. Finally, as RAL surgery has a steep learning curve, operative times may initially be longer until surgeons become more facile with the technique, and thus patients with severe illness may benefit more from an open procedure with a shorter duration of anesthesia [1]. This benefit should be considered against the cost of potential respiratory complications during the postoperative recovery for open surgery with more severe pain and poor respiratory efforts in more ill patients.

Preoperative Considerations/Studies/Tests

During the preoperative evaluation for MAPV, patients should receive videourody-namic studies and renal ultrasound, with a DMSA renal scan as necessary [10]. Videourodynamic studies allow for the evaluation of bladder function and bladder neck competency, while the renal imaging allows for the assessment of renal anatomy. The DMSA renal scan contributes additional information about the patient's renal morphology and function [1]. If the indication for the MACE stoma is for functional constipation, colonic manometry and a contrast enema may be required to guide surgical planning [11].

Equally important to the imaging studies is family and caregiver education in advance of the operation about the surgery and postoperative care. This process is improved by the involvement of a clinical nurse educator, who can help teach catheterization skills and aid in setting appropriate expectations throughout the process [12]. While both of these procedures aim to achieve social continence, they are neither perfectly successful nor without potential complications, for which patients and families must be prepared [3, 13, 14]. Placement of the stomas should also be discussed as the MAPV can be routed to either the umbilicus or the right iliac fossa, while the MACE is most commonly a right-sided stoma [1, 3]. Finally, patients and family members must be given adequate time to address their questions and concerns, since the MAPV may alleviate some of the physical barriers to intermittent self-catheterization but may not address all of the psychological barriers that lead to noncompliance, such as anxiety and fear [15].

Prior to the preoperative period, a urine culture should be performed to diagnose and treat any existing urinary tract infections prior to surgery. Bowel preparation has not been shown to be necessary for MAPV alone, and we also avoid bowel preparation for concurrent MAPV-MACE procedures [16]. Patients can be admitted on the day of surgery. Prophylactic antibiotics should be administered 1 hour prior to the start of surgery, with the specific combination tailored to patient allergies, institutional guidelines, and local resistance patterns. Our protocol includes cefazolin, gentamicin, and metronidazole, with vancomycin replacing cefazolin for patients with ventriculoperitoneal shunts [1]. In general, antibiotic prophylaxis should be targeted toward skin and gram-negative intestinal flora pathogens [17].

Surgical Technique

(1) Patient positioning

Patient positioning is critical to ensure patient and provider safety and a wide range of movement of the robotic arms. We place patients in the dorsal lithotomy position, with a Trendelenburg of 10–15°. This allows access to control bladder filling and keeps the small bowel away from the operating field, while still allowing for identification of the appendix [1, 18].

(2) Port/camera placement

For improved access to the appendix and bowel, we recommend placing the camera port in a supraumbilical position. We use a 12 mm blunt tip balloon trocar for the camera port, where the advantages of this port are improved anchoring with the balloon and the trocar has a short intra-abdominal length, which maximizes space in the small, crowded surgical field. We place the camera port using an open Hassan's technique.

For the robotic arms, we use the 8 mm ports. We recommend using the impression of the port without its obturator to guide placement. This prevents the trocar from dislodging during the procedure and minimizes any gas leak. We use local anesthesia at the port sites to minimize postoperative pain.

We insert the left arm port 8 cm lateral to the umbilicus; the right is inserted 9–10 cm lateral to the umbilicus; and the fourth arm is placed 7–8 cm lateral to the right arm port. We place a 5 mm assistant port in the left upper quadrant, which is equidistant from the camera and left working port. For children taller than 5 ft., one can use a fourth robotic arm, which aids in traction and counter-traction during critical steps [1].

(3) Appendix identification

Upon entry to the peritoneal cavity, we first identify the appendix and place a stay suture at the distal end for later identification and manipulation (Fig. 24.1). We recommend routine use of diagnostic laparoscopy prior to docking the robot. This is especially critical in patients with a VP shunt. If the appendix is not of sufficient length, we recommend conversion to an open approach and to perform a Monti catheterizable channel instead [18].

(4) Foley catheter placement

We place a Foley catheter in the bladder, which allows control of bladder volumes to aid in cystotomy and tunnel creation.

Fig. 24.1 A stay suture is placed on the distal end of the appendix for later identification and manipulation of the appendix

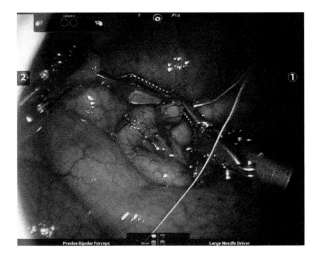

(5) Appendix mobilization

First, the appendix is mobilized at the appendicular/cecal junction (Fig. 24.2a). It is critical to maintain its blood supply during mobilization. The appendix should be sufficiently mobile to reach the bladder and anterior abdominal wall without tension. At this point, additional mobilization of the cecum and right colon can be performed, if necessary.

If performing only MAPV, we place a 3-0 polyglactin purse-string suture at the appendicular base and separate the appendix from the cecum. The purse-string suture is tied and the cecal opening is closed in a second layer with the same suture. We prefer to take part of the cecum in cases where the appendix length is short, where a longer cecal flap can be taken to bridge the distance from the bladder to the cutaneous stoma.

For concurrent MACE procedures, if there is a sufficiently long appendix (10–12 cm), we use the proximal 2–4 cm for the MACE channel, while the distal appendix is utilized for the MAPV. The appendix is then split, while keeping the mesentery intact for the MAPV (Fig. 24.2b, c). In patients with a

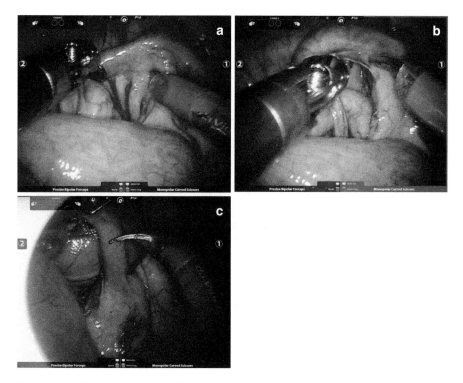

Fig. 24.2 (**a**) The appendix is mobilized at the appendicular/cecal junction, while maintaining its blood supply. (**b**) The mesentery of the appendix is dissected without interrupting its blood supply. (**c**) The appendix is split with the proximal 2–4 cm for the MACE channel and the distal appendix for MAPV

short appendix who required both channels, we prefer to use the entire appendix for the MAPV and to create a cecal flap tubularization for the MACE.

(6) Bladder tunnel creation

If no additional procedures are being performed, such as augmentation ileocystoplasty, then we prefer the anterior bladder wall for the insertion site for implantation of the appendix. The advantages are that this is technically easier than posterior anastomosis, especially in patients with a large bladder, and that the distance to the abdominal wall is shorter, decreasing the required length of the appendix.

Next, we add 60 mL of normal saline to the Foley catheter to partially fill the bladder (Fig. 24.3a, b). A stay stitch is then passed from the bladder through the anterior abdominal wall (Fig. 24.4a). Using electrocautery, the detrusor layer of the bladder wall is incised to expose the bladder mucosa (Fig. 24.4b,c). We recommend a minimum tunnel length of 4 cm. The direction of the tunnel is according to the location of the stoma (craniocaudal for umbilical stomas, oblique for right lower quadrant stomas) (Fig. 24.5a, b).

(7) Appendix spatulation and bladder anastomosis

Once the submucosal tunnel is created, the appendix should be broad in size. It is then anchored to the bladder with two 4-0 PDS sutures on either side, and the spatulation is created (Fig. 24.6a, b). Next, the anterior wall of the appendix is matured to the bladder mucosa with interrupted 4-0 PDS sutures. Following this, the bladder mucosa is approximated over the appendix so as to create the submucosal tunnel of about 4 cm in length (Fig. 24.7). Then, an 8 French feeding tube is brought through the stoma into the bladder, and the feeding tube is secured to the bladder mucosa with interrupted 4-0 PDS suture (Fig. 24.8).

(8) Suprapubic catheter placement

Two suprapubic catheters are inserted using the Seldinger technique on either wall of the bladder and inflated with the primary balloon (Fig. 24.9a, b).

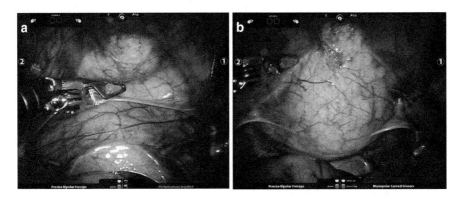

Fig. 24.3 (**a**) The bladder prior to filling. (**b**) The bladder after filling of the Foley

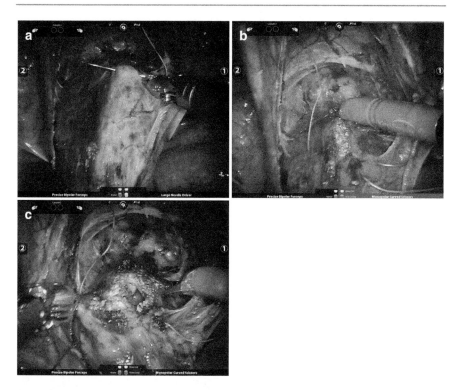

Fig. 24.4 (**a**) Stay stitch is passed through the anterior bladder wall. (**b** and **c**) The bladder is incised using electrocautery

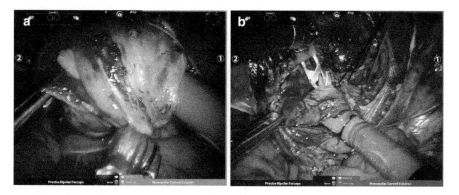

Fig. 24.5 (**a** and **b**) Bladder mucosa tunnel is created with a minimum length of 4 cm

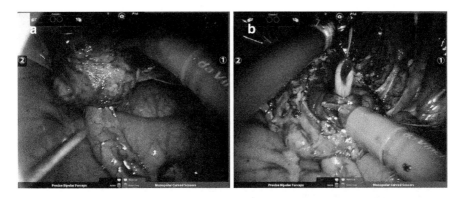

Fig. 24.6 (**a** and **b**) The appendix is spatulated with two 4-0 PDS sutures on either side

Fig. 24.7 The bladder mucosa is approximated over the appendix

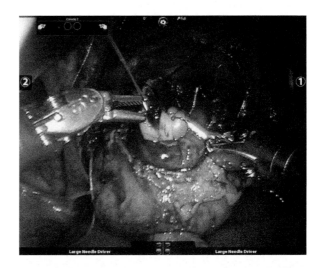

Fig. 24.8 Feeding tube is placed through the stoma

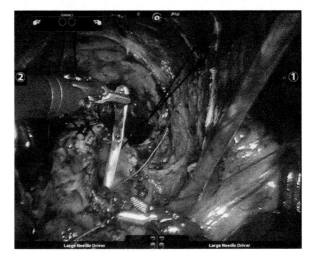

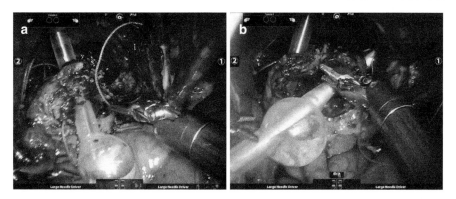

Fig. 24.9 (**a** and **b**) Suprapubic catheter placement

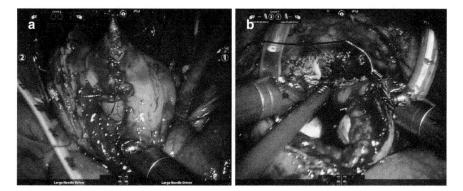

Fig. 24.10 (**a**) View of MAPV prior to bladder closure. (**b**) Closure of the bladder beginning at bladder neck

(9) Bladder closure

Following this, the bladder can be closed with a 2-0 Quill suture or standard 2-0 Vicryl sutures, starting with a single pseudomuscular layer, beginning from the bladder neck to the dome of the bladder (Fig. 24.10a, b). The patency is checked with 4 mL of saline injected into the Foley catheter.

(10) Maturation of stomas

For MACE, the remaining portion of proximal appendix that was previously split is identified (Fig. 24.11a). A stay suture is placed through the proximal appendix to bring it to the skin for stomal creation (Fig. 24.11b–d).

The proximal end of the appendix is then brought through the 12 mm umbilical port site or to the right lower quadrant through the 8 mm right robotic arm port. A V-, VQ-, or VQZ-shaped skin flap is created at the stoma site, and the MAPV is spatulated, allowing the flap to be placed into the more proximal portion of the

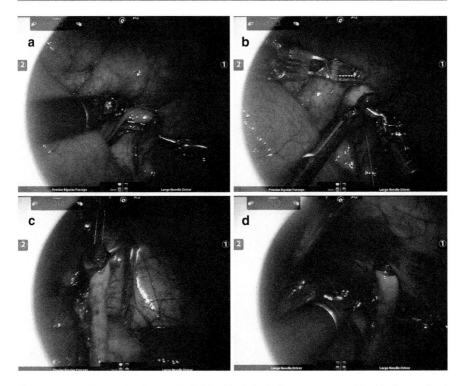

Fig. 24.11 (**a**) The proximal appendix is identified. (**b–d**) Stay sutures are placed in the proximal appendix and used to bring the appendix to the skin

MAPV. The rest of the skin is approximated with interrupted 6-0 PDS sutures. An 8 French feeding tube is then placed inside the channel and secured to the skin with the previous suture.

(11) Closure

The port sites are closed with 2-0 Vicryl. Subcutaneous tissues are approximated with 4-0 Vicryl, and the skin is approximated with subcuticular 5-0 PDS sutures. The suprapubic catheter is left open for gravity drainage and is secured to the skin while the urethral catheter is clamped.

Special Considerations

In all patients with ventriculoperitoneal shunts, the end of the shunt is placed in an ENDOPOUCH RETRIEVER® specimen retrieval bag to avoid contamination of the shunt with bowel contents.

Intraoperative Adjunct Procedures

Bladder Augmentation

For patients undergoing simultaneous bladder augmentation, we recommend cystoscopy and bilateral stent placement to aid in the intraoperative identification of the ureters. We no longer routinely perform these procedures, but we highly recommend them for those performing their initial cases.

The main difference in approach with simultaneous bladder augmentation is the use of the posterior wall for anastomosis. Following placement of the appendicular anastomosis, the bladder is incised coronally, allowing identification of both ureteral orifices. Next, a feeding tube is inserted through the appendix, while avoiding any injury to the ureters. Then, an 18F Foley suprapubic catheter is introduced through the left lower abdominal wall and into the bladder through its anterior wall.

The ileal de-tubularization is then performed with an incision along the antimesenteric border using a Harmonic scalpel. Next, the proximal and distal ends are sutured to the left lateral and right lateral apices of the cystotomy, respectively. After that, the posterior edge of the cystotomy is anastomosed to the ileal segment first, suturing from inside the bladder. The anterior portion of the cystotomy is then sutured to the opposite edge of ileum with an extravesical view of the bladder. We recommend using a 2-0 braided absorbable suture and a Mega™ needle driver (Intuitive Surgical), as well as Lapra-Ty clips (Ethicon Endo-surgery) to reduce the tension on the continuous suture line [1].

Bladder Neck Reconstruction

Similarly, to patients undergoing bladder augmentation, we perform cystoscopy and bilateral stent placement to aid in ureteral identification intraoperatively. We perform the bladder neck reconstruction after identification of the appendix, through which we place a stay suture.

After identification, the bladder is reflected down and 60 mL of normal saline is injected. Then, cystotomy is performed. The two stay sutures are placed with a Keith needle on either side to keep the bladder open. The ureteral orifices are then identified with the previously placed stents. The cystotomy is performed into the bladder neck and urethral areas.

Next, the infratrigonal area in the bladder neck region is identified. A new bladder neck is chosen along the posterior wall below the ureteral orifice. The length should be about 2 cm. A thin strip is then mapped on each side laterally using a 6F feeding tube. The lateral wings are created, after which the de-mucosalization of the lateral wings is performed. Then, over the 6 French feeding tube, the first layer of bladder mucosa is closed, including the seromuscular layer, with 4-0 PDS tied as tightly as possible. A second layer is then created after excising the lateral wings to bring the right lateral wall of the bladder muscle to the left side, again with continuous 4-0 PDS sutures. Once this is done, the left lateral wing, after minimal excision, is brought on to the right side and again with continuous 4-0 PDS sutures. Then, we return our focus to the MAPV.

4-Week Postoperative Algorithm

The immediate postoperative goals for patients are to resume full diet, to have sufficient pain control, and for patients and family to feel comfortable with home care of drainage tubes. Once these are met, patients are then discharged home. The MAPV and suprapubic catheters remain in place for 4 weeks. Afterward, the MAPV catheter is removed in the clinic, and the patient/family are taught clean intermittent catheterization (CIC) through the appendiceal stoma. In case it is needed, the suprapubic catheter is maintained for an additional week or until the family is comfortable performing CIC.

Patients are seen in the clinic at the 2- and 4-week marks after the removal of the catheters. The first visit is to assess for perioperative complications and reinforce the CIC education. The next visit is at the 4-week mark after surgery for a renal ultrasound (RUS) and examination. If the patient has an uneventful postoperative course, follow-up visits are scheduled on a yearly basis with a RUS and basic metabolic panel. At the 5-year mark, we also measure the vitamin B12 levels for those who had an augmentation cystoplasty.

For the MACE channel follow-up, the catheter is maintained for 4 weeks, after which flushes are initiated with 100 ml normal saline and then gradually increasing to 300 ml if necessary for bowel management.

Managing Complications

Previous studies have shown that the robot-assisted laparoscopic approach for MAPV and MACE is both safe and effective. In our previously published series of 18 cases, there were 5 immediate postoperative complications (all of which were Clavien grade I) with no intraoperative complications [19]. There were three cases of ileus, defined as delayed oral intake, though none required surgical intervention. There was one case of stomal site infection and one poorly draining suprapubic catheter due to a mucus plug. Four patients developed delayed complications. One developed stomal incontinence, which was attributed to a short appendiceal length and suboptimal tunnel length. The incontinence resolved after one dextranomer/hyaluronic acid injection (Deflux; Palette Life Sciences, Santa Barbara, CA, USA). The overall continence rate was 94.4%. Another developed a parastomal hernia, requiring surgical revision. The third suffered from recurrent keloid formation leading to stomal stenosis, which required dilatations and stoma revision at the skin level. The fourth patient developed stomal stenosis at the skin level due to noncompliance. The family declined treatment and the patient is catheterized via the urethra.

In a multi-institutional study that included 88 patients with a median follow-up of 29.5 months, 26/88 (29.5%) of patients suffered a complication within 90 days of the procedure [9]. The most common complications were ileus (11.4%), surgical site infection (7.9%), UTI (6.8%), and small bowel obstruction (3.4%). Only six patients experienced a Clavien grade III or higher complication, which included suprapubic tube placement, nephrostomy tube placement, and operative management of ileus and small bowel obstruction. Seventy-five (85.2%) patients were continent after the initial procedure alone. In total, 11 follow-up procedures were performed in 9 patients (10.2%) for MAPV. Six were injections of bulking agents, and five were surgical revisions. After these additional procedures, 81 patients (92.0%) were continent at their last follow-up.

Historically, the most common complication following MAPV is cutaneous scarring at the stoma. A large series of 112 continent channels reported a cutaneous level scarring rate of 31% [20]. In a series of 11 robot-assisted laparoscopic cases, 3 required open revision for cutaneous level scarring, with 2 having a previous history of severe keloid formation [21]. Thus, rates of cutaneous revisions based on approach do not seem to differ. Potential options to minimize cutaneous scarring are surgical modifications which maximize the mucocutaneous junction (V-shaped flap, VQZ plasty, and VQ plasty). Additionally, the appendix can be harvested with a small cecal cuff [22]. Lastly, it is critical to minimize tension on the channel, while preserving its blood supply.

Overall, MACE stomas have incredibly high patient satisfaction rates, where patients after the procedure feel more hygienic and sociable and describe improvements in their quality of life [23–25]. Common postoperative complications of MACE include stomal leakage, stomal site infection, and stomal stenosis. In a series of 26 laparoscopic MACE procedures, the authors found that stomal stenosis occurred in 4/26 (14%) cases and stomal leakage occurred in 13/26 (50%) of cases. When compared to the open approach, the odds ratio of stomal stenosis was significantly less with laparoscopy (OR = 0.0438; $p = 0.045$), and the increase in stomal leakage with laparoscopy was not statistically significant (OR = 3.89; $p = 0.12$). Of note, the open cases had a significantly higher rate of stomal site infections (OR = 25.2; $p = 0.014$) [24].

Conclusion

There are several key techniques that enable successful completion of the MAPV and MACE procedures. First, proper patient positioning and port placement are critical to maximize space and dexterity in a small operating field. Next, it is critical to determine the length of the appendix via diagnostic laparoscopy prior to docking the robot, especially in patients with a VP shunt. Additionally, creation of a submucosal detrusor tunnel of at least 4 cm is important to maintain stomal continence. Lastly, patient education for CIC is necessary to promote long-term continence through the channels.

References

1. Barashi NS, Rodriguez MV, Packiam VT, Gundeti MS. Bladder reconstruction with bowel: robot-assisted laparoscopic ileocystoplasty with mitrofanoff appendicovesicostomy in pediatric patients. J Endourol. 2018;32(S1):S119–26.
2. Cameron AP, Rodriguez GM, Gursky A, He C, Clemens JQ, Stoffel JT. The severity of bowel dysfunction in patients with neurogenic bladder. J Urol. 2015;194(5):1336–41.
3. Gor RA, Katorski JR, Elliott SP. Medical and surgical management of neurogenic bowel. Curr Opin Urol. 2016;26(4):369–75.
4. Veeratterapillay R, Morton H, Thorpe AC, Harding C. Reconstructing the lower urinary tract: the Mitrofanoff principle. Indian J Urol. 2013;29(4):316–21.
5. Faure A, Cooksey R, Bouty A, Woodward A, Hutson J, O'Brien M, et al. Bladder continent catheterizable conduit (the Mitrofanoff procedure): long-term issues that should not be underestimated. J Pediatr Surg. 2017;52(3):469–72.
6. Merenda LA, Duffy T, Betz RR, Mulcahey MJ, Dean G, Pontari M. Outcomes of urinary diversion in children with spinal cord injuries. J Spinal Cord Med. 2007;30(Suppl 1):S41–7.
7. Kudela G, Smyczek D, Springer A, Korecka K, Koszutski T. No appendix is too short-simultaneous Mitrofanoff catheterizable vesicostomy and Malone Antegrade Continence Enema (MACE) for children with spina bifida. Urology. 2018;116:205–7.
8. Wille MA, Jayram G, Gundeti MS. Feasibility and early outcomes of robotic-assisted laparoscopic Mitrofanoff appendicovesicostomy in patients with prune belly syndrome. BJU Int. 2012;109(1):125–9.
9. Gundeti MS, Petravick ME, Pariser JJ, Pearce SM, Anderson BB, Grimsby GM, et al. A multi-institutional study of perioperative and functional outcomes for pediatric robotic-assisted laparoscopic Mitrofanoff appendicovesicostomy. J Pediatr Urol. 2016;12(6):386.e1–5.
10. Razmaria AA, Marchetti PE, Prasad SM, Shalhav AL, Gundeti MS. Does robot-assisted laparoscopic ileocystoplasty (RALI) reduce peritoneal adhesions compared with open surgery? BJU Int. 2014;113(3):468–75.
11. Gasior A, Reck C, Vilanova-Sanchez A, Diefenbach KA, Yacob D, Lu P, et al. Surgical management of functional constipation: an intermediate report of a new approach using a laparoscopic sigmoid resection combined with Malone appendicostomy. J Pediatr Surg. 2018;53(6):1160–2.
12. Bray L, Callery P, Kirk S. A qualitative study of the pre-operative preparation of children, young people and their parents' for planned continence surgery: experiences and expectations. J Clin Nurs. 2012;21(13–14):1964–73.
13. Leslie B, Lorenzo AJ, Moore K, Farhat WA, Bägli DJ, Pippi Salle JL. Long-term followup and time to event outcome analysis of continent catheterizable channels. J Urol. 2011;185(6):2298–302.
14. Yerkes EB, Cain MP, King S, Brei T, Kaefer M, Casale AJ, et al. The malone antegrade continence enema procedure: quality of life and family perspective. J Urol. 2003;169(1):320–3.
15. Seth JH, Haslam C, Panicker JN. Ensuring patient adherence to clean intermittent self-catheterization. Patient Prefer Adherence. 2014;8:191–8.
16. Gundeti MS, Godbole PP, Wilcox DT. Is bowel preparation required before cystoplasty in children? J Urol. 2006;176(4):1574–7.
17. Cohen A.J., Gundeti M.S. (2018) Robotic Surgery for Neuropathic Bladder. In: Hemal A., Menon M. (eds) Robotics in Genitourinary Surgery. Springer, Cham. https://doi.org/10.1007/978-3-319-20645-5_63.
18. Famakinwa O, Gundeti MS. Robotic assisted laparoscopic Mitrofanoff appendicovesicostomy (RALMA). Curr Urol Rep. 2013;14(1):41–5.
19. Famakinwa OJ, Rosen AM, Gundeti MS. Robot-assisted laparoscopic Mitrofanoff appendicovesicostomy technique and outcomes of extravesical and intravesical approaches. Eur Urol. 2013;64(5):831–6.

20. McAndrew HF, Malone PSJ. Continent catheterizable conduits: which stoma, which conduit and which reservoir? BJU Int. 2002;89(1):86–9.
21. Wille MA, Zagaja GP, Shalhav AL, Gundeti MS. Continence outcomes in patients undergoing robotic assisted laparoscopic mitrofanoff appendicovesicostomy. J Urol. 2011;185(4):1438–43.
22. Keating MA, Rink RC, Adams MC. Appendicovesicostomy: a useful adjunct to continent reconstruction of the bladder. J Urol. 1993;149(5):1091–4.
23. Malone PS, Ransley PG, Kiely EM. Preliminary report: the antegrade continence enema. Lancet Lond Engl. 1990;336(8725):1217–8.
24. Saikaly SK, Rich MA, Swana HS. Assessment of pediatric Malone antegrade continence enema (MACE) complications: effects of variations in technique. J Pediatr Urol. 2016;12(4):246.e1–6.
25. Hoekstra LT, Kuijper CF, Bakx R, Heij HA, Aronson DC, Benninga MA. The Malone antegrade continence enema procedure: the Amsterdam experience. J Pediatr Surg. 2011;46(8):1603–8.

Part VIII

Introduction for Simple Prostatectomy

Daniel D. Eun

In this section, we address evolving robotic techniques for simple prostatectomy. Although open surgical approaches for symptomatic patients with significantly enlarged prostate has been around for decades, simple prostatectomy has been associated with significant risk for bleeding, both intraoperatively and postoperatively. With the popular emergence of laparoscopic and robotic prostate surgery, it became quickly evident that one great advantage of the closed abdomen was significant improvement in intraoperative blood loss. As a growing number of robotic surgeons well versed in radical prostatectomy began mimicking the previously described approaches to simple prostatectomy, their patients also enjoyed the benefits of improved intraoperative blood loss, but still had to deal with the implications of postoperative hematuria that is inherent in the technical design of operation. Large bore three-way catheters, catheter traction, and continuous bladder irrigation were still necessary components of postoperative management, often to the dismay of the patients and their surgeons.

In 2013, I fundamentally altered the approach to robotic simple prostatectomy by (1) sparing the space of Retzius and approaching the adenoma dissection through a posterior bladder incision and (2) completing a watertight, circumferential anastomosis of the bladder neck to the apical prostatic urethra. In doing so, we quickly realized that the postoperative hematuria could be greatly reduced, thereby significantly reducing the amount of postoperative bleeding and greatly simplifying the postoperative pathway. Almost 10 years later and nearly 300 prostates later, we have learned much and have vastly improved the outcomes and care of these patients. Our transfusion rate is <3% and we routinely place 18 French, two-way catheters postoperatively without continuous irrigation and send patients home same day from the recovery room.

I hope that you will read this section with great interest and apply what we have learned and adapted to your practice. Ultimately, my wish is that it will improve your outcomes and overall patient's experience.

Prostate: Robotic-Assisted Simple Prostatectomy

25

Kevin K. Yang and Daniel D. Eun

Introduction and Patient Selection

Simple prostatectomy for patients with bladder outlet obstruction from large prostatic glands has been well described in the urology literature. While the definition of "large" glands has been subjective, with the EAU guidelines describing sizes ≥80 g [1] and the AUA guidelines describing sizes ≥60 g [2], the decision ultimately comes down to surgeon comfort and patient preference. Most of the comparative data of the simple prostatectomy technique comes from the historic open cohorts. While patients had significant AUA symptom score improvements, open simple prostatectomy (OSP) saw longer hospitalization courses, higher transfusion rates, and longer times of catheterization than the transurethral enucleation techniques that later emerged [3, 4].

Robotic-assisted simple prostatectomy (RASP) emerged as the logical successor to OSP and addressed the latter's concerns of blood loss, morbidity, and length of stay. After the initial report in 2008 [5], subsequent adoption by high-volume robotic institutions demonstrated feasibility, reproducibility, and improved outcomes with a progressing learning curve. Umari et al. compared RASP to holmium laser enucleation of the prostate (HoLEP) showing similar operative times, symptom score improvements, and postoperative hemoglobin [6]. Median hospitalization was 4 days, while median catheterization time was 3 days. As the technique permeated, reports noted a shorter learning curve of 10–12 cases for RASP compared to 40–60 cases for HoLEP [7, 8].

Supplementary Information The online version of this chapter (https://doi.org/10.1007/978-3-030-50196-9_25) contains supplementary material, which is available to authorized users.

K. K. Yang · D. D. Eun (✉)
Department of Urology, Lewis Katz School of Medicine at Temple University, Philadelphia, PA, USA
e-mail: Daniel.Eun@tuhs.temple.edu

© Springer Nature Switzerland AG 2022
M. D. Stifelman et al. (eds.), *Techniques of Robotic Urinary Tract Reconstruction*, https://doi.org/10.1007/978-3-030-50196-9_25

In our experience, we select patients with gland size >80 grams, who have significant lower urinary tract symptoms refractory to medical management or prior surgical treatment, or patients requiring repeat or prolonged catheterization due to refractory urinary retention. Preoperative workup includes a focused history and physical examination, prostate sizing (cross-sectional imaging or transrectal ultrasound), post-void residual, AUA symptom scores, sexual health inventory for men scores, PSA, and prostate biopsy whenever clinically appropriate. Preoperative urine cultures should be obtained and treated if positive. Flexible cystoscopy should be performed prior to RASP to rule out bladder stones, bladder diverticula, or suspicious bladder lesions. If needed, plan for RASP can also include concurrent bladder diverticulectomy and cystolithotomy [9, 10]. We do not routinely perform urodynamic studies as a preoperative prerequisite to RASP.

Approaches to the Prostate Adenoma

Although OSP afforded a wide array of approaches to the adenoma (retropubic, suprapubic, perineal), RASP was initially described and performed transabdominally mimicking OSP techniques. Most of the literature has described a traditional retropubic maneuver after dropping the bladder: the medial umbilical ligaments and median umbilical ligaments are incised to enter the space of Retzius similar to the robotic radical prostatectomy technique followed by an anterior capsulotomy or cystotomy just cranial to the bladder neck in order to access the adenoma.

We describe a more contemporary, robotic Retzius-sparing technique where the bladder is not mobilized and a vertical, midline cystotomy is created at the dome, extended posteriorly and stopped prior to reaching the trigone. The adenectomy is performed through this posterior cystotomy. Instead of a traditional posterior trigonal advancement, which was popularized by the open technique, we prefer to completely and circumferentially anastomose the entire bladder neck to the apical prostatic urethra, thereby excluding the raw resection bed, in a watertight fashion. This 360° anastomosis greatly improves postoperative symptoms, decreases postoperative hematuria, and negates the need for a large three-way catheter and continuous bladder irrigation. The raw resection bed remains extraperitoneal since the space of Retzius is not opened. This technique is described in the section below.

Step-by-Step Technique

Patient Positioning and Access

Patients undergoing RASP are placed in a supine Trendelenburg position with the Intuitive Surgical da Vinci Xi robotic platform® being docked from the side. If the Si platform is used, patients are placed in a low lithotomy position, and the robot is docked between the legs. A new 16 or 18 French Foley catheter is inserted on the surgical field to drain the bladder. We obtain pneumoperitoneum using a Veress needle with the camera port placed periumbilically and a 12 mm assistant port placed 3 fingerbreadths cranial to the right iliac crest. 8 mm left and right robotic ports are inserted 8–10 cm lateral to the camera port. The fourth arm robotic port is placed on the left side mirroring the 12 mm assistant port. Finally, a 5 mm assistant port is inserted in the right upper quadrant between the camera port and right robotic port (Fig. 25.1).

Retzius-Sparing Cystotomy

Using a 0° camera, the pelvis is cleared of bowel contents, and a generous, midline cystotomy is extended from the dome to posterior wall before reaching the trigone (Fig. 25.2). Care is taken to avoid extending the cystotomy near the trigonal ridge or ureters. If the edges of the bladder wall obscure visualization, suture or self-retaining clips can be used to retract the bladder flaps on each side. We do not routinely use a retraction technique since the camera spends the majority of the case inside the bladder walls and find that retraction is not usually necessary.

Dissection of Prostate Adenoma

The vertical cystotomy should be large enough not only for exposure of the median lobe and ureteral orifices but also to accommodate the three arms of the robot and camera. The ureteral orifices must be identified prior to adenoma incision. With upward retraction, the adenoma dissection starts by initially incising the bladder mucosa at 6 o'clock (posterior aspect of the median lobe, if present) to reveal the "shiny white" posterior adenoma plane (Fig. 25.3). Care is taken to start this

Fig. 25.1 Port placements for Si console. For the Xi, the 12 mm camera port is replaced by an 8 mm trocar

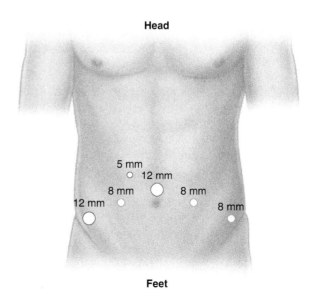

Fig. 25.2 View of prostate adenoma with a prominent median lobe via a Retzius-sparing, vertical cystotomy fashion

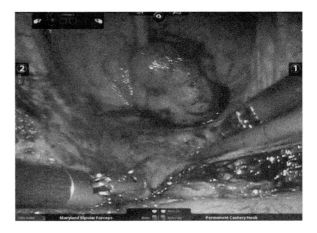

Fig. 25.3 Initial dissection of the adenoma starts at 6 o'clock, 1–2 cm away from the ureteral orifices (yellow arrows) which are readily identified on the trigonal ridge

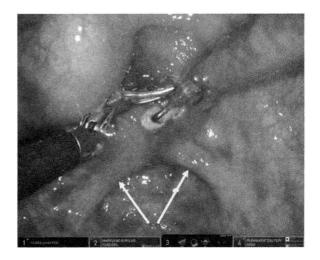

dissection at least 1–2 cm away from the ureteral orifices to allow enough room for wide anastomotic sutures at the end of the case. At the beginning of the case, bleeding is typically from the bladder mucosa and can be controlled with cautery using caution to avoid injuring the ureteral orifices. With a combination of blunt and precise cautery dissection, this plane is extended in the adenoma plane posteriorly as far as possible toward the prostatic apex. Once the distal limit has been reached, the posterior bladder neck mucosal incision is sequentially extended laterally and then anteriorly, with progressive posterior and lateral dissection of the adenoma plane resulting in increased exposure (Fig. 25.4). It is important to address focused hemostatic control as one progresses to maintain visualization. Arterial bleeding from the prostatic pedicles may occur at the 5 o'clock and 7 o'clock position. If needed, persistent bleeding at any point in the case can be over sewn using absorbable figure-of-eight sutures.

Fig. 25.4 After completing the deep posterior dissection, the posterior bladder neck mucosal incision is sequentially extended laterally and then anteriorly

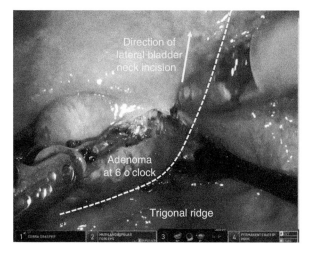

It is also imperative to confirm visual presence of prostate parenchyma, and not wispy fat and vessels, just outside of the dissection plane, to ensure that one is not dissecting on the capsular or "nerve-sparing" plane. Optimal retraction of the prostate adenoma and bladder neck using the fourth arm or assistant grasper is essential for efficient progression during dissection. We prefer to utilize an Intuitive Surgical EndoWrist® cobra grasper instrument as the fourth arm for its small profile and grasping jaws. A robotic tenaculum can also be used in a similar fashion.

Once the posterior and lateral dissection is completed, the circumferential dissection plane at the bladder neck is completed anteriorly, and dissection is deepened to the anterior aspect of the prostate. At this point, it is critical to keep the anterior prostatic dissection on the adenoma plane and under the dorsal venous complex (DVC) to avoid unnecessary bleeding. The anterior commissure is a reliably identifiable structure with longitudinally oriented fibers that run in a deep groove that is clearly seen between the lateral adenoma lobes anteriorly. It is important that this landmark is visually confirmed to correctly judge the dissection plane before furthering the dissection to the apex (Fig. 25.5). If the plane anterior to the lateral apices appears horizontally flat, the dissection plane is most likely on or outside the capsular plane, and the dissection plane needs to be slightly deepened to the adenoma plane before proceeding. Inadvertent dissection along the anterior prostatic capsular plane may risk unnecessary dissection and possible injury to the urethral sphincter complex.

Once the apical adenoma planes are separated circumferentially, the distal prostatic urethra at the level of the verumontanum is incised and the catheter identified. With an intentional and controlled approach at the prostatic apex, identification of the catheter can be calculated, and inadvertent disruption to the membranous urethra and sphincter complex can be reliably avoided (Fig. 25.6).

Once the adenoma is removed, the prostatic fossa can be packed with lap sponges and held in place for several minutes before addressing any significant bleeding points with controlled cautery or oversewn with sutures.

Fig. 25.5 The anterior commissure (dotted line) is reliably identifiable with longitudinally oriented fibers that run in a deep groove in between the bilateral anterior adenoma lobes and must be visually confirmed before furthering the dissection to the apex

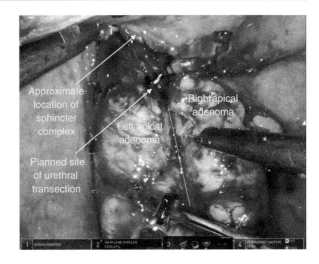

Fig. 25.6 A controlled and planned anterior urethral incision (arrow, catheter is seen) at the apical adenoma avoids inadvertent injury to the membranous urethra and sphincter complex. The verumontanum lies in the posterior urethra on the opposite side of the exposed catheter

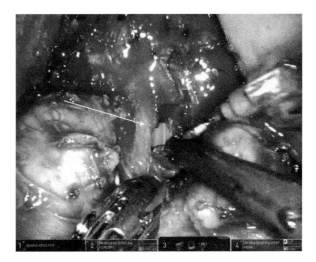

360 Degree Vesicourethral Reconstruction

We routinely perform a complete 360° vesicourethral anastomosis on all patients who undergo RASP. This allows for significantly improved postoperative hemostasis without the need for a large bore hematuria catheter, catheter-based traction maneuvers, or continual bladder irrigation (CBI). Since the prostatic fossa is sealed over with an anastomosis, the surgical site remains extraperitoneal and greatly reduces the possibility for postoperative hemorrhage. Lastly, the exclusion of the raw surgical bed from the urinary tract and reduction of the urethral gap result in improved postoperative irritative voiding symptoms. Since the hematuria typically

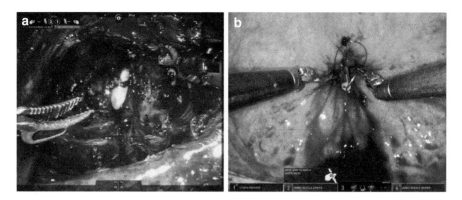

Fig. 25.7 Prostatic defect before (**a**) and after (**b**) 360° vesicourethral anastomosis reconstruction

resolves quickly due to exclusion of the raw prostatic fossa, we routinely place an 18 French, two-way Foley catheter without CBI at the completion of the anastomosis and without any other drains. Patients per our pathway are discharged home on postoperative day 1, similar to our radical prostatectomy patients, with plans to remove the catheter 1 week after surgery without a cystogram.

A 12 inch absorbable 3-0 monofilament barbed suture on a CV-23 needle (Covidien V-Loc™) is used starting at the 5 o'clock position on the bladder mucosa. This is then approximated to the same starting position on the prostatic urethra, and the posterior plate is created by running the suture clockwise. The anastomosis is continued until there is a complete circumferential, mucosal-to-mucosal approximation and exclusion of the raw prostatic fossa from the urinary tract (Fig. 25.7a, b). If the defect is especially large, additional sutures are sometimes needed. Prior to completing the anastomosis, a thrombin-based matrix such as FLOSEAL© (Baxter International Inc.) or SURGIFLO® (Johnson & Johnson) is injected through the anastomotic suture line into the prostatic fossa dead space for further hemostasis. This is delivered through the assistant port, using sterile arterial line tubing (Fig. 25.8).

Specimen Extraction and Closure

Bladder retraction sutures, if present, are removed, and the vertical midline cystotomy is closed with a running 12 inch, absorbable 3-0 monofilament barbed suture in two layers. An 18 French two-way urethral catheter is inserted with 20 cc of sterile water in the balloon. The bladder closure is tested with 300 mL of sterile saline to identify any leakage points. The prostatic adenoma is removed via an Endo Catch™ bag (Medtronic) through an extended camera port incision. No intra-abdominal drain is placed.

Fig. 25.8 Post-
anastomotic injection of
thrombin-based hemostatic
agent into prostatic fossa
dead space using sterile
arterial line tubing

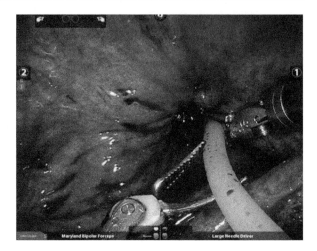

Postoperative Care and Management

Perioperative antibiotics and venous thromboembolism are continued during the
hospitalization, which should be typically one night. As mentioned, continuous
bladder irrigation and Foley traction are not utilized in our pathway. The urethral
catheter is typically removed on an outpatient basis between postoperative days 5
and 7 without a cystogram.

Complications and Management

Common adverse events such as urinary or incisional infections are managed expec-
tantly. Our transfusion rates for RASP have been comparable to endoscopic procedures (3%). Rare instances of cystotomy closure dehiscence are managed with
prolonged catheterization or robotic operative repair if the defect is large. Despite
this, cystogram evaluations prior to Foley catheter removal are not routinely performed as small leaks into the closed prostatic fossa space are self-limiting and the
cystotomy closure is vigilantly tested intra-operatively. Although often discussed in
the radical prostatectomy literature, the worrisome complications of incontinence
and impotence are exceedingly uncommon in a properly performed RASP where
the adenoma plane is followed within the prostatic capsule. Our experience has not
noted a bladder neck contracture or urethral stricture, which the risk may be mitigated by the 360° vesicourethral anastomosis.

References

1. Gravas S, Cornu JN, Drake MJ, Gacci M, Gratzke C, Herrmann TRW, Madersbacher S, Mamoulakis C, Tikkinen K. EAU guidelines on management of non-neurogenic male lower urinary tract symptoms (LUTS), incl. Benign Prostatic Obstruction (BPO). EAU Uroweb 2018.
2. Foster HE, Dahm P, Kohler TS, Lerner LB, Parsons JK, Wilt TJ, McVary KT. Surgical management of lower urinary tract symptoms attributed to benign prostatic hyperplasia: AUA guideline amendment 2019. J Urol. 2019;202(3):592–8.
3. Moody JA, Lingeman JE. Holmium laser enucleation for prostate adenoma greater than 100 gm.: comparison to open prostatectomy. J Urol. 2001;165(2):459–62.
4. Kuntz RM, Lehrich K, Ahyai SA. Holmium laser enucleation of the prostate versus open prostatectomy for prostates greater than 100 grams: 5-year follow-up results of a randomised clinical trial. Eur Urol. 2008;53(1):160–6.
5. Sotelo R, Clavijo R, Carmona O, Garcia A, Banda E, Miranda M, Fagin R. Robotic simple prostatectomy. J Urol. 2008;179(2):513–5.
6. Umari P, Fossati N, Gandaglia G, Pokorny M, De Groote R, Geurts N, Goossens M, Schatterman P, De Naeyer G, Mottrie A. Robotic assisted simple prostatectomy versus holmium laser enucleation of the prostate for lower urinary tract symptoms in patients with large volume prostate: a comparative analysis from a high volume center. J Urol. 2017;197(4):1108–14.
7. Johnson B, Sorokin I, Singla N, Roehrborn C, Gahan JC. Determining the learning curve for robot-assisted simple prostatectomy in surgeons familiar with robotic surgery. J Endourol. 2018;32(9):865–70.
8. Brunckhorst O, Ahmed K, Nehikhare O, Marra G, Challacombe B, Popert R. Evaluation of the learning curve for holmium laser enucleation of the prostate using multiple outcome measures. Urology. 2015;86(4):824–9.
9. Magera JS, Adam Childs M, Frank I. Robot-assisted laparoscopic transvesical diverticulectomy and simple prostatectomy. J Robot Surg. 2008;2(3):205–8.
10. Matei DV, Brescia A, Mazzoleni F, Spinelli M, Musi G, Melegari S, Galasso G, Detti S, de Cobelli O. Robot-assisted simple prostatectomy (RASP): does it make sense? BJU Int. 2012;110(11 Pt C):E972–9.
11. Lee Z, Lee M, Keehn AY, Asghar AM, Strauss DM, Eun DD. Intermediate-term Urinary Function and Complication Outcomes After Robot-Assisted Simple Prostatectomy. Urology. 2020;141:89–94

Part IX

Urethra

Lee Zhao

The section covers some new applications of robotic surgery—reconstruction of the posterior urethra, bladder neck, and placement of artificial urinary sphincter.

The reach and dexterity of the robot is an enabling technology that allows the surgeon to perform surgery that may not be possible with open techniques. Visualization of the space under the bladder allows for safe dissection of the vagina and rectum, thus allowing for placement of artificial urinary sphincter. The deep reach of the robot allows for precise suture placement, enabling reconstruction of the bladder neck and posterior urethra.

Robot-Assisted Laparoscopic Bladder Neck Reconstruction

26

Angelena B. Edwards and Micah Jacobs

Indications

Pediatric and adolescent patients with neurogenic bladder who continue to experience incontinence despite maximum medical management with anticholinergic therapy and intermittent catheterization can be considered for further surgical intervention. Most patients will have a voiding cystourethrogram available for review to characterize their bladder shape, capacity, bladder neck anatomy, and the presence or absence of trabeculations. A patient's expected bladder capacity can be calculated by the formula [volume in milliliters = (age + 2) × 30] [1], but the capacity is often reduced in children with neurogenic bladder. For this reason, urodynamic testing with attention directed at capacity, detrusor leak point pressure, Valsalva leak point pressure, and bladder compliance is extremely helpful in preparation for reconstruction. In addition, videourodynamic testing often can display potential inaccuracies when judging capacity, compliance, or peak detrusor pressures if the patient has high-grade vesicoureteral reflux (VUR). Large volumes of instilled fluid refluxing into the upper tracts can provide false reassurance that the upper tracts are not at risk.

Supplementary Information The online version of this chapter (https://doi.org/10.1007/978-3-030-50196-9_26) contains supplementary material, which is available to authorized users.

A. B. Edwards (✉)
Department of Urology, Division of Pediatric Urology, Children's Health System Texas, University of Texas Southwestern, Dallas, TX, USA

Department of Urology, Division of Pediatric Urology, University of Iowa, Iowa City, IA, USA
e-mail: Angelena-edwards@uiowa.edu

M. Jacobs
Department of Urology, Division of Pediatric Urology, Children's Health System Texas, University of Texas Southwestern, Dallas, TX, USA
e-mail: Micah.jacobs@childrens.com

© Springer Nature Switzerland AG 2022
M. D. Stifelman et al. (eds.), *Techniques of Robotic Urinary Tract Reconstruction*, https://doi.org/10.1007/978-3-030-50196-9_26

If a recent voiding cystourethrogram (VCUG) is available, this can accomplish a similar goal when paired with the results of a multichannel urodynamic study.

When evaluating bladder neck competency, it is important to consider that this is a dynamic process that can be impacted by other aspects of the bladder properties and not just leakage at a certain pressure. The outlet is often judged incompetent if the bladder neck is open on fluoroscopy, the sphincter is denervated on electromyography, or leak point pressures are less than 30–40 cm H20 [2]. However, using a supraphysiologic detrusor leak point pressure to determine the need for bladder outlet surgery is problematic. Although leak point pressures below this level may be associated with a lower risk for upper tract changes, this does not justify surgically reconstructing the bladder neck to raise the leak point pressure in order to achieve continence. The patient's bladder compliance and capacity should be established first. If an appropriate bladder capacity with high compliance cannot be established prior to surgery, bladder outlet surgery without augmentation is likely to result in high bladder filling pressures with persistent urinary leakage (now at high pressures), new or worsening VUR, and potential upper tract deterioration [3]. This can be prevented by performing a bladder augmentation concurrently with, or instead of, a bladder outlet procedure if there appears to be a low capacity and poorly compliant bladder.

Upper tract imaging should also be performed prior to bladder neck reconstruction to rule out pathology that can occur in neuropathic bladder patients prior to outlet manipulation. Renal ultrasound is an effective initial assessment of upper tract changes along with VCUG. If there is concern for renal injury, radionuclide scintigraphy is warranted.

When discussing potential surgery with the patient and family, it is important to focus on renal preservation and the minimization of future risk to the kidneys but also to establish the goals of surgical intervention, the mechanism of continence, and the need for catheterization. When considering bladder outlet surgery, it is critical to establish that patients have stable family and caregiver support, since, without a dedicated catheterization schedule and maintenance of a catheterizable channel, children are at grave risk of raising outlet pressures in a bladder that is not being emptied. Other important preoperative considerations for minimally invasive bladder reconstruction are prior abdominal surgeries (including bowel resection and prior surgery of the urinary tract) as well as the presence of a VP shunt. The patient should be informed of potential complications that can arise during surgery prior to consent. Preoperative planning should include urine culture and treatment of urinary tract infections prior to surgical intervention.

Perioperative Preparation

All patients should receive a preoperative urine culture 2–3 weeks prior to scheduled surgical intervention to allow a complete treatment course if a urinary tract infection is present. Formal bowel prep can be considered on an individual patient basis. Current management trends are leaning toward the use of enhanced recovery after surgery (ERAS) protocol pathways with minimal bowel preparation [4]. The surgical team may consider an abdominal X-ray prior to reconstructive intervention to assess stool burden and the administration of preoperative enemas as indicated. If a stoma is planned outside of the umbilicus, preoperative stoma marking should be considered to facilitate catheterization after the surgery.

Review of Surgical Approaches for Bladder Neck Reconstruction

When determining which type of bladder outlet procedure is desired, there are multiple patient factors that can play a role in the decision. These include body habitus, ambulatory status, manual dexterity, and the gender of the patient. Many ambulatory patients that catheterize through the urethral meatus will prefer to continue doing so. In such cases, a formal bladder neck reconstruction, which might result in difficulty with urethral catheterization, may be a poor choice for those patients. In contrast, a female who is a full-time wheelchair user and may not be able to catheterize via urethra may prefer a catheterizable channel for improved independence. In this case, formal reconstruction with concomitant sling may provide the highest likelihood for urethral continence.

This chapter focuses on the neurogenic bladder patient who will be managed with clean intermittent catheterization via appendicovesicostomy (APV) as a means of bladder emptying as well as bladder neck reconstruction to address stress urinary incontinence by increasing bladder neck resistance.

As with open surgery, several different minimally invasive techniques have been described in the literature for reconstruction of the bladder neck in order to achieve urethral continence. The Young-Dees-Leadbetter approach focuses on increasing resistance by urethral lengthening which creates a narrow and longer urethra. This chapter describes a similar technique dedicated to urethral lengthening and narrowing, modified to a robotic approach. Other techniques that have been described focus on construction of a flap valve mechanism (Kropp procedure), suspension, and/or coaptation of the urethra with sling placement, artificial urinary sphincter placement, or periurethral injection of bulking agents.

Robot-Assisted Laparoscopic Bladder Neck Reconstruction

Instrumentation and Equipment Required

Equipment for the da Vinci Si Surgical System (Intuitive Surgical, Inc. Sunnyvale, CA) (Table 26.1)
- EndoWrist Maryland dissector, 8 mm (Intuitive Surgical, Inc. Sunnyvale, CA)
- EndoWrist curved monopolar scissors, 8 mm (Intuitive Surgical, Inc. Sunnyvale, CA)

Table 26.1 Robotic instrument configuration

Surgical instrumentation			
Right arm	Left arm	Camera	Assistant
• Monopolar scissors • Needle driver	• Maryland dissector	**Endoscopic lens: 30° down**	• Suction-irrigator

344   A. B. Edwards and M. Jacobs

- EndoWrist needle driver, 8 mm (Intuitive Surgical, Inc. Sunnyvale, CA)
- InSite Vision system with 30° lens (Intuitive Surgical, Inc. Sunnyvale, CA)
- Laparoscopic suction irrigator
- Laparoscopic needle driver
- Laparoscopic Maryland grasper
- Laparoscopic monopolar scissors
- Endovascular stapler with vascular load

Trocars
- 12 mm camera trocar
- Two 8 mm robotic trocars
- 12 mm assistant trocar

Recommended Suture and Materials
- 2-0 Vicryl for port site facial closure
- 4-0 or 5-0 Monocryl suture for skin closure and maturation of stoma
- Bladder neck sling: pericardium allograft tissue (Tutoplast ®) or porcine small intestinal submucosa (SIS)
- 2-0 PDS suture for sling placement
- 4-0 and 3-0 Monocryl suture for urethral closure
- 3-0 Monocryl suture for anterior bladder closure
- 4-0 and 5-0 Monocryl suture for APV to bladder anastomosis
- 4-0 PDS suture to secure APV externally to detrusor tunnel
- 12F catheter into the APV
- 8F catheter into the urethra
- 4F or 5F open-ended ureteral catheters

Patient Positioning

Cystoscopy is performed in lithotomy to place externalized ureteral catheters prior to the start of the laparoscopic portion of the case. This facilitates identification of the ureteral orifices during the bladder neck reconstruction.

If the length from the umbilicus to the foot is less than 36 inches, the patient is then repositioned supine. Taller patients are positioned in low lithotomy with robotic docking to occur between the legs for the remainder of the case. All pressure points are padded, and the patient is secured to the bed with tape and padding across the chest and lower thighs with an additional towel and tape securing the arms to the bed. Patients in lithotomy should have stirrup heights adjusted intermittently throughout the case. The patient is then prepped and draped in a sterile fashion including the perineum.

Port Placement

Pneumoperitoneum is established using a modified Hasson technique [5] in prepubertal children and using a Veress needle [6] in pubertal patients in an infraumbilical location [7]. The umbilical incision is made in a V shape to serve as the future skin flap for advancement into the APV which is expected to be located in the umbilicus but will also serve as the location for the 12 mm camera port. Under direct visualization, two additional 8 mm robotic ports are placed in the midclavicular line just inferior to the umbilical site, followed by a 12 mm assistant port in the left upper quadrant midway between the umbilical and left robotic port (superior to the umbilical port) [8] (Fig. 26.1). The patient is placed in Trendelenburg.

Surgical Approach

1. *Laparoscopic Mobilization of the Right Colon and Appendix*
   The initial step is to harvest the appendix and mobilize the right colon to the hepatic flexure via standard laparoscopic technique. This portion of the procedure can be completed laparoscopically since the da Vinci Si Surgical System (Intuitive Surgical, Inc. Sunnyvale, CA) does not have the multisite ability of the da Vinci Xi Surgical System, and therefore the upward extent of the dissection

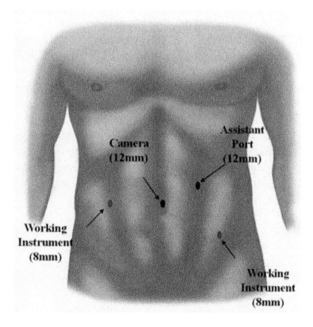

Fig. 26.1 Port placement for laparoscopic mobilization of the right colon and appendix and robot-assisted laparoscopic bladder neck reconstruction

required for mobilization with the given trocar configuration chosen for this pelvic-based operation is limited. The appendix is harvested using an endoscopic stapler with a vascular load. Special attention is given to preserving the mesoappendix. The staple line can also be extended along the antimesenteric side of the cecum to augment the length of the harvested appendix if needed. Once the appendix is free, the robot is docked to the ports.

2. *Bladder Neck Exposure*

The bladder neck can be exposed from a posterior or anterior approach initially. When starting with the posterior approach, a crescent-shaped incision is made on the posterior bladder peritoneum to mobilize the rectum in males or the vagina in females away from the operative field. The goal of this mobilization is to expose the path at which the bladder neck sling will lie and ensure no injury to the rectum or vagina will occur during its placement. Therefore, the dissection can be carried down to the posterior bladder neck and proximal urethra. This can be more easily identified by placing gentle traction on the Foley to observe where the balloon sits against the bladder neck.

The bladder is then mobilized anteriorly by developing the space of Retzius starting with an incision through the urachal remnant. The dissection should be carried down to the puboprostatic ligaments/anterior bladder neck with control of the dorsal vein complex. The dissection is carried laterally to expose the endopelvic fascia, which is incised to allow placement of the bladder neck sling under direct visualization.

The bladder neck can also be exposed through an anterior approach by starting with an incision in the peritoneum and median umbilical ligament. The space of Retzius is then developed and the bladder neck identified along with transection/ligation of the dorsal vein, transection of the puboprostatic ligaments, and exposure and incision of the endopelvic fascia [9].

3. *Sling Preparation and Placement*

Once the exposure of the bladder neck and proximal urethra is complete, the sling is prepared. On the back table, a 10 cm × 1 cm strip of SIS or bovine pericardium is prepared. Once in the abdomen, the sling is either passed from posterior to anterior (for a bladder that has been mobilized from behind) or simply around the bladder neck (if only an anterior dissection has been performed). The passage of the sling from the posterior approach can be facilitated by attachment of a 10F subclavian line tunneling device cut to 2.5 cm to either end of the cadaveric strip [10].

4. *Bladder Neck Reconstruction*

After the sling has been passed behind the bladder neck, it can be used as a retractor, lifting the bladder neck and proximal urethra into view to facilitate the reconstruction. The proximal urethra is then incised just below the bladder neck from the 3 o'clock to the 9 o'clock position. This incision is then extended superiorly along the bladder neck to a position just below the ureteral orifices. Both ureteral orifices can then be identified easily due to the preplaced ureteral catheters. The urethra is then retubularized with a two-layer closure using 4-0 Monocryl followed by 3-0 Monocryl suture over an 8F catheter. The bladder closure is then completed with 3-0 Monocryl suture in two layers. Integrity of the repair can be visualized by filling the bladder through the urethral catheter with saline. The sling is then wrapped 360° around the bladder neck and sutured to the pubic bone using 2-0 PDS. Nonabsorbable materials such as hernia tacks should be avoided, due to the potential for migration into the bladder or vagina and future stone formation.

5. *Creation of Appendicovesicostomy*

The freed appendix is then intubated with an 8F feeding tube secured at the proximal end with 3-0 PDS suture. The distal 5 mm of the appendix is amputated. The anterior bladder is then hitched to the anterior abdominal wall, with a 3-0 PDS suture, to allow a tension-free APV anastomosis and to assist with exposure of the posterior bladder for the remainder of the procedure. A 5 cm detrusorrhaphy is created in the posterior bladder using monopolar electrocautery. Once this window of bladder mucosa is exposed, an incision is made in its most inferior aspect. A 4-0 Monocryl suture is used to secure the distal end of the appendix to the detrusor muscle at the inferior apex of the detrusorrhaphy to prevent the channel from retracting into the future tunnel. The anastomosis between the distal end of the appendix and the bladder mucosa is then performed with interrupted 5-0 Monocryl suture. The appendix is then placed into the previously created detrusor tunnel, and the detrusor is closed over the appendix using interrupted 4-0 Vicryl suture. A 4-0 PDS suture is used to secure the appendix to the detrusor muscle at the point at which it exits the tunnel. The proximal end of the appendix is delivered under direct vision through the umbilical port site. It is secured at the fascial level with 4-0 PDS suture. The appendix is spatulated and then circumferentially sutured to the fascia and skin using 4-0 or 5-0 Monocryl suture. The V-shaped skin flap from the initial umbilical port is advanced into the appendiceal spatulation during skin closure. The prior 3-0 PDS suture used to secure the appendix to the feeding tube is cut, and the feeding tube is removed. A 12F Foley catheter is inserted and secured to the skin [10–12].

6. *Port Site Closure*

The remaining port sites are closed with 2-0 Vicryl suture at the level of the fascia, and 5-0 Monocryl is used to close the skin. Care is taken to ensure that the APV and urethral catheters can be irrigated and drain freely.

7. *Postoperative Care*

Patients are admitted postoperatively to the medical-surgical ward, and their diet is advanced as tolerated. The majority of patients are discharged home within 3–4 days after they are tolerating a regular diet. The catheters stay in place for 3–4 weeks and are removed during an outpatient visit. Patients remain on prophylactic antibiotic prophylaxis while the catheters are in place. Each patient will undergo individual clean intermittent catheterization education with the nursing staff and urodynamic testing at the 2–3 month postop mark.

Complications

Patients undergoing this surgical procedure can experience numerous complications including, but not limited to, recurrent urinary incontinence, stomal stenosis [13], bladder stone formation, urinary tract infections, wound dehiscence, bowel obstruction, urine leak or bladder rupture, de novo vesicoureteral reflux, and port site hernias [14]. Recurrent urinary incontinence may be related to mechanical bladder neck reconstruction failure but also could be due to poor bladder dynamics in patients that, in hindsight, would have benefited from simultaneous bladder augmentation due to high bladder pressures, low bladder compliance, and low bladder capacity [15, 3].

References

1. Berger RM, Maizels M, Moran GC, Conway JJ, Firlit CF. Bladder capacity (ounces) equals age (years) plus 2 predicts normal bladder capacity and aids in diagnosis of abnormal voiding patterns. J Urol. 1983;129(2):347–9.
2. Elder JS, Pippi-Salle JL. Bladder outlet surgery for congenital incontinence. In: Gearhart, Rink, Mouriquand: Pediatric Urology, 2nd ed., Elsevier 2009;761–74.
3. Grimsby GM, Menon V, Schlomer BJ, Baker LA, Adams R, Gargollo PC, et al. Long-term outcomes of bladder neck reconstruction without augmentation cystoplasty in children. J Urol. 2016;195(1):155–61.
4. Rove KO, Brockel MA, Saltzman AF, Dönmez MI, Brodie KE, Chalmers DJ, et al. Prospective study of enhanced recovery after surgery protocol in children undergoing reconstructive operations. J Pediatr Urol. 2018;14(3):252.e1–9.
5. Hasson HM. A modified instrument and method for laparoscopy. Am J Obstet Gynecol. 1971;110(6):886–7.
6. Patel DN, Parikh MN, Nanavati MS, Jussawalla MJ. Complications of laparoscopy. Asia Oceania J Obstet Gynaecol. 1985;11(1):87–91.
7. Toro A, Mannino M, Cappello G, Di Stefano A, Di Carlo I. Comparison of two entry methods for laparoscopic port entry: technical point of view. Diagn Ther Endosc. 2012;2012:305428.
8. Grimsby GM, Jacobs MA, Gargollo PC. Comparison of complications of robot-assisted laparoscopic and open appendicovesicostomy in children. J Urol. 2015;194(3):772–6.
9. Dajusta D, Ching C, Fuchs M, Brown C, Sanchez A, Levitt M, et al. V09-08 robotic assisted neo-malone, bladder neck reconstruction with sling and mitrofanoff in a patient with myelomeningocele. J Urol. 2018; https://doi.org/10.1016/j.juro.2018.02.2180.
10. Bagrodia A, Gargollo P. Robot-assisted bladder neck reconstruction, bladder neck sling, and appendicovesicostomy in children: description of technique and initial results. J Endourol. 2011;25(8):1299–305.
11. Liard A, Séguier-Lipszyc E, Mathiot A, Mitrofanoff P. The Mitrofanoff procedure: 20 years later. J Urol. 2001;165(6 Pt 2):2394–8.
12. Mitrofanoff P. Trans-appendicular continent cystostomy in the management of the neurogenic bladder. Chir Pediatr. 1980;21(4):297–305.
13. Cain MP, Casale AJ, King SJ, Rink RC. Appendicovesicostomy and newer alternatives for the Mitrofanoff procedure: results in the last 100 patients at Riley Children's hospital. J Urol. 1999;162(5):1749–52.

14. Thomas JC, Dietrich MS, Trusler L, DeMarco RT, Pope JC, Brock JW, et al. Continent catheterizable channels and the timing of their complications. J Urol. 2006;176(4 Pt 2):1816–20; discussion 20.
15. Grimsby GM, Jacobs MA, Menon V, Schlomer BJ, Gargollo PC. Perioperative and short-term outcomes of robotic vs open bladder neck procedures for neurogenic incontinence. J Urol. 2016;195(4 Pt 1):1088–92.

Robot-Assisted Bladder Neck Artificial Urinary Sphincter Implantation

27

Benoit Peyronnet, Frank Van Der Aa, Grégoire Capon, Aurélien Descazeaud, Olivier Belas, Xavier Gamé, Adrien Vidart, Vincent Cardot, and Georges Fournier

Indications

Female Patients

Stress urinary incontinence (SUI) is common in women and increases with age with a reported prevalence of up to 30–60% in elderly women [1]. Over the past two decades, the use of synthetic mid-urethral slings (MUS) has become the gold standard surgical

Supplementary Information The online version of this chapter (https://doi.org/10.1007/978-3-030-50196-9_27) contains supplementary material, which is available to authorized users.

B. Peyronnet (✉)
Department of Urology, University of Rennes, Rennes, France

F. Van Der Aa
Department of Urology, University of Leuven, Leuven, Belgium

G. Capon
Department of Urology, University of Bordeaux, Bordeaux, France

A. Descazeaud
Department of Urology, University of Limoges, Limoges, France

O. Belas
Department of Urology, Polyclinique Le Mans Sud, Le Mans, France

X. Gamé
Department of Urology, University of Toulouse, Toulouse, France

A. Vidart
Department of Urology, Foch Hospital, Suresnes, France

V. Cardot
Department of Urology, Clinique Bizet, Paris, France

G. Fournier
Department of Urology, University of Brest, Brest, France

treatment of SUI in female patients [1, 2]. However, MUS fail in about 15% of women with SUI [3]. Female patients with a lack of urethral mobility [4, 5] and, to a lesser extent, those with low urethral closure pressure have an increased risk of persistent SUI after MUS, as high as 75% [4, 6]. The mechanism causing SUI in these patients is often termed "intrinsic sphincter deficiency" (ISD) as opposed to SUI related to urethral hypermobility [4, 7]. There is no worldwide consensual definition of SUI due to ISD [4]. The ISD definition used in France is a combination of clinical and urodynamic criteria, the former being the key determinants: demonstrable SUI on cough stress test with lack of urethral mobility, negative Marshall/Bonney test (i.e., still leaking on cough stress test despite urethral support), and a low maximum urethral closure pressure [4]. Fixed urethra is the core feature of this definition which makes the indication of female AUS highly dependent on clinical judgment and expertise as standardized measurement of urethral mobility such as the Q-tip test or urethral ultrasound has not been widely adopted for various reasons [8, 9]. However, visual urethral mobility evaluation, when performed by experienced clinicians, has been reported to strongly correlate with the Q-tip test [10]. Other clinical criteria such as failure of a first anti-incontinence procedure, high SUI scores, constant leakage for any daily activity, and leakage with abdominal straining may reinforce the clinical suspicion of ISD [4]. In female patients with SUI due to ISD, as defined above, AUS is recommended as the gold standard treatment in the French guidelines [4]. In daily practice, SUI due to ISD most commonly occurs in two different populations: female patients with neurogenic stress urinary incontinence (usually due to spinal cord injury, spina bifida, or pelvic trauma) or patients who failed previous anti-incontinence surgical procedures [11]. However, there are considerable discrepancies in the role and use of AUS in female patients from one country to another, and the situation in France has for long been pretty unique with a much wider use than in any other country in the world [12, 13]. According to the European Association of Urology guidelines, AUS should be implanted only as a last resort procedure and only in expert centers, while the International Consultation on Incontinence recommends to use AUS only in selected female patients [14, 15]. Because AUS in female patients is not approved by the Food and Drug Administration (FDA), it is not mentioned as an option in the American Urological Association (AUA) guidelines on SUI [16], and its use has been very limited in the United States of America (USA) over the past years [17]. The indications of AUS in female patients in various international guidelines are summarized in Table 27.1.

Table 27.1 Indications of female artificial urinary sphincter in current guidelines

	French Association of Urology (AFU) [4]	International Consultation on Incontinence (ICI/ICS) [15]	European Association of Urology (EAU) [14]	American Urological Association (AUA) [16]
Indications of female artificial urinary sphincter	Gold standard treatment for SUI due to ISD, especially lack of urethral mobility	In selected patients	Complicated stress urinary incontinence, as a last resort option, only in expert centers	Not mentioned

ISD intrinsic sphincter deficiency; *SUI* stress urinary incontinence

Male Patients

The AUS is the gold standard treatment of SUI due to ISD in male patients [14]. In the vast majority of the cases, SUI in male patients result from radical prostatectomy, and in this scenario, the AUS cuff is placed at the bulbar urethra [18]. When male SUI is not post-prostatectomy, another possible option is to place the AUS cuff at the bladder neck. The strongest rationale to do so is for spina bifida and spinal cord-injured patients with neurogenic SUI. The theoretical benefits of bladder neck implantation in this patient population are as follows. (1) It may reduce the risk of erosion from retrograde instrumentation such as cystoscopy and clean intermittent catheterization. (2) A perineal approach might increase the risk of poor wound healing and pressure sores in paraplegic patients. (3) In patients with lumbosacral lesion, an open bladder neck is a common occurrence, and the prostatic urethra may fill with stagnant urine above a closed bulbar cuff, which may represent a potential source of infection. (4) Bladder neck cuff placement might spare antegrade ejaculation [19]. In a recent multicenter retrospective series of adult spina bifida patients, one of these theoretical advantages was partially confirmed with a trend toward longer explantation-free survival in the bladder neck group compared to the peribulbar group [19]. In its 2015 consensus statement, the International Continence Society (ICS) recommended to favor bladder neck AUS over bulbar urethra AUS in neurological patients [18]. Bladder neck implantation might also be used as an alternative to bulbar urethra in patients with SUI resulting from radiation therapy or benign prostatic obstruction (BPO) surgery.

Preoperative Evaluation

The preoperative work-up we perform before male and female robotic AUS is roughly similar and is summarized in Table 27.2. It includes a thorough medical history, paying special attention to history of previous anti-incontinence surgery and more globally of previous pelvic surgery. Many of the female AUS patients have undergone mid-urethral sling insertion, and the question of excising the tape before scheduling the AUS implantation should always be raised, especially in those with voiding dysfunction or other mesh-related complications. History of

Table 27.2 Preoperative must dos

Robotic AUS preoperative work-up
Thorough medical history
Physical examination
Pencil test
Questionnaires (e.g., USP, ICIQ-SF,UDI, etc.)
Uroflowmetry and post-void residual (except in self-catheterizing neurogenic patients)
Urethrocystoscopy
Urodynamics

pelvic radiation therapy should also be sought because it has been proven to increase the risk of AUS erosion in female patients in open series [20], and, as of now, we never performed robotic AUS implantation in irradiated women. During the clinical interview, subclinical cognitive dysfunction should be sought, especially in elderly women as it may hinder device handling. Physical examination should investigate whether the patient will be able to easily manipulate the device, especially in women, making sure they can grab their labia majora which can be challenging in obese patients. A pencil test is useful to assess patients' cognitive function and manual dexterity. Physical examination will also strive to demonstrate SUI using a cough stress test in the lithotomy position. In female patients, the urethral mobility is assessed, and a Marshall/Boney test is performed, evaluating whether SUI is corrected when supporting the mid-urethra. When urine leakage is not demonstrated with the patient laying, having the patient cough while standing may help unmask SUI. Pelvic organ prolapse is also sought and, when present, can lead to offer concomitant sacrocolpopexy [21]. In case vulvovaginal atrophy is noted, topical estrogen therapy preoperatively is prescribed. Validated self-administered questionnaires are done to further explore and gauge lower urinary tract symptoms (LUTS) as well as their impact on patients' quality of life. We typically use the Urinary Symptom Profile (USP) [22] and International Consultation on Incontinence Questionnaire Short-Form (ICIQ-SF) [23], but any other validated questionnaires can be used. A free uroflowmetry and post-void residual (PVR) are performed to rule out voiding dysfunction which could prompt to perform mid-urethral sling excision/urethrolysis before scheduling the AUS implantation. A urethrocystoscopy is also part of the systematic preoperative work-up to rule out mid-urethral sling perforation and bladder stone. Finally, urodynamics is routinely done preoperatively and absolutely mandatory in neurological patients to detect detrusor overactivity (DO) or poor compliance bladder that could worsen and result in upper urinary tract deterioration postoperatively. In patients with constant leakage, defunctionalized bladder can mimic DO and poor compliance [24].

Review of Surgical Approaches

The challenge of AUS implantation in females lies in the dissection of the bladder neck. As stated by Scott, one of the fathers of AUS, this surgery is difficult because there is no natural plane between the urethra and vagina [25] and the bladder neck is located deep in the pelvis. The open approach has been the most largely reported for AUS implantation in female patients, yielding deceiving perioperative outcomes in most series with up to 43.8% of intraoperative bladder neck injury, up to 25% of intraoperative vaginal injury, and up to 45.3% of explantation [26]. This relatively high morbidity has lead surgeons to explore other approaches aiming to minimize the technical difficulty of AUS implantation. Vaginal AUS implantation was described as a first alternative to the open approach in the 1980s but with very few series published and none for almost 30 years now [26]. The theoretical risk of device infection due to the high bacterial load in the vagina has likely been the main cause of abandonment of this approach. In the late 2000s, laparoscopic AUS implantation in female patients was described with encouraging outcomes in experienced hands [27, 28]. More recently, several series have reported the use of a robotic approach for female AUS implantation, which may combine minimal invasiveness and lower technical complexity compared to the laparoscopic route thanks to the enhanced dexterity with the EndoWrist technology allowing multiple dimension mobility of the instruments, the magnified 3D image, the physiologic tremor filtering, and motion scaling of the surgical robot [21, 29–31]. In a preliminary series of six cases, Fournier et al. reported promising outcomes with no explantation/erosion and 83.3% of patients fully continent postoperatively [29]. Using the same robotic technique with a paramount role of the assistant's finger placed in the vaginal fornix to expose the vesicovaginal plane, Peyronnet et al. later reported their eight first robotic cases and observed a significantly decreased postoperative complication rate compared to their open cohort (25% vs. 75%; $p = 0.02$) with a reduced length of hospital stay (3.8 vs. 9.3 days; $p = 0.09$) [30]. The excellent outcomes of this technique were further confirmed in a multicenter series of 49 cases with a minimum 12 months of follow-up. In this complex patient population with 85.7% having a history of previous anti-incontinence surgery, the authors reported only one explantation (2%) with 81.6% of patients fully continent after a median follow-up of 18.5 months [21]. Using a slightly different technique, without the help of the assistant's finger and with the cuff placed more distally toward the midurethra, Biardeau et al. reported 9 cases with less favorable outcomes, especially 22.2% of erosions, highlighting the need of standardized surgical steps in addition to the robotic approach to decrease female AUS implantation surgical morbidity [31]. Despite the high level of evidence, studies are still lacking to support its use [27]; female AUS might become in the near future a well-established therapeutic option thanks to the easier implantation through a robotic approach and the newer generation of implants, electromechanical and with no pump to place in the labia majora.

In the initial descriptions of AUS implantation in the 1970s, the cuff was systematically placed at the bladder neck in male patients, because radical prostatectomy was not described yet and the main cause of male SUI was neurogenic ISD [32]. For long, the open approach was the only one described for bladder neck AUS implantation in male patients. In 2013, Yates et al. reported the six first cases of robot-assisted bladder AUS implantation in neurogenic male patients with excellent short-term outcomes [33]. Since then, two small sample series have stressed the occurrence of early bladder neck atrophy requiring revision (cuff downsizing) and a relatively high rate of perioperative complications, highlighting a possibly longer learning curve for this procedure than for female bladder neck AUS [34, 35].

Step by Step of Procedure

Female

The procedure is performed by two surgeons: a surgeon at the console and another surgeon (or a surgeon in training in some cases) to provide assistance on the surgical field.

Patient's Positioning, Ports Placement, and Robot Docking

The patient is placed in a 23° Trendelenburg position with spread legs (Fig. 27.1). The procedure is performed using a transperitoneal approach with a 0° lens. Five ports are placed: one 12 mm camera port at the umbilicus, three 8 mm robotic ports (one in the right flank and two at the lateral edge of right and left rectus abdominis muscles), and an additional 12 mm port in the left flank for the assistant. A minimum 7 cm space is maintained between each port. The four-arm da Vinci Si robot is placed in a right-side-docking position (Fig. 27.1). Only three robotic instruments are used for the whole procedure: a bipolar ProGrasp forceps in the left robotic arm, scissors in the internal right robotic, arm and a regular ProGrasp forceps in the external right robotic arm.

Access to the Bladder Neck

A 14 Fr urethral catheter is inserted, and the bladder is filled with 100–300 ml of saline to identify its boundaries. The bladder is dropped down from the abdominal wall, and the Retzius space is dissected until the bladder neck and the endopelvic fascia are individualized. Before starting the dissection of the vesicovaginal space, it is paramount to locate accurately the bladder neck as in this technique the AUS cuff will be inserted around the bladder neck and not at the level of the urethra. The bladder neck is larger than the urethra, and its wall is thicker allowing the use of a larger cuff, minimizing the risk of erosion. The bladder neck contours are identified thanks to the saline instilled in the bladder, and if needed the catheter balloon can also be gently moved back and forth by the assistant.

Vesicovaginal Dissection

Once the space of Retzius has been dissected down to the endopelvic fascia, the assistant surgeon places one finger in the vagina. This is a key point of this technique. The assistant finger is placed in one of the lateral fornix in order to push it upward and laterally, toward the ipsilateral shoulder (Fig. 27.2). It allows to start the dissection of the vesicovaginal plane "on" the tip of the assistant's finger, laterally, away from the bladder neck minimizing the risk of bladder neck injury. The additional benefit of pushing the vaginal fornix laterally is that, after the dissection has been sufficiently initiated, it enables direct vision of the vesicovaginal space posterior to the bladder neck. This requires to largely mobilize the lateral side of the bladder so that the bladder neck could be rotated. The plane is initiated with cold scissors. In our early cases, we incised the endopelvic fascia to open it, but we realized that if the fascia is sufficiently stretched by the assistant finger, it can be opened

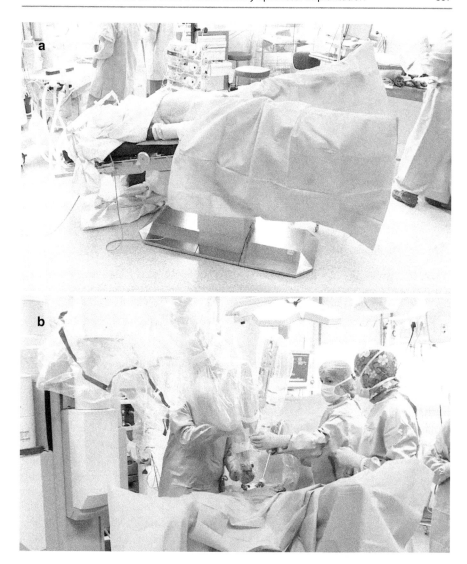

Fig. 27.1 Patient's positioning for robotic female artificial urinary sphincter implantation. **a.** Trendelenburg position with spread legs. **b.** Right-side docking to allow easy access to the vagina

simply by gently spreading it with the edge of the scissors. This allows to perform a purely blunt dissection of the bladder neck (i.e., no incision by electrocautery is used at any point during this step) to minimize the risk of bladder neck or vaginal injury. While performing these subtle moves with the scissors, the perivesical fascia is entered, and the vaginal wall appears progressively as a shiny white plane (called in France the bald plane as it looks like a bald head). This is the plane where the dissection around the bladder neck has to be carried out. The breach in the endopelvic fascia is extended cranially and caudally, by cutting with the scissors parallel to

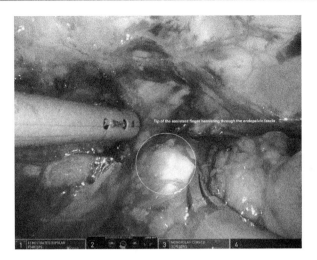

Fig. 27.2 Assistant finger pushing into the right vaginal fornix upward and laterally toward the ipsilateral shoulder, therefore creating a hernia into the endopelvic fascia and exposing progressively the intervesicovaginal plane

the vaginal wall, to avoid traction on the bladder neck and vaginal wall during the dissection and to allow the assistant finger pushing more thoroughly. Using the edge of the scissors, all the small fibers of the endopelvic and perivesical fascia are reclined medially, carrying on the dissection of the white shiny vaginal wall (the bald plane). Once the plane has been sufficiently developed, dissection is pursued behind the bladder neck using the ProGrasp forceps, sliding on the assistant finger while gently opening the blades tangentially to the bladder neck and vaginal walls to separate them. At this step the contralateral ProGrasp forceps is used as a retractor to gently push the bladder neck medially and upward (Fig. 27.3). Once the median line has been reached, the same maneuvers are performed on the other side of the bladder neck. The two dissected spaces are thus joined, with often a remaining veil of perivesical fascia to be opened on the tip of the ProGrasp forceps after the assistant surgeon has ensured with his/her finger that the vaginal wall is intact and has not been pinched by the tip of the ProGrasp forceps. At the end of the dissection, the bladder is filled with methylene blue to verify the integrity of the bladder neck.

The bladder dome is intentionally opened only in a few cases when the vesicovaginal dissection is felt very challenging, to allow monitoring of the dissection from inside the bladder, in order to minimize the risk of bladder neck injury.

Cuff and Balloon Placement

The bladder neck circumference is measured using a measuring tape introduced through the 12 mm port. The cuff chosen is intended to be a bit loose, on purpose, to prevent bladder outlet obstruction (Fig. 27.4). The cuff is then introduced through

Fig. 27.3 Dissection of the posterior part of the bladder neck under direct vision using the contralateral ProGrasp forceps as a retractor to move the bladder neck upward and medially

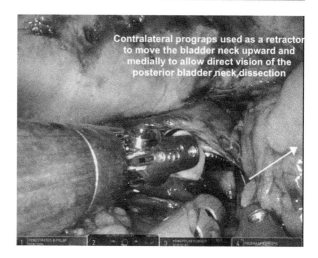

Fig. 27.4 When measuring the bladder neck, the cuff is intended to be a bit loose, on purpose to prevent bladder outlet obstruction

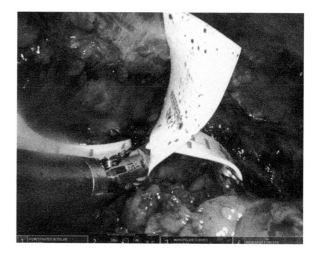

the same 12 mm port and positioned around the bladder neck. The device is manipulated cautiously to avoid any damage. The 61–70 cmH2O pressure-regulating balloon is implanted in the prevesical space via a 3 cm suprapubic incision and filled with saline. The peritoneum is then closed with barbed suture.

Pump Placement and Connections
The pump is implanted in one of the labia majora by creating a subcutaneous passage starting from the short suprapubic incision used to introduce the balloon and using a long instrument (e.g., scissors or Kelly clamp) (Fig. 27.5). The connections

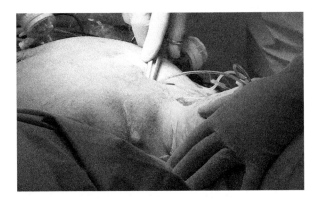

Fig. 27.5 Creation of the space for the future cuff in the labia majora using long scissor inserted through the subinguinal incision

are made through the suprapubic incision. The incisions are closed. At the end of the procedure, the device is deactivated.

Male

The two main differences between the female and the male techniques are as follows:

- The dissection is conducted at the posterior part of the bladder neck first in the male technique.
- The dissection is not guided by the assistant finger in the male technique.
- Patient's positioning, port placement, and robot docking parallel exactly what is done in the female technique.

Then the procedure starts by opening the peritoneum at the level of the seminal vesicles. The seminal vesicles are dropped down to create a space between the posterior part of the bladder neck and the seminal vesicles. The dissection is then carried out on both sides of the bladder neck, being very cautious to avoid any ureteral injury and to spare the neurovascular bundles. The bladder is then dropped down to go anteriorly. A ProGrasp forceps is placed in the space dissected on one side of the bladder neck and found anteriorly. A surgical loop is passed through this dissected space. The same maneuver is done on the other side of the bladder neck allowing to pass the surgical loop all around the bladder neck. This loop is replaced by the measuring tape to size the bladder neck. The passage is enlarged so that the cuff would apply perfectly on all its circumference. The cuff size usually ranges from 6 cm to 10 cm. The cuff is inserted through the 12 mm port and placed around the bladder neck. As in the female technique, a 3 cm subinguinal incision is made to insert the pressure-regulating balloon (PRB). A 61–70 cm H2O PRB is generally used. The peritoneum is then closed using barbed sutures after the PRB has been filled. The robot is undocked, and the pump is placed in the scrotum through the subinguinal incision. The connections are made through this incision and the skin incisions are closed. At the end of the procedure, the device is deactivated.

Managing Complications

Erosion, Infection

As with bulbar urethra AUS in male patients, the most serious complications that can occur after robotic bladder neck AUS implantation are device erosion or infection. Everything shall be done to minimize those risks, performing cautious dissections intraoperatively, getting sterile preoperative urine culture, and using intraoperative antibiotic prophylaxis. These complications are seen more rarely using the robotic approach (<3% in the largest series available) [21]. When device erosion occurs, either vesical or vaginal, explantation should be performed. Reimplantation after a minimum 3-month period can be discussed on a case by case basis bearing in mind that, despite there is currently no data to support this assertion, we know by experience that reimplantation procedure is more challenging with a higher risk of failure. In case of device infection, the gold standard is to explant the whole AUS as well, although conservative management with bacteriological samples and targeted antibiotics might be successful in very selected cases.

Urinary Retention

Urinary retention has been reported in up to 18.8% of female patients after AUS implantation [26]. This is usually transient, lasting a few days after the implantation. Rather than leaving an indwelling urinary catheter, teaching the patient to perform self-catheterization until it resolves might decrease the risk of infection and erosion and help track resumption of spontaneous voiding. In case urinary retention persists, AUS explantation may be discussed with the patient, weighting the harms of self-catheterization vs. the burden of previous SUI. A urethrocystoscopy should also be performed in case of persistent urinary retention to rule out cuff erosion.

Overactive Bladder Symptoms

Overactive bladder (OAB) symptoms have been reported in up to 43.8% of female patients after AUS implantation. A urethrocystoscopy should be performed to rule out cuff erosion. The whole OAB armamentarium could then be used, starting with antimuscarinics and/or beta 3 agonists. When these pharmaceutical treatments fail, posterior tibial nerve stimulation, sacral neuromodulation, and intradetrusor botulinum toxin A could be offered. In the latter case, great care should be taken when performing the injection, deactivating the sphincter during the procedure and using a flexible cystoscope or a pediatric cystoscope (Chap. 17) whenever possible, to minimize the risk of causing damages to the AUS cuff.

Nonmechanical and Mechanical Failure

In case of mechanical and/or nonmechanical failure, surgical revision should be offered. In case of mechanical failure, the failing component should be replaced if the device is recent, and the whole device should be changed when the device is in place for a long time (e.g., >5 years). In case of nonmechanical failure, higher PRB should be placed, or cuff should be downsized depending upon the preoperative work-up and intraoperative observations.

References

1. Cox A, Herschorn S, Lee L. Surgical management of female SUI: is there a gold standard? Nat Rev Urol. 2013;10(2):78–89.
2. Syan R, Brucker BM. Guideline of guidelines: urinary incontinence. BJU Int. 2016;117(1):20–33.
3. Tommaselli GA, Di Carlo C, Formisano C, Fabozzi A, Nappi C. Medium-term and long-term outcomes following placement of midurethral slings for stress urinary incontinence: a systematic review and meta-analysis. Int Urogynecol J. 2015;26(9):1253–68.
4. Cour F, Le Normand L, Lapray JF, et al. Intrinsic sphincter deficiency and female urinary incontinence. Prog Urol. 2015;25(8):437–54.
5. Wlaźlak E, Viereck V, Kociszewski J, et al. Role of intrinsic sphincter deficiency with and without urethral hypomobility on the outcome of tape insertion. Neurourol Urodyn. 2017;36(7):1910–6.
6. Lo TS, Pue LB, Tan YL, Wu PY. Risk factors for failure of repeat midurethral sling surgery for recurrent or persistent stress urinary incontinence. Int Urogynecol J. 2016;27(6):923–31.
7. Osman NI, Li Marzi V, Cornu JN, Drake MJ. evaluation and classification of stress urinary incontinence: current concepts and future directions. Eur Urol Focus. 2016;2(3):238–44.
8. Pirpiris A, Shek KL, Dietz HP. Urethral mobility and urinary incontinence. Ultrasound Obstet Gynecol. 2010;36(4):507–11.
9. Caputo RM, Benson JT. The Q-tip test and urethrovesical junction mobility. Obstet Gynecol. 1993;82(6):892–6.
10. Robinson BL, Geller EJ, Parnell BA, Crane AK, Jannelli ML, Wells EC, et al. Diagnostic accuracy of visual urethral mobility exam versus Q-Tip test: a randomized crossover trial. Am J Obstet Gynecol. 2012;206(6):528.e1–6.
11. Freton L, Tondut L, Enderle I, Hascoet J, Manunta A, Peyronnet B. Comparison of adjustable continence therapy periurethral balloons and artificial urinary sphincter in female patients with stress urinary incontinence due to intrinsic sphincter deficiency. Int Urogynecol J. 2018 in press; https://doi.org/10.1007/s00192-017-3544-8.
12. Matsushita K, Chughtai BI, Maschino AC, et al. International variation in artificial urinary sphincter use. Urology. 2012;80(3):667–72.
13. Peyronnet B, Hascoet J, Scailteux LM, Gamé X, Cornu JN. The changing face of artificial urinary sphincter use in France: the future is female. Eur Urol Focus. 2018; in press pii: S2405-4569(18)30404-8
14. Lucas MG, Bosch RJ, Burkhard FC, et al. EAU guidelines on surgical treatment of urinary incontinence. Eur Urol. 2012;62(6):1118–29.
15. Herschorn S, Bruschini H, Comiter C, et al. Committee of the international consultation on incontinence. Surgical treatment of stress incontinence in men. Neurourol Urodyn. 2010;29(1):179–90.

16. Kobashi KC, Albo ME, Dmochowski RR, et al. Surgical treatment of female stress urinary incontinence: AUA/SUFU guideline. J Urol. 2017;198(4):875–83.
17. Lee R, Te AE, Kaplan SA, Sandhu JS. Temporal trends in adoption of and indications for the artificial urinary sphincter. J Urol. 2009;181(6):2622–7.
18. Biardeau X, Aharony S, the AUS Consensus Group, et al. Artificial urinary sphincter: report of the 2015 consensus conference: artificial urinary sphincter. Neurourol Urodyn. 2016;35:S8–S24.
19. Khene ZE, Paret F, Perrouin-Verbe MA, et al. Artificial urinary sphincter in male patients with spina bifida: comparison of perioperative and functional outcomes between bulbar urethra and bladder neck cuff placement. J Urol. 2018;199(3):791–7.
20. Costa P, Poinas G, Ben Naoum K, et al. Long-term results of artificial urinary sphincter for women with type III stress urinary incontinence. Eur Urol. 2013;63(4): 753–8.
21. Peyronnet B, Capon G, Belas O, et al. Robot-assisted ams-800 artificial urinary sphincter bladder neck implantation in female patients with stress urinary incontinence. Eur Urol. 2019;75(1):169–75.
22. Haab F, Richard F, Amarenco G, Coloby P, Arnould B, Benmedjahed K, Guillemin I, Grise P. Comprehensive evaluation of bladder and urethral dysfunction symptoms: development and psychometric validation of the urinary symptom profile (USP) questionnaire. Urology. 2008;71(4):646–56.
23. Kerry A, Donovan J, Peters TJ, Shaw C, Gotoh M, Abrams P. ICIQ: a brief and robust measure for evaluating the symptoms and impact of urinary incontinence. Neurourol Urodyn. 2004;23(4):322–30.
24. Peyronnet B, Brucker BM. Management of overactive bladder symptoms After radical prostatectomy. Curr Urol Rep. 2018;19(12):95.
25. Scott FB. The use of the artificial sphincter in the treatment of urinary incontinence in the female patient. Urol Clin North Am. 1985;12(2):305–15.
26. Peyronnet B, O'Connor E, Khavari R, et al AMS-800 artificial urinary sphincter in female patients with stress urinary incontinence: asystematic review. Neurourol Urodyn. 2018 in press.
27. Mandron E, Bryckaert PE, Papatsoris AG. Laparoscopic artificial urinary sphincterimplantation for female genuine stress urinary incontinence: technique and 4-year experience in 25 patients. BJU Int. 2010;106(8):1194–8.
28. Rouprêt M, Misraï V, Vaessen C, et al. Laparoscopic approach for artificial urinary sphincter implantation in women with intrinsic sphincter deficiency incontinence: a single-centre preliminary experience. Eur Urol. 2010;57(3):499–504.
29. Fournier G, Callerot P, Thoulouzan M, et al. Robotic-assisted laparoscopic implantation of artificial urinary sphincter in women with intrinsic sphincter deficiency incontinence: initial results. Urology. 2014;84(5):1094–8.
30. Peyronnet B, Vincendeau S, Tondut L, Bensalah K, Damphousse M, Manunta A. Artificial urinary sphincter implantation in women with stress urinary incontinence: preliminary comparison of robot-assisted and open approaches. Int Urogynecol J. 2016;27(3):475–81.
31. Biardeau X, Rizk J, Marcelli F, et al. Robot-assisted laparoscopic approach for artificial urinary sphincter implantation in 11 women with urinary stress incontinence: surgical technique and initial experience. Eur Urol. 2015;67(5):937–42.
32. Scott FB, Bradley WE, Timm GW. Treatment of urinary incontinence by implantable prosthetic sphincter. Urology. 1973;1(3):252–9.
33. Yates DR, Phé V, Rouprêt M, et al. Robot-assisted laparoscopic artificial urinary sphincter insertion in men with neurogenic stress urinary incontinence. BJU Int. 2013;111(7): 1175–9.
34. Hervé F, Lumen N, Goessaert AS, Everaert K. Persistent urinary incontinence after a robot-assisted artificial urinary sphincter procedure: lessons learnt from two cases. BMJ Case Rep. 2016;2016. pii: bcr2016216971
35. Encatassamy F, Hascoet J, Brierre T, et al. Robot-assisted bladder neck artificial urinary sphincter implantation in male patients with neurogenic stress urinary incontinence: a multicenter study. Eur Urol Suppl. 2019;18(1):e1055. https://doi.org/10.1016/S1569-9056(19)30762-6.

Rectourethral and Colovesical Fistula

Kirtishri Mishra, Min Suk Jan, and Lee C. Zhao

Abbreviations

RUF	Rectourethral fistula
XRT/AB	Radiation and ablative therapy
EBRT	External beam radiation therapy
HIFU	High-intensity focused ultrasound
RUG	Retrograde urethrogram

Introduction

Rectourethral fistula (RUF) is an uncommon but devastating complication with significant deterioration in quality of life [1, 2]. RUFs may result from surgical injury, including low anterior resection (LAR), abdominoperineal resection (APR), prostatectomy, transurethral resection of the prostate (TURP), and ablative therapies (AT).

Supplementary Information The online version of this chapter (https://doi.org/10.1007/978-3-030-50196-9_28) contains supplementary material, which is available to authorized users.

K. Mishra
Urology Institute, University Hospitals of Cleveland and Case Western Reserve University School of Medicine, Cleveland, OH, USA
e-mail: kirtishri.mishra@uhhospitals.org

M. S. Jan
Crane Center for Transgender Surgery, Greenbae California, New York, NY, USA

L. C. Zhao (✉)
NYU Langone Health, New York, NY, USA
e-mail: Lee.zhao@nyulangone.org

Other significant etiologies include external beam radiotherapy (EBRT), brachytherapy (BT), and congenital cause. In the United States, the most common causes of RUF are iatrogenic (radiation, ablative therapy, and prostatectomy) related to oncologic treatment for prostate cancer and occur from 0.1% to 3.0% of prostate cancer treatment [3]. A 2010 study by Thomas et al. cited an RUF rate of 0.53% after prostatectomy. A perineal approach exhibited a 3.06-fold higher risk of RUF versus a retropubic approach [4]. Robotic radical prostatectomy further decreases the incidence of RUF to 0.04% [5, 6]. With improvement in oncologic outcomes from prostate cancer (15-year relative survival rate > 90%), it is extremely important to preserve patient quality of life [7].

Colovesical fistulas most commonly arise from diverticulitis, colorectal or bladder malignancy, and inflammatory bowel disease [8]. Initial treatment is conservative as long as there is no sign of peritonitis, especially in the setting of IBD [9]. For those refractory to conservative management, colonic resection and cystorrhaphy are the treatment of choice. One might consider colonic diversion in cases of gross contamination, significant inflammation, cancer, or abscess. After colon resection, primary bladder closure is typically uncomplicated. Since RUF is the more difficult entity to treat, it will be the focus of this chapter.

Simple RUFs are defined as less than 1.5 cm and result from surgical etiology [8]. Alternatively, complex fistulas are those that are larger than 1.5 cm and are preceded by nonsurgical causes such as EBRT, BT, or AT, which include high-intensity focused ultrasound (HIFU), cryotherapy, and microwave [8]. The etiology of RUF is crucial in the management of the condition. Simple fistulas have a higher chance of successful repair or spontaneous resolution with appropriate urine and stool diversion, whereas, complex fistulas often occur in the setting of compromised tissue quality and tend toward less successful repair or spontaneous resolution [10–12]. In a study of 210 patients undergoing treatment for fistula, Harris et al. described a 99% successful treatment rate for postsurgical fistulas compared to an 86.5% for fistulas caused by EBRT or AT [10].

In 2018, Martini et al. proposed a novel staging system for RUF. They proposed classification of RUF by stage (size less than or greater than 1.5 cm), position (urethral sphincter involvement), and grade (etiology) of the fistula (Table 28.1) [13].

Table 28.1 Classification of rectourethral fistula (RUF) based on stage (size), grade (etiology), and position (involvement of urethral sphincter)

Stage	Size
I	Fistula diameter < 1.5 cm
II	Fistula diameter > 1.5 cm
III	Any diameter with urethral sphincter damage
Grade	Etiology
Grade 0	Intraoperative accidental rectal injury (with no prior nonsurgical treatment)
Grade 1	Primary nonsurgical treatment (radiation therapy, CrT, brachytherapy, high-intensity focused ultrasound) or adjuvant treatment that uses physical agents
Grade 2	Salvage prostatectomy or salvage prostatic ablation
Additional info	Recurrent fistula

Adopted from Martini et al. [17]

Likely owing to the relative rarity of RUF, this classification has not enjoyed widespread use, and a standard by which to categorize fistula is lacking. Similarly, timing of intervention, surgical methodology, and management of complications await standardization [14–18].

In general, if an injury is identified intraoperatively, immediate repair is indicated. If an injury goes unrecognized and the fistula presents in the early postoperative period, then fecal and urinary diversion may be performed. A small percentage of the fistulas (primarily simple) may self-resolve with this alone. However, if identified after the tract epithelializes (generally 6–8 weeks), then chances of spontaneous resolution is significantly lower. Fecal and urinary diversion are also indicated in patients who present with sepsis [4, 16, 19].

There are over 40 different techniques described for RUF repair [20]. These repairs range from endoscopic minimally invasive approaches, transabdominal, transanal, transperineal, abdominoperineal, anterior and posterior transsphincteric, and transsacral [11, 18, 20–23]. A 2013 meta-analysis evaluated the most common approaches used for RUF and found no significant benefit for any one approach over another. The rates of successful closure were similar despite the approach (~90%) [24]. Two traditional methods for the treatment of RUF include the transperineal and York-Mason technique. The transperineal technique is perhaps the most commonly utilized technique [25]. The patient is placed in a high-lithotomy position, and an inverted U-incision is made. The plane between the anal sphincter and the bulbospongiosus muscle is developed, while preserving the anal sphincter. The fistula is identified and excised, with a subsequent rectal repair in one or two layers. The fistula is then closed primarily or with a buccal mucosal graft. Interposition of well-vascularized tissue such as gracilis flap should be considered, especially in complex fistulas [8, 23]. Alternatively, the York-Mason repair is a trans-anosphincteric approach in which the rectum is entered from the posterior wall while the patient is in a prone jackknife position [26]. The anal sphincter is divided after reapproximating sutures are placed. The fistula is identified and excised on the anterior wall, and then an advancement flap is performed to close the defect in multiple layers. Once the repair is performed, the sphincter is approximated utilizing the stay sutures. In a study by Renschler et al., 92% of patients treated with this approach maintained stool continence at 30 years [26]. Interposition of healthy tissue is limited with the York-Mason as one is generally restricted to the use of local tissue. When dealing with radiation-induced RUF, local tissue may also be damaged from radiation. These techniques have been well described and will not be discussed in this chapter. The robotic approach, which allows the surgeon to access deep narrow spaces, appears to be particularly well suited to RUF repair.

Preoperative Evaluation

The workup for RUF begins with a detailed history [27]. Patients should be asked about symptoms of passage of urine per rectum, pneumaturia, fecaluria, watery stool, incontinence, perineal pain/pressure, UTI, and rectal bleeding [8, 28]. One objective evaluation of pneumaturia is to have the patient void with the penis sub-merged in a clear cup of water – pneumaturia will manifest as air bubbles. It is important to assess for external urinary sphincter function by noting the presence or absence of stress urinary incontinence and the ability to disrupt a urinary stream. Every effort should be taken to preserve either an intact internal or external urinary sphincter. In patients without an internal urinary sphincter, such as after radical prostatectomy, dissection through the pelvic floor and the external urinary sphincter via a perineal approach may cause de novo incontinence. Thus, the abdominal approach may be preferred for fistulas above the pelvic floor [29]. A focused history would elicit the etiology of RUF, especially a history of radiation and prior surgery. It is also important to rule out radiation cystitis as this represents a relative contra-indication to RUF repair.

A thorough physical exam is mandatory. A digital rectal exam (DRE) should be performed to evaluate the anterior rectal wall, the location of the RUF in relation to the anal sphincter, the mobility of the rectum, and the character of the surrounding tissue. Evaluation of the anal sphincter is imperative, as involvement of the anal sphincter may render the patient fecally incontinent even after a successful repair of the RUF; therefore, strong consideration should be made to perform a permanent bowel diversion in these patients. Anal manometry may also offer further insight into a patient's ability to maintain stool continence after repair [16, 21]. Often, an exam under anesthesia (EUA) is required to more accurately assess the patient. A more thorough DRE with or without proctoscopy or sigmoidoscopy may be performed.

Cystourethroscopy should also be performed at the time of EUA to examine the entire urethra and directly visualize the fistula and note its location relative to the external urinary sphincter [9]. Other than assessing the bladder for a fistulous tract (which may not have been visible on imaging), the provider must rule out other pathologies such as urethral stricture, bladder neck contracture, and cavitation [15]. Importantly, bladder capacity should be measured as this may limit reconstructive options [15, 16]. Due to leakage of urine from the bladder, urodynamics is nearly impossible in the setting of an RUF or colovesical fistula. We prefer to fill the bladder under gravity with the Foley balloon under tension to measure bladder capacity. For patients with a bladder capacity less than 200 ml, serious discussion regarding cystectomy with urinary diversion must be had, as even with repair of the fistula, the patient may have intolerable voiding dysfunction. Patients who are not accepting of the possibility of a staged procedure to restore continence with artificial urinary sphincter should also consider cystectomy with urinary diversion.

Retrograde urethrogram (RUG) and cystogram are important tools to identify the location of the fistula and its relation to the sphincter [15, 21, 30]. One can also fill the rectum with contrast through the fistula, allowing one to visualize the fistula location in relation to the anal sphincter (Fig. 28.1). While CT with rectal contrast or MRI may be utilized, we find that in our practice it is not necessary in most cases of RUF.

Fig. 28.1 Fistulogram of rectourethral fistula. (Note the location proximal to the anal sphincter, which is functional)

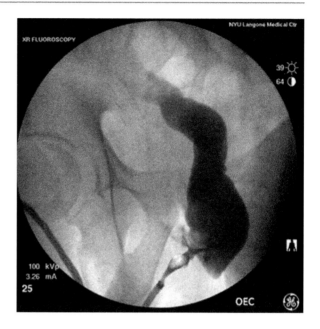

Fecal diversion before reconstruction is recommended in cases of recurrent UTI, perineal sepsis, abscess, or complex fistulas [1, 8]. This not only accomplishes the immediate goal of minimizing fistulous output but also allows the inflammation in the involved tissue to diminish, which may optimize chances for a successful repair. A repeat workup may be performed after 3–4 months of urine and stool diversion to assess for resolution. If progress is evident, then a longer period of observation may be warranted; however, if there is little to no improvement, then a reconstructive effort should be undertaken [27].

Overall, the decision to pursue a repair for RUF needs to be a shared decision between the patient and provider with careful management of expectations. The patient must understand that the overall treatment process from the onset may take 6 months or longer. Depending on the location of the RUF, the patient could have urinary incontinence. The reversal of fecal diversion can be performed once the patient has demonstrated that the fistula has resolved. Management of urination incontinence, such as with AUS implantation, is typically deferred until after reversal of fecal diversion [27]. The patient must be counseled on the possibility of failure of RUF repair and subsequent cystectomy with urinary diversion.

While urine culture can help treat specific organisms preoperatively, perioperative antibiosis should be broad, covering for gram-positive, gram-negative, and anerobic organisms. A type and screen is usually sufficient, as major bleeding is rare.

Operative Equipment

In the past, we preferred the da Vinci robotic system (Intuitive Surgical, Sunnyvale, CA) Xi since it can more easily be side docked to better facilitate perineal access. More recently, we have shifted to the SP (single port) system as its narrow profile better facilitates access deep into the pelvis with less interference from the pelvic wall. Furthermore, the articulating camera allows one to see around corners, which is more helpful the deeper one travels into the pelvis. Additionally, the SP robot allows for more vertical clearance at the perineum, facilitating simultaneous perineal surgery. AirSeal (ConMed, Utica, NY) is a key component to combined abdominoperineal cases as it allows for the maintenance of pneumoperitoneum even with a large air leak. Because the open perineum is the site of escaping pressurized air, the perineal surgeon is subject to aerosolized blood. We have found an orthopedic surgical hood useful for personal protection against blood-borne pathogens, while allowing for continued visualization. A cystoscope can be used to localize the fistula and external urinary sphincter. Placement of a wire or ureteral catheter at the beginning of the case can help with fistula identification.

Surgical Technique

Sequential compression devices are placed, and 5000 units of subcutaneous heparin is administered in patients with moderate to high risk for venous thromboembolism. Broad-spectrum antibiotics covering for skin, urinary, and gastrointestinal pathogens are administered 1 hour preoperatively. Patients are placed in dorsal lithotomy with arms tucked to the sides. All pressure points are well padded, and the patient is secured to the table for safe steep Trendelenburg position.

With the Xi system, pneumoperitoneum is established using a Veress needle or Hasson technique. If fecal diversion has not already been performed, the case begins with the colorectal surgeon performing laparoscopic diversion. Additional 8 mm robotic trocars are placed in the same configuration as a robotic prostatectomy. Instruments may be chosen at the discretion of the surgeon – our preferences using the Xi robot are monopolar scissors, bipolar Maryland forceps, and ProGrasp forceps. An 8 mm AirSeal (ConMed, Utica, NY) port is used for assistance. Alternatively, a 2.7 cm vertical supraumbilical Hasson access technique is required when using the SP system. The robot is docked from the side to allow for perineal access.

All cases begin with flexible cystoscopy. A guidewire or ureteral catheter is placed across the fistula. When feasible, the wire is grasped and externalized through the rectum for through-and-through access from the urethra to the anus. Methylene blue may be injected at the surgeon's discretion into the fistula to aid in identification. If the ureteral orifices are in close proximity to the fistula, it may behoove one to place ureteral stents at the beginning of the case. One may also place these at a later time using the robotic instruments when the bladder has been opened.

The robotic dissection begins with a posterior approach. The vas deferens is identified and used to guide dissection to Denonvilliers' fascia. Sharp dissection with judicious bipolar electrocautery is used to separate the rectum from the urinary tract. An EEA sizer can provide downward tenting of the rectum, aiding in the separation of the rectum from the bladder neck and prostate. If using the Xi system, the Firefly™ camera can aid in identifying the urethra since the white light of the cystoscope emits in the near-infrared spectrum, which penetrates a modest amount of tissue (Fig. 28.2).This essentially provides "X-ray vision" to the surgeon. As one nears the fistula, the assistant can perform a DRE to help guide the final approach. The fistula is then divided. One will see the wire, stent, or blue dye placed at the beginning of the case. The edges of the rectum are then freshened and closed primarily with barbed, absorbable suture. An air leak test is then performed to ensure a watertight closure. If the rectum does not appear to be salvageable, resection of the disease rectum followed by colo-anal anastomosis has been reported as a possible alternative [31]. Attention is then turned to the urinary reconstruction.

If the prostate is in situ and the fistula is small, one can attempt a primary closure. In situations where there is fistulization into a prostate with radionecrosis, primary closure may be impossible. A salvage prostatectomy is often necessary to remove the necrotic tissue to allow for watertight closure. The space of Retzius should be opened to be able to perform salvage prostatectomy. Bladder advancement flaps may provide

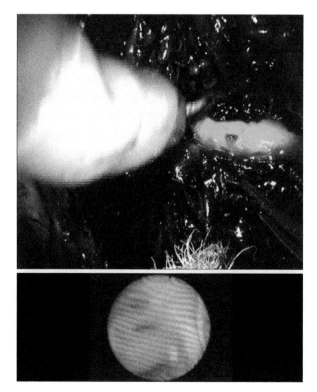

Fig. 28.2 The Firefly camera mode is able to visualize the near-infrared light of the flexible cystoscope, which more readily penetrates tissue. In this case, the scope is highlighting the location of the rectourethral fistula

distal advancement of the bladder neck to allow for anastomosis to the urethral stump. If a gap remains between the healthy bladder and urethra, a perineal approach may be performed for bulbar urethral mobilization. The mobilized bulbar urethra can then be advanced proximally. A holding suture is placed on the urethral stump and delivered to the awaiting robotic surgeon, and a "pull through" analogous to the technique described by Badenoch is performed [32, 33]. If possible, a circumferential anastomosis is performed. Otherwise, an augmented anastomotic urethroplasty may be performed with buccal mucosa graft. One must be cognizant that urethral dissection will increase the risk of urethral erosion after AUS placement [34].

Interposition with healthy, well-vascularized tissue is a necessary step in complex RUF repair. Several options exist. If the fistula is distal, a gracilis flap may be harvested and tunneled into the pelvis and fixed in place between the rectum and the urinary anastomosis. It has been shown to be effective with little morbidity [35]; however, it does add another surgical site and incision. Alternatively, since the surgeon already has abdominal access, an omental or rectus flap may be more practical. Omentum is in abundant supply and will reach into the pelvis with mobilization. In proximal and/or large fistulas, the rectus abdominis flap is a useful technique to provide an interposing layer between the bladder and rectum. Traditionally, the rectus abdominis flap required a large midline incision from xiphoid to pubis; however, robotic harvest has eliminated the need for this incision. Furthermore, the anterior rectus sheath is left intact, reducing the risk of incisional hernia. The robot is redocked contralateral to the rectus to be harvested (Fig. 28.3). If there is a colostomy,

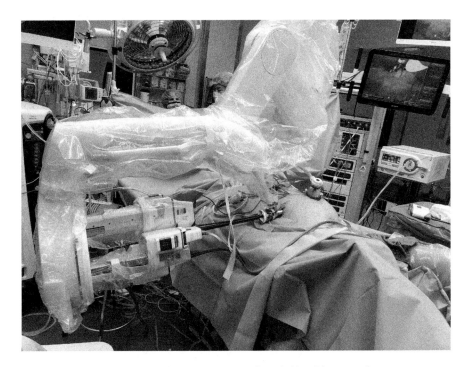

Fig. 28.3 The single port robot docked on the contralateral side of the rectus harvest

the robotic arms should be carefully positioned to avoid injury. The posterior rectus sheath is incised at the level of the inferior epigastric artery taking care not to injure the pedicle. The posterior sheath incision is then advanced to the costal margin. The rectus flap is then dissected circumferentially, and a Penrose drain is passed around it to aid in retraction. Circumferential dissection is then carried superiorly to the level of the costal margin (Fig. 28.4). Close attention is required at the tendinous inscriptions to avoid violation of the anterior sheath. Bipolar cautery is used to control perforating vessels. The rectus muscle is then amputated at the costal margin, and two holding stitches are placed with two long tails for each suture. The Carter-Thomason suture passer (CooperSurgical, Trumbull, CT) is then passed through the lateral perineum, entering the pelvis between the rectum and urethra where a single suture is grasped and externalized. The other tail is passed separately, and the two tails are tied over a Xeroform bolster to fix the rectus flap as far distally as possible. This is done on the left and right side of the perineum. The posterior rectus sheath is then anastomosed to the anterior sheath to reduce the risk of intra-abdominal adhesions.

Another promising technique is robotic transanal minimally invasive surgery (TAMIS) for use in cases of simple RUF where interposition of remote tissue is not necessary. An access channel (Applied Medical, Rancho Santa Margarita, CA) is placed across the anus. Sutures can be placed to fix the access channel to the patient. Trocars are preloaded onto the GelSeal cap, which is then attached to the access channel (Fig. 28.5). With the robot now docked, the fistula is circumscribed sharply, and a full-thickness rectal flap is developed. A plane is then developed between the prostate and rectum. The urethra is closed with absorbable suture. A biologic material such as AlloDerm can be placed over the closed urethra. The rectum is then closed over the mesh with absorbable suture [36].

Fig. 28.4 The rectus muscle has been circumferentially dissected and a Penrose drain placed for retraction

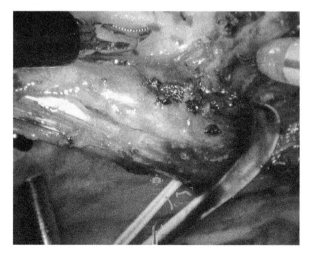

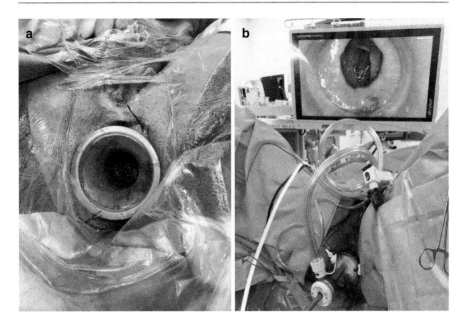

Fig. 28.5 TAMIS. **a**. The access channel has been placed. Note the sutures that help prevent channel dislodgement. **b**. The GelSeal has been attached and the laparoscope used to visualize the rectum

Conclusion

Rectourethral fistulas are difficult entities to treat due to their location deep in the pelvis and morbidity in gaining access. Robotic surgery has facilitated better visualization and exposure. Combined with classic reconstructive techniques of repair and interposition of healthy tissue, we are now seeing a new era of minimally invasive reconstruction for rectourethral fistulas.

References

1. Choi JH, Jeon BG, Choi S-G, Han EC, Ha H-K, Oh H-K, et al. Rectourethral fistula: systemic review of and experiences with various surgical treatment methods. Ann Coloproctol. 2014;30(1):35–41.
2. Chen S, Gao R, Li H, Wang K. Management of acquired rectourethral fistulas in adults. Asian J Urol. 2018;5(3):149–54.
3. Siegel RL, Miller KD, Jemal A. Cancer statistics, 2016. CA Cancer J Clin. 2016;66(1):7–30.
4. Thomas C, Jones J, Jäger W, Hampel C, Thüroff JW, Gillitzer R. Incidence, clinical symptoms and management of rectourethral fistulas after radical prostatectomy. J Urol. 2010;183(2):608–12.
5. Wedmid A, Mendoza P, Sharma S, Hastings RL, Monahan KP, Walicki M, et al. Rectal injury during robot-assisted radical prostatectomy: incidence and management. J Urol. 2011;186(5):1928–33.

6. Lance RS, Freidrichs PA, Kane C, Powell CR, Pulos E, Moul JW, et al. A comparison of radical retropubic with perineal prostatectomy for localized prostate cancer within the uniformed services urology research group. BJU Int. 2001;87(1):61–5.
7. Faris SF, Milam DF, Dmochowski RR, Kaufman MR. Urinary diversions after radiation for prostate cancer: indications and treatment. Urology. 2014;84(3):702–6.
8. Zinman L. The management of the complex recto-urethral fistula – Zinman – 2004 – BJU International – Wiley Online Library [Internet]. 2004. [cited 2020 Jan 18]. Available from: https://onlinelibrary-wiley-com.ezproxy.med.nyu.edu/doi/epdf/10.1111/j.1464-410X.2004.05225.x
9. Lichtenstein GR, Loftus EV, Isaacs KL, Regueiro MD, Gerson LB, Sands BE. ACG clinical guideline: management of crohn's disease in adults. Am J Gastroenterol. 2018;113(4):481–517.
10. Harris CR, McAninch JW, Mundy AR, Zinman LN, Jordan GH, Andrich D, et al. Rectourethral fistulas secondary to prostate cancer treatment: management and outcomes from a multi-institutional combined experience. J Urol. 2017;197(1):191–4.
11. Evans LA, Ferguson KH, Foley JP, Rozanski TA, Morey AF. Fibrin sealant for the management of genitourinary injuries, fistulas and surgical complications. J Urol. 2003;169(4):1360–2.
12. Nicita G, Villari D, Caroassai Grisanti S, Marzocco M, Li Marzi V, Martini A. Minimally invasive transanal repair of rectourethral fistulas. Eur Urol. 2017;71(1):133–8.
13. Martini A, Gandaglia G, Nicita G, Montorsi F. A novel classification proposal for rectourethral fistulas after primary treatment of prostate cancer. Eur Urol Oncol. 2018;1(6):510–1.
14. Golabek T, Szymanska A, Szopinski T, Bukowczan J, Furmanek M, Powroznik J, et al. Enterovesical fistulae: aetiology, imaging, and management. Gastroenterol Res Pract [Internet]. 2013 [cited 2020 Feb 29];2013. Available from: https://www.ncbi.nlm.nih.gov/pmc/articles/PMC3857900/
15. Munoz MMD, Nelson HMD, Harrington JMD, Tsiotos GMD, Devine RMD, Engen DMD. Management of acquired rectourinary fistulas: outcome according to cause. Dis Colon Rectum. 1998;41(10):1230–8.
16. Scozzari G, Arezzo A, Morino M. Enterovesical fistulas: diagnosis and management. Tech Coloproctol. 2010;14(4):293–300.
17. Mandel P, Linnemannstöns A, Chun F, Schlomm T, Pompe R, Budäus L, et al. Incidence, risk factors, management, and complications of rectal injuries during radical prostatectomy. Eur Urol Focus. 2018;4(4):554–7.
18. Keller DS, Aboseif SR, Lesser T, Abbass MA, Tsay AT, Abbas MA. Algorithm-based multidisciplinary treatment approach for rectourethral fistula. Int J Color Dis. 2015;30(5):631–8.
19. Venkatesan K, Zacharakis E, Andrich DE, Mundy AR. Conservative management of urorectal fistulae. Urology. 2013;81(6):1352–6.
20. Bukowski TP, Chakrabarty A, Powell IJ, Frontera R, Perlmutter AD, Montie JE. Acquired rectourethral fistula: methods of repair. J Urol. 1995;153(3):730–3.
21. Shin PR, Foley E, Steers WD. Surgical management of rectourinary fistulae11No competing interests declared. J Am Coll Surg. 2000;191(5):547–53.
22. Davis JW, Schellhammer PF. Prostatorectal fistula 14 years following brachytherapy for prostate cancer. J Urol. 2001;165(1):189.
23. Samplaski MK, Wood HM, Lane BR, Remzi FH, Lucas A, Angermeier KW. Functional and quality-of-life outcomes in patients undergoing transperineal repair with gracilis muscle interposition for complex rectourethral fistula. Urology. 2011;77(3):736–41.
24. Hechenbleikner EM, Buckley JC, Wick EC. Acquired rectourethral fistulas in adults: a systematic review of surgical repair techniques and outcomes. Dis Colon Rectum. 2013;56(3):374–83.
25. Voelzke BB, McAninch JW, Breyer BN, Glass AS, Garcia-Aguilar J. Transperineal management for postoperative and radiation rectourethral fistulas. J Urol. 2013;189(3):966–71.
26. Renschler TD, Middleton RG. 30 years of experience with york-mason repair of recto-urinary fistulas. J Urol. 2003;170(4, Part 1):1222–5.
27. Lane BR, Stein DE, Remzi FH, Strong SA, Fazio VW, Angermeier KW. Management of radiotherapy induced rectourethral fistula. J Urol. 2006;175(4):1382–8.

28. Kaufman DA, Zinman LN, Buckley JC, Marcello P, Browne BM, Vanni AJ. Short- and long-term complications and outcomes of radiation and surgically induced rectourethral fistula repair with buccal mucosa graft and muscle interposition flap. Urology. 2016;98:170–5.

29. Nikolavsky D, Blakely SA, Hadley DA, Knoll P, Windsperger AP, Terlecki RP, et al. Open reconstruction of recurrent vesicourethral anastomotic stricture after radical prostatectomy. Int Urol Nephrol. 2014;46(11):2147–52.

30. Martins FE, Martins NM, Pinheiro LC, Ferraz L, Xambre L, Lopes TM. Management of iatrogenic urorectal fistulae in men with pelvic cancer. Can Urol Assoc J. 2017;11(9):E372–8.

31. Netsch C, Bach T, Gross E, Gross AJ. Rectourethral fistula after high-intensity focused ultrasound therapy for prostate cancer and its surgical management. Urology. 2011;77(4):999–1004.

32. Badenoch AW. A pull-through operation for impassable traumatic stricture of the urethra. Br J Urol. 1950;22(4):404–9.

33. Simonato A, Gregori A, Lissiani A, Varca V, Carmignani G. Use of Solovov–Badenoch principle in treating severe and recurrent vesico-urethral anastomosis stricture after radical retropubic prostatectomy: technique and long-term results. BJU Int. 2012;110(11b):E456–60.

34. McKibben MJ, Shakir N, Fuchs JS, Scott JM, Morey AF. Erosion rates of 3.5-cm artificial urinary sphincter cuffs are similar to larger cuffs. BJU Int. 2019;123(2):335–41.

35. Zmora O, Potenti FM, Wexner SD, Pikarsky AJ, Efron JE, Nogueras JJ, et al. Gracilis muscle transposition for iatrogenic rectourethral fistula. Ann Surg. 2003;237(4):483–7.

36. Robotic TAMIS for local repair of acquired rectovaginal and rectourethral fistulae [Internet]. [cited 2020 Feb 29]. Available from: https://www.youtube.com/watch?v=eIsrFVE8TBI

Part X

Robotic Fistula Introduction

Lee Zhao

In this section of the book, repair of the urinary fistula is discussed. Adjunctive technology is a theme throughout this book, but is particularly useful for fistula repair. Cystoscopy during the time of robotic dissection can help identify the location of a colovesical fistula, placement of indocyanine green (ICG) into the urine (off-label use) can help delineate bowel used for urinary reconstruction from innocent bystanders, and intravascular injection of ICG allows for identification of viable tissue. Thus, as the authors in the following chapters describe, robotic technology is ideal for identification of the fistula, delineating viable tissue, and facile suturing for closure.

Uretero-vaginal Fistula

Marcio Covas Moschovas, Paolo Dell'Oglio,
Alessandro Larcher, and Alexandre Mottrie

Introduction

The uretero-vaginal fistula is a connection between the ureter and the vagina that usually results in complete incontinence. These types of fistulas are uncommon surgical complications after ureteral injury during pelvic procedures. Ureteral lesions range between 0.5% and 2.5% during obstetric or gynaecological surgeries, and the most common damages reported in fistula cases are ureteral lacerations, ischemic devitalization, accidental ligation, avulsion and crushing [1]. Other risk factors are represented by obesity, endometriosis, pelvic inflammatory disease, radiation therapy and pelvic malignant disease. The most conventional ureteral site affected in uretero-vaginal fistulas is the lower third portion of the ureter [1].

There is an aetiology difference between the developed and the undeveloped countries. Obstetric procedures, as hysterectomies and caesarean sections, are the most common causes of uretero-vaginal fistulas in underdeveloped countries with 25 and 38% of the cases, respectively, while gynaecological surgery represents the first cause in developed countries [2, 3].

Supplementary Information The online version of this chapter (https://doi.org/10.1007/978-3-030-50196-9_29) contains supplementary material, which is available to authorized users.

M. C. Moschovas · A. Mottrie (✉)
ORSI Academy, Melle, Belgium

Department of Urology, OnzeLieve Vrouw Hospital, Aalst, Belgium

P. Dell'Oglio · A. Larcher
ORSI Academy, Melle, Belgium

Department of Urology, OnzeLieve Vrouw Hospital, Aalst, Belgium

Unit of Urology, Division of Oncology, Urological Research Institute, IRCCS Ospedale San Raffaele, Milan, Italy

© Springer Nature Switzerland AG 2022
M. D. Stifelman et al. (eds.), *Techniques of Robotic Urinary Tract Reconstruction*, https://doi.org/10.1007/978-3-030-50196-9_29

Preoperative Evaluation

In patients with a suspicion for genitourinary fistula, it is essential to rule out some differential diagnosis as urinary incontinence, ectopic ureters, aqueous vaginal discharge and vesico-vaginal fistulas [4].

Complete physical examination with manual and specular vaginal evaluation is mandatory. The vaginal liquids can be collected using urine test strip for urea [5], and a microscopic examination can be performed with culture to address the proper antibiotic to use in case of urinary tract infection.

During the diagnostic process of urogenital fistula, it is imperative to describe the location, size and number of fistulas [6]. Therefore, cystoscopy is strongly recommended. This diagnostic test allows the physicians also to exclude other fistulas [7]. Indeed, 12% of uretero-vaginal fistulas are associated with vesico-vaginal fistulas [8]. Moreover, the internal bladder wall visualization allows the surgeon to preoperatively plan the ureter reimplantation choosing the best bladder section.

Some authors described [4] the use of intra-vesical methylene blue injection (dye test) to diagnose and locate the urogenital fistula site. Blue vaginal discharge on vaginal tampons suggests vesico-vaginal fistula, while colourless discharge raises the suspicion for uretero-vaginal fistula [4]. However, the colourless discharge does not rule out the vesico-vaginal fistula. In 1990 O'Brien [9] described a double dye test. On this technique the patient receives oral pyridium, and as soon as the urine turns orange, a vaginal tampon is placed. If the proximal tampon tip is coloured by orange, the result is suggestive of ureteral fistula, whereas the blue colour at the mid or lower part of the tampon suggests vesicle fistula.

Cystogram, CT scan, IV pyelogram, retrograde pyelogram and cystourethrogram (micturition) are all radiological exams that can be performed to assess the fistula location, extension and its relation with surrounding organs. However, the risks and benefits should be individualized to each patient due to radiation exposure in all these methods. One alternative to avoid the radiation exposure during the fistula investigation is represented by the colour Doppler ultrasound where the contrast agent is injected into the bladder and trans-rectal or transvaginal ultrasound is performed [10].

Preoperative Patient Management

The time from diagnosis to surgery usually depends on the time needed to repair the fistula. Once the patient is diagnosed with uretero-vaginal fistula, the treatment of choice to repair the fistula is represented by the ureteric stent (double-J stent) positioning to decrease the vaginal urinary leakage and avoid the ureteric stricture and obstruction. In the presence of a complete ureteric obstruction, a nephrostomy should be placed until the fistula repair [11].

To date, no data is available regarding the perfect timing for uretero-vaginal fistula repair. Data assessing genitourinary fistula in general are controversial. Cruikshank et al. [12] and Shelbaia et al. [13] reported a late fistula repair after

35 days of surgery with a success rate of 91 and 100%, respectively. Waaldijk et al. reported two series of fistula repair success related to the timing of surgery. In the first study, the success rate was 91.8% for 170 patients who underwent fistula repair after 3 months [14]. In the second study, 1716 patients underwent fistula repair before 3 months with a success rate of 95.2% after the first attempt and 98.5% after the second one.

In most of the cases, the choice between early and late repair is driven by the fistula aetiology. For example, in patients with previous radiotherapy exposure, general consensus was reached that the late repair is the most appropriate approach. Although in clinical setting the majority of the fistulas is treated in a later time, a trend towards earlier repair approach (1 or 2 weeks) has been observed [14–16].

Patients with uretero-vaginal fistulas can suffer from cystitis, dermatitis and vaginitis due to the continuous urinary leakage. These conditions should be treated appropriately in the preoperative care to avoid complications during or after the procedure and to increase the patient quality of life. It is essential to dry the perineal skin as much as possible to avoid dermatitis and fungal infections. Perineal pads are the most common solution adopted in patients with urinary leakage. However, sometimes the lost urine volume can be large, and the perineal pads might not be enough. In this case, patient must be encouraged to use continence products such as vaginal prosthesis [17]. Perineal dermatitis can be managed with a periodic pad change to avoid the daily skin aggression. Some topic agents can also be used to protect and heal the local oedema and inflammation.

Another step in the preoperative care described in the literature is the oestrogen use. Some Authors [4] reported the use of topical oestrogen for postmenopausal patients or those with vaginal dryness. The rationale stems in the fact that hormone helps tissue vascularization before the surgical repair.

Step-by-Step Reproducible Method

The combination of preoperative imaging studies and the intraoperative anatomy while dissecting the tissues is mandatory for uretero-vaginal fistula surgical planning. The current available imaging studies enable the fistula location, size and relation with other organs. However, those exams do not predict the attachment and tissue vascularization found intraoperative.

Different approaches and techniques to repair uretero-vaginal fistula are described in the literature. The fistula can be repaired through an intra-abdominal or a combination of intra-abdominal and vaginal approach [18]. The benefits of the minimally invasive procedure are well established in the literature in terms of lower incision size, less blood loss and abdominal pain, lower postoperative complications such as chest infections and deep vein thrombosis [19].

The most common procedure in the uretero-vaginal fistula repair is the distal ureter dissection, resection and reimplantation in a healthy part of the bladder. The first step is the ureter finding and dissection distally until its vaginal attachment. Once the fistula is found, a ureteral resection is performed proximally and distally to the fistula in the ureter portion without fibrosis or oedema. The remaining distal ureter can be resected until its insertion on the bladder or ligated after the fibrotic part extraction. The vaginal fibrous tissue is resected until the visualization of well-vascularized borders for the primary suture and vaginal closing. With the ureter released, it is crucial to have a good bladder exposure and mobilization to plan the type of ureteral reimplantation to be performed. It is mandatory that the uretero-vesical anastomosis has a tension-free suture (Figs. 29.1, 29.2 and 29.3).

Fig. 29.1 Direct implantation in the bladder dome if there is no tension

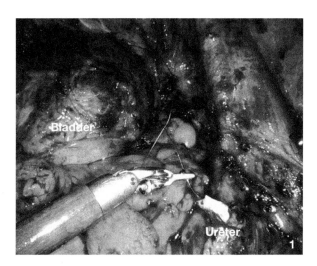

Fig. 29.2 Psoas hitch technique

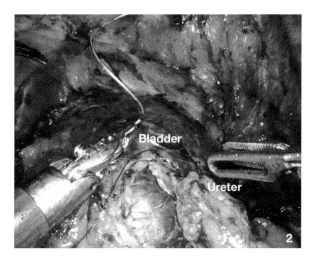

Fig. 29.3 Boari flap in
cases that the ureter length
is not enough to reach
the bladder

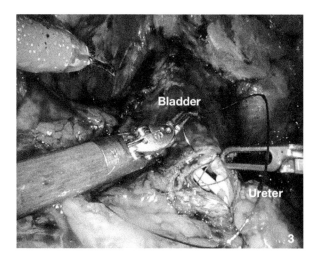

There are three common reimplantation options: (1) direct implantation in the
bladder dome if there is no tension, (2) psoas hitch technique and (3) Boari flap
in cases that the ureter length is not enough to reach the bladder. The anastomosis
is performed with absorbable running suture after the double-J stent placement.
Alberts et al. [20], in a systematic review regarding the ureteral reimplantation techniques and its relation with complications, found no difference in ureteral strictures
between the three most common used techniques (Lich-Gregoir, Politano-Leadbetter
and U-stitch). However, the lowest urological complication rate described was associated with Lich-Gregoir technique.

Symmonds et al. [21] published some critical steps to have a better outcome in
the genitourinary fistula repair. The authors described the importance of the fistular
scar tissue excision to revitalize the borders for a primary suture. Another aspect
that the authors described was the bladder mobilization before the ureter reimplantation to grant a tension-free uretero-vesical anastomosis.

Currently, different from the recto-vaginal and recto-vesical fistula repair, there
is no data available to support the use of biological agents, and interposition of
adjunct tissues in the uretero-vaginal fistula repair [22].

The robotic-assisted approach performed with the da Vinci robotic platform
starts with the patient in dorsal lithotomy or dorsal decubitus position with Foley
catheter. The usual procedure has five trocars (4 for the robot and 1 for the assistant)
although an extra auxiliary 5 mm trocar can be placed for the table assistant in more
complex cases. The camera port is placed above the umbilicus, 20 cm from the
pubic bone. Two other trocars are placed 9 cm bilaterally from the camera. The last
robot trocar is placed 9 cm from one of the previous two trocars mentioned in the
step before (on the left or right side; Fig. 29.4). The last trocar (assistant) is placed
4 cm above the (right or left) upper iliac crest.

Fig. 29.4 The last trocar (assistant) is placed 4 cm above the (right or left) upper iliac crest

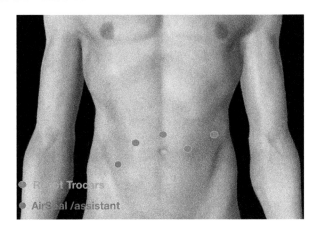

One Month Postoperative Care

The adequate postoperative care is crucial for a satisfactory ureteric reimplantation healing. The bladder Foley catheter is essential to avoid detrusor distension and traction in the anastomosis, and it usually remains from 3 to 5 days after the surgery. The double-J stent placed in the ureter drains the urine appropriately until the complete uretero-vesical attachment. Usually, it is removed from 7 to 15 days after the procedure, and a cystogram exam is performed to review the anastomosis [4].

Some authors [4] supported the use of suprapubic catheter drainage to lower the intra-vesical pressure and protect the anastomosis. However, there is lack of evidence to extensively use this approach in all patients who undergo uretero-vaginal fistula repair.

Postoperative Complications and Management

The most common postoperative complications reported are urgency, urge incontinence, recurrence and ureteral and bowel obstruction. However, only few studies evaluated intraoperative and postoperative morbidity in this specific setting, and all these reports are limited by the small sample size and did not report complications in agreement with standardized criteria, such as Martin criteria [23]. Therefore, this may lead to an underestimation of the complication rates reported.

Regarding the postoperative management, each case must be individualized, and a ureteral, bladder and kidney evaluation is mandatory to guide the appropriate treatment [4].

References

1. Murtaza B, Mahmood A, Niaz WA, et al. Ureterovaginal fistula – etiological factors and outcome. J Pak Med Assoc. 2012;62:999–1003.
2. Ozumba BC, Attah CA. Ureteral injury in obstetric and gynecologic operations in Nigeria. Int J Gynaecol Obstet. 1991;36:131–5.
3. Randawa A, Khalid L, Abbas A. Diagnosis and management of ureterovaginal fistula in a resource-constrained setting: experience at a district hospital in northern Nigeria. Libyan J Med. 2009;4:41–3.
4. Ghoniem GM, Warda HA. The management of genitourinary fistula in the third millennium. Arab J Urol. 2014;12:97–105.
5. Urogynecology and Reconstructive Pelvic Surgery 4th Edition.Published Date: 25th November 2014. eBook ISBN: 9780323262576.
6. Mallikarjuna C, Nayak P, Reddy KP, et al. The AINU technique for laparoscopic vesicovaginal fistula repair: a preliminary report. Urol Int. 2015;95:357–60.
7. Hampel C, Neisius A, Thomas C, et al. Vesicovaginal fistula. Incidence, etiology and phenomenology in Germany. Der Urologe Ausg A. 2015;54:349–58.
8. Goodwin WE, Scardino PT. Vesicovaginal and ureterovaginal fistulas: a summary of 25 years of experience. J Urol. 1980;123:370–4.
9. O'Brien WM, Lynch JH. Simplification of double-dye test to diagnose various types of vaginal fistulas. Urology. 1990;36:456.
10. Volkmer BG, Kuefer R, Nesslauer T, et al. Colour Doppler ultrasound in vesicovaginal fistulas. Ultrasound Med Biol. 2000;26:771–5.
11. Mandal AK, Sharma SK, Vaidyanathan S, Goswami AK. Ureterovaginal fistula: summary of 18 years' experience. Br J Urol. 1990;65:453–6.
12. Cruikshank SH. Early closure of posthysterectomy vesicovaginal fistulas. South Med J. 1988;81:1525–8.
13. Shelbaia AM, Hashish NM. Limited experience in early management of genitourinary tract fistulas. Urology. 2007;69:572–4.
14. Waaldijk K. The immediate surgical management of fresh obstetric fistulas with catheter and/or early closure. Int J Gynaecol Obstet. 1994;45:11–6.
15. Witters S, Cornelissen M, Vereecken R. Iatrogenic ureteral injury: aggressive or conservative treatment. Am J Obstet Gynecol. 1986;155:582–4.
16. Collins CG, Pent D, Jones FB. Results of early repair of vesicovaginal fistula with preliminary cortisone treatment. Am J Obstet Gynecol. 1960;80:1005–12.
17. Green DE, Phillips GL Jr. Vaginal prosthesis for control of vesicovaginal fistula. Gynecol Oncol. 1986;23:119–23.
18. Nezhat CH, Nezhat F, Nezhat C, Rottenberg H. Laparoscopic repair of a vesicovaginal fistula: a case report. Obstet Gynecol. 1994;83:899–901.
19. Agha R, Muir G. Does laparoscopic surgery spell the end of the open surgeon? J R Soc Med. 2003;96:544–6.
20. Alberts VP, Idu MM, Legemate DA, et al. Ureterovesical anastomotic techniques for kidney transplantation: a systematic review and meta-analysis. Transpl Int. 2014;27:593–605.
21. Symmonds RE. Incontinence: vesical and urethral fistulas. Clin Obstet Gynecol. 1984;27:499–514.
22. Rivadeneira DE, Ruffo B, Amrani S, Salinas C. Rectovaginal fistulas: current surgical management. Clin Colon Rectal Surg. 2007;20:96–101.
23. Martin RC 2nd, Brennan MF, Jaques DP. Quality of complication reporting in the surgical literature. Ann Surg. 2002;235:803–13.

Robotic Management of Vesicovaginal Fistulas

30

Luis G. Medina, Jullet Han, and Rene Sotelo

Introduction

Vesicovaginal fistula (VVF) is a distressing condition that affects 0.3–2% of women worldwide, with developing countries representing a disproportionate 95% of the cases [1, 2]. An estimated 30,000–130,000 new cases occur each year; however, the causes of VVFs vary geographically [3]. Prolonged obstructed labor in the setting of young age, poor nutrition, and inadequate access to healthcare dominate the landscape in developing countries. VVFs in industrialized countries, in contrast, are commonly the sequelae of pelvic surgery, radiation, malignant disease, trauma, or foreign bodies [4]. Patients commonly present with continuous leakage of urine from the vagina, resulting in significant impairment in quality of life, physical disability, and psychosocial isolation.

The basic tenets of a VVF repair include adequate mobilization of tissues, tension-free but watertight approximation of the tissues, multilayered closure with nonoverlapping suture lines, and maximal bladder drainage. The two conventional approaches include transvaginal for low-lying fistulas and transabdominal for more complex fistulas, supratrigonal fistulas, concomitant ureteral involvement, or poor vaginal access.

Supplementary Information The online version of this chapter (https://doi. org/10.1007/978-3-030-50196-9_30) contains supplementary material, which is available to authorized users.

L. G. Medina · J. Han · R. Sotelo (✉)
USC Institute of Urology, Norris Comprehensive Cancer Center, Keck School of Medicine, University of Southern California, Los Angeles, CA, USA
e-mail: Luis.Medina@med.usc.edu; jullet.han@med.usc.edu; rene.sotelo@med.usc.edu

Transabdominal techniques in VVF repairs have evolved since it was first described in 1852 [5] and now include minimally invasive approaches due to the already known advantages of these regarding its morbidity. The first laparoscopic repair was described in 1994 [6], but it was not widely accepted due to a difficult pelvic access, long instruments with limited degrees of freedom, fulcrum effect, and a bidimensional visual field [7]. A decade later in 2005, the first robotic-assisted laparoscopic repair was reported, which quickly superseded traditional and laparoscopic approaches. Owing to its superior three-dimensional anatomic visibility, more precise dissections, and enhanced dexterity in tissue manipulation, robotics provided a platform for managing complex VVFs [8]. Herein, we describe the evaluation and management of VVFs using a robotic-assisted laparoscopic repair.

Evaluation and Diagnosis

Once a VVF is suspected, a thorough pelvic exam with diagnostic cystoscopy to assess the size and location of the fistula should be performed. Adjunctive testing such as methylene blue instillation into the bladder with simultaneous examination of the vaginal vault can help delineate the location of the fistula if it is not apparent on initial exam. A computed tomography (CT) cystogram may aid with localization of the fistula and its relation to its surrounding structures, especially if the patient has a prior history of pelvic surgery [9]. A CT urogram can determine if there is a concomitant ureteral injury, which is reported in up to 12% of cases [3]. A biopsy is warranted if pelvic malignancy is evident.

Preoperative Preparation

Surgical intervention should be considered if a fistula is complex or fails to heal with conservative management. The timing of surgical repair has been debated among many experts, with recommendations ranging from 4 weeks to 12 weeks from the time of initial presentation with conservative management to allow the inflammation to settle. In cases were the fistula presented immediately after a surgical procedure, some have recommended prompt surgical repair, as delaying it could result in fibrosis and loss of tissue planes [10].

The general consensus is that repairs should take place in an aseptic environment with minimal tissue edema and inflammation. Therefore, infections should be adequately treated with appropriate antibiotics. Drainage catheters should be removed weeks prior to the surgery to minimize inflammatory edema of the bladder mucosa. Patients should use continent pads and impermeable barrier creams, such as zinc oxide, to minimize irritative effects of incontinence on surrounding perineal and vulva skin. Nutritional status can be assessed with prealbumin levels and optimized accordingly. Comorbidities such as diabetes mellitus and hypertension should be well controlled prior to surgical repairs.

Robotic Surgical Approaches

The surgical principles for the minimally invasive management of VVFs are standardized among the literature; however, different approaches have been reported based on the plane used to identify the fistulous tract for its repair.

The transvesical approach is an adaptation of the mini O'Connor procedure, where it involves an intentional vertical cystotomy toward the fistula. This allows for direct visualization of the fistula tract and ureteral orifices. However, the cystotomy may result in detrusor dysfunction, decreased bladder capacity, and recurrent urinary tract infections. Furthermore, this approach has increased bleeding risks and longer operative times [9, 11].

The retrovesical approach involves accessing the fistulous tract in an extravesical manner. This was proposed as safer approach yet as it causes less trauma to the bladder; however, the dissection planes can be more difficult to delineate and can lead to inadvertent injuries of the cervical canal or ureters. This is especially true in cases when the uterus is present, which happens in cases in which the VVF is a consequence of iatrogenia during a c-section. Cases associated with malignancies or radiation are also considered to have an increased risk for iatrogenia if a retrovesical approach is undertaken [8, 9].

The transvaginal approach involves opening the vagina toward the fistula defect. It is deemed useful in patients in which the vesicovaginal space is difficult to dissect. This approach seeks to overcome the difficulties of transvesical and retrovesical approaches. However, few cases have been reported [7].

Despite all this controversy, the transvesical approach is still widely used because it allows an easy identification of the fistulous tract with adequate visualization of the ureteric orifices in most of cases. Additionally, no differences in terms of functional outcomes have been shown in any study between the different approaches. Prospective and randomized studies are needed on this regard. As of now, the decision of the surgical approach to be used relies on surgeon's preference. In this chapter, we describe the steps of transvesical approach [7].

Step-by-Step Description of the Technique

The patient is placed in lithotomy position with all pressure points padded to avoid neuropathic complications. The vaginal vault and abdomen are prepped in a standard aseptic fashion.

A cystoscopy is performed at the beginning of the case to identify the ureteral orifices (UOs) and fistula tract. The UOs are cannulated with open-ended catheters or double-J stents to facilitate ureteral identification and reduce the risk of inadvertent injuries. This step can also be performed after the initial cystotomy. An open-ended stent is inserted into the fistulous tract and pulled through the vaginal canal in an antegrade fashion. If the fistulous tract is not easily identified, the bladder can be filled with methylene blue, and a vaginoscopy can be performed to identify and cannulate the tract in a retrograde fashion.

After the ureters and fistula are identified, intra-abdominal access is established using the Hasson technique given the high suspicion for intra-abdominal adhesions in this patient population [12]. Pneumoperitoneum is set to 15 mmHg, and a 12 mm camera port is placed 3–5 cm above the umbilicus. A 0-degree lens is used to assess for adhesions or bowel injuries that may have occurred during the initial access. The remaining ports are placed under direct vision, which include two 8-mm ports positioned 1 cm below the level of the umbilicus at the left and right midclavicular lines. Another 5- or 10-mm assistant port is placed at the right or left side of the 8-mm port, which is used for suction-irrigation and the AirSeal insufflator system (SurgiQuest Inc., Milford, CT, USA) (Fig. 30.1).

To perform the laparoscopic omental flap harvesting, the patient is repositioned to supine position during this step. The flap is harvested using the same principles of the open omentoplasty technique [13] and mobilized to the area of the VVF without tension. In cases when the omentum is not long enough, additional length can

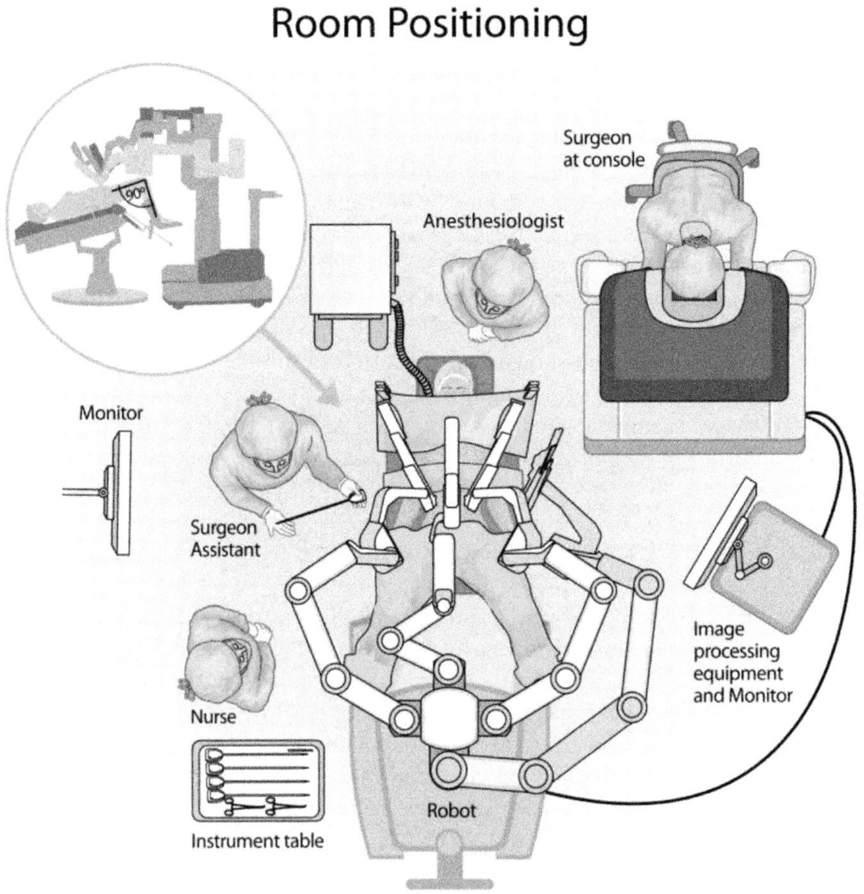

Room Positioning

Fig. 30.1 Operative room setup and patient positioning for the performance of a vesicovaginal fistula

be gained by separating it from the greater curvature of the stomach at the level of the right gastroepiploic arcade and the stomach. The omental flap can be also prepared and harvested in a robotic fashion if the da Vinci Xi Surgical System (Intuitive Surgical, Sunnyvale, CA, USA) is being used using the same principles previously described.

After that, the patient is then placed in extreme Trendelenburg, and the da Vinci Surgical System (Intuitive Surgical, Sunnyvale, CA, USA) is docked. The Si system is docked between the patient's legs, while the Xi system can be docked from the patient side. Adhesiolysis is performed using a combination of sharp and blunt dissection with Maryland fenestrated bipolar forceps and/or monopolar curved scissors. The uterus (if present), the superior aspect of the bladder, and the pouch of Douglas are subsequently identified and exposed.

A cystotomy is made starting 3–4 cm above the retrovesical space and extended posteriorly; the catheters identifying the ureters and the fistulous tract should come into view at this moment. The cystotomy is carefully extended distal to the fistulous tract with monopolar scissors, and the vesicovaginal plane around the fistula is carefully dissected. The borders of the fistula are excised to viable tissue to enhance the success rate of the repair. If AirSeal (SurgiQuest Inc., Milford, CT, USA) is not used, pneumoperitoneum can be maintained by clamping a Foley catheter filled with 70 cc of saline solution inside the vagina or by packing the vagina with a moist lap pad (Figs. 30.2 and 30.3).

The catheter cannulating the fistula is subsequently removed, and the plane between the bladder and the vagina is widely dissected with sharp dissection until there is adequate mobilization of the bladder to perform a tension-free closure. The vaginal defect is reapproximated with a transverse closure using a 3-0 V-Loc suture. It is important that the both suture lines are aligned perpendicular to each other, which reduces risk of refistulization. If it is not possible, it is highly recommended that an omental flap is interposed between the two suture lines. This scenario is

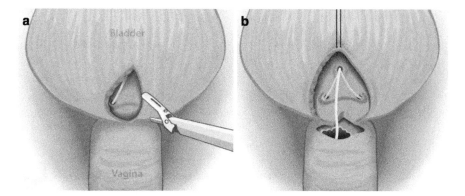

Fig. 30.2 Steps to perform a vesicovaginal fistula repair. **a**: The bladder is opened intentionally in the above fistulous defect. **b**: The cystotomy is extended toward the defect, and the catheters identifying the ureteric orifices and the fistulous tract are seen

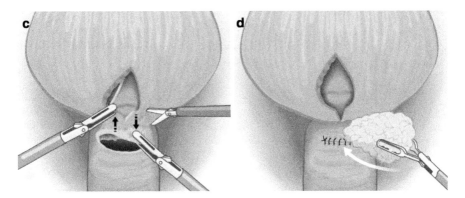

Fig. 30.3 Steps to perform a vesicovaginal fistula repair. **c**: The plane between the vagina and the bladder is carefully dissected. **d**: Previously harvested omentum flap is interposed and fixed in place

Fig. 30.4 Steps to perform a vesicovaginal fistula repair. **e**: A longitudinal cystorrhaphy is performed using barbed suture in a running continuous fashion

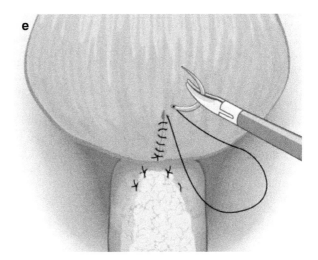

common in robotic VVF repairs with uterine preservation, in which the uterus can impose tension over the reconstruction.

Once the vaginal fistula is closed, the omental flap is interposed and anchored to the anterior vaginal wall at midline with a 3-0 V-Loc suture. Next, the bladder edges are reapproximated with a tension-free closure. In patients with a prior history of radiation, the bladder may be noncompliant and result in too much tension on the closure. In these cases, the paravesical space can be dissected laterally to increase mobility of the bladder edges. A cystorrhaphy is performed with a longitudinal closure using a barbed suture in a running continuous fashion, beginning at the distal end of the cystotomy and extending proximally, while making sure that the UOs are visualized at all times (Figs. 30.3 and 30.4).

If it is not possible to perform the cystorrhaphy with a single suture, a second suture is started at the proximal end of the cystotomy. Placing the suture on traction can improve exposure, which is crucial to avoid injury to the ureteric orifices. The integrity of the closure is assessed by filling the bladder with saline solution to ensure a watertight closure.

A Jackson-Pratt drain is introduced into rectouterine space and secured to the skin. Hemostasis is confirmed after the pneumoperitoneum is reduced below 10 mmHg, and all trocars are removed under direct visual guidance. Fascia and port sites are closed in a standard fashion. Finally, ureteral catheters are removed without resistance; the surgeon should make sure that the catheter is not included into the suture line if resistance is encountered.

Postoperative Management

The Jackson-Pratt drain is removed after 2–3 days if the output is <50 ml in a 24-hour period. The urethral catheter should be maintained for 10 days or longer and irrigated as needed to maintain patency. The catheter can be maintained for longer if the tissue quality was deemed poor during reconstruction. A retrograde cystogram can be done to confirm that there is no contrast extravasation prior to catheter removal. Appropriate prophylactic antibiotics are generally given for 10 days or until all tubes are removed. Urine cultures are ordered at the moment of the catheter removal and 2 weeks after that [14]. Vaginal intercourse, tampon usage, and douching are prohibited for up to 2 months postoperatively. If double-J stents were left in place, they are removed under cystoscopic guidance after 21 days.

Adjunct Tissue or Biologics to Improve Outcomes

VVFs present a significant anatomic challenge for its repair. Additional factors such as radiation, large fistula size, recurrent fistulas, or involvement of the urethra or ureter can increase the complexity of the surgical management and compromise the success of the repair in the first attempt. Approaches including interposition tissue have been utilized to improve surgical outcomes of VVF repairs. These flaps, such as the omental flap, function not only as an anatomical barrier, but it also introduces vascular and lymphatic flow into the surgical bed that could potentially augment tissue growth and promote healing [9]. Biologic tissues such as amniotic membranes or fibrin glue have also gained popularity in VVF repairs [15]. Amniotic membranes can also be used as interposition flap, but it is thought to enhance VVF repairs via an immunomodulatory effect on angiogenesis and inflammation [16, 17]. Transvaginal injection of fibrin into the fistulous tract has also been reported. It works by forming an elastic coagulum that acts as a barrier [18]. Cyanoacrylate injection is another interposition material that has been reported for management of recurrent VVF, which is a substance that polymerizes after contact with tissue or water and promotes epithelialization over it [19]. Currently, there is a lack of randomized clinical trials or large data series on the utility of biological tissues in VVF repairs, and future studies are needed to elucidate its effectiveness. As of now, we only recommend its use as an adjunct to other surgical management strategies.

Postoperative Outcomes and Complications

The overall success rate for all non-radiated VVF repairs is 92%, yet lower for cases associated to radiation. However, there is considerable variability reported in the literature between the two approaches, with the transvaginal approach ranging from 40% to 100% and the transabdominal approach between 70% and 100% [20]. Refistulization may occur within the first 3 months after index repair, with the success rates decreasing with subsequent repairs. Cromwell et al. reported success rates of 88.1% after an index repair and 68.9% after a second operation [21]. However, this data was based on conventional approaches to VVF repair. The long-term outcomes of robotics in VVF repairs are still in its infancy; however preliminary studies have demonstrated excellent results, with up to 93.3% success rate after the index repair [22].

Gupta et al. compared robotic approaches to open repairs and have found no differences regarding complications or success rates [23]. However, they commented that robotics probably is the best treatment modality for recurrent fistulas [24, 25].

Patients should be counseled on the risk of refistulization based on their personal attributes using tools such as the Bengtson risk score [21].

Acute urinary retention due to a blockage of the Foley catheter can also occur, and therefore urine output and all tubing need to be carefully monitored postoperatively. Other possible complications can be vaginal bleeding or hematuria coming from the suture lines located in the vagina and bladder, respectively.

Conclusion

While none of the approaches used for VVF repairs have been shown to be superior due to the lack of randomized data and small number of patients, management and surgical approach of VVFs should be tailored to the individual patient, as well as surgeon experience and expertise. While the use of robotic surgery in VVF repairs is still in its infancy, it has consistently demonstrated superiority over open repairs in terms of visibility, dexterity, and precision of dissection. Hence, this approach is especially useful in the setting of complex VVFs.

References

1. Eilber KS, Kavaler E, Rodriguez LV, Rosenblum N, Raz S. Ten-year experience with transvaginal vesicovaginal fistula repair using tissue interposition. J Urol. 2003;169(3):1033–6.
2. Bragayrac LAHD, Sotelo RJ. Urinary fistulas. In: Sotelo RAM, Arriaga J, editors. Complications in robotic urologic surgery. Cham: Springer; 2018. p. 285–97.

3. Moses RA, Ann Gormley E. State of the art for treatment of vesicovaginal fistula. Curr Urol Rep. 2017;18(8):60.
4. Roth R. Vesicovaginal and urethrovaginal fistulas. In: Howard Jones JR, editor. Te-Linde's operative gynecology. Philadelphia: JB Lippincott; 2011. p. 973–93.
5. JM S. On the treatment of vesicovaginal fistula. Am J Med Sci. 1852;23:50.
6. Nezhat CH, Nezhat F, Nezhat C, Rottenberg H. Laparoscopic repair of a vesicovaginal fistula: a case report. Obstet Gynecol. 1994;83(5 Pt 2):899–901.
7. Bragayrac LA, Azhar RA, Fernandez G, Cabrera M, Saenz E, Machuca V, et al. Robotic repair of vesicovaginal fistulae with the transperitoneal-transvaginal approach: a case series. Int Braz J Urol. 2014;40(6):810–5.
8. Medina LG, Hernandez A, Sevilla C, Cacciamani GE, Winter M, Ashrafi A, et al. Robotic uterine-sparing vesicovaginal fistula repair. Int Urogynecol J. 2018;29(12):1845–7.
9. Ramphal SR. Laparoscopic approach to vesicovaginal fistulae. Best Pract Res Clin Obstet Gynaecol. 2018;54:49–60.
10. Nagraj HK, Kishore TA, Nagalaksmi S. Early laparoscopic repair for supratrigonal vesicovaginal fistula. Int Urogynecol J Pelvic Floor Dysfunct. 2007;18(7):759–62.
11. Melamud O, Eichel L, Turbow B, Shanberg A. Laparoscopic vesicovaginal fistula repair with robotic reconstruction. Urology. 2005;65(1):163–6.
12. Sanchez AML, Husain F, Sotelo R. Complications of robotic surgical access. In: Hubert JWP, editor. Robotic urology. 3th ed. Stockholm: Springer; 2018. p. 517–28.
13. Paparel P, Caillot JL, Perrin P, Ruffion A. Surgical principles of omentoplasty in urology. BJU Int. 2007;99(5):1191–6.
14. Sotelo R, Moros V, Clavijo R, Poulakis V. Robotic repair of vesicovaginal fistula (VVF). BJU Int. 2012;109(9):1416–34.
15. Bodner-Adler B, Hanzal E, Pablik E, Koelbl H, Bodner K. Management of vesicovaginal fistulas (VVFs) in women following benign gynaecologic surgery: a systematic review and meta-analysis. PLoS One. 2017;12(2):e0171554.
16. Barski D, Gerullis H, Ecke T, Varga G, Boros M, Pintelon I, et al. Repair of a vesico-vaginal fistula with amniotic membrane – step 1 of the IDEAL recommendations of surgical innovation. Cent European J Urol. 2015;68(4):459–61.
17. Price DT, Price TC. Robotic repair of a vesicovaginal fistula in an irradiated field using a dehydrated amniotic allograft as an interposition patch. J Robot Surg. 2016;10(1):77–80.
18. Daley SMLC, Swanson SK, Novicki DE, Itano NB. Fibrin sealant closure of a persistent vesicovaginal fistula after failed transabdominal closure. J Pelvic Med Surg. 2006;12(4):229–30.
19. Sawant AS, Kasat GV, Kumar V. Cyanoacrylate injection in management of recurrent vesicovaginal fistula: our experience. Indian J Urol. 2016;32(4):323–5.
20. Angioli R, Penalver M, Muzii L, Mendez L, Mirhashemi R, Bellati F, et al. Guidelines of how to manage vesicovaginal fistula. Crit Rev Oncol Hematol. 2003;48(3):295–304.
21. Cromwell D, Hilton P. Retrospective cohort study on patterns of care and outcomes of surgical treatment for lower urinary-genital tract fistula among English National Health Service hospitals between 2000 and 2009. BJU Int. 2013;111(4 Pt B):E257–62.
22. Bora GS, Singh S, Mavuduru RS, Devana SK, Kumar S, Mete UK, et al. Robot-assisted vesicovaginal fistula repair: a safe and feasible technique. Int Urogynecol J. 2017;28(6):957–62.
23. Gupta NP, Mishra S, Hemal AK, Mishra A, Seth A, Dogra PN. Comparative analysis of outcome between open and robotic surgical repair of recurrent supra-trigonal vesico-vaginal fistula. J Endourol. 2010;24(11):1779–82.
24. Medina LG, Cacciamani GE, Hernandez A, Landsberger H, Doumanian L, Ashrafi AN, et al. Robotic management of rectourethral fistulas after focal treatment for prostate cancer. Urology. 2018;118:241.
25. Sotelo R, Medina LG, Husain FZ, Khazaeli M, Nikkhou K, Cacciamani GE, et al. Robotic-assisted laparoscopic repair of rectovesical fistula after Hartmann's reversal procedure. J Robot Surg. 2018;339–43.

Posterior Urethroplasty

Min Suk Jan and Lee C. Zhao

Introduction

The posterior urethra is composed of the bladder neck, prostatic urethra, and the membranous urethra, which is surrounded by the external urinary sphincter. Stenosis of these regions arises from various etiologies, including pelvic fracture urethral injury (PFUI), post-prostatectomy vesicourethral anastomotic stenosis (VUAS), post-transurethral resection of the prostate (TURP), bladder neck contracture (BNC), and radiation-induced stenosis (RIS). Traditional open surgery can be challenging due to difficulty accessing the deep pelvis. Understanding these difficulties and unique challenges posed by each etiology is necessary to recognize how the surgeon can best leverage the advantages of robot assistance. This chapter will outline current techniques to approach each etiology of posterior urethral stenosis.

Pelvic Fracture Urethral Injury

Blunt injury to the pelvis may cause pelvic fracture and destabilization of the pelvic ring, leading to injuries to the urethra ranging from the partial to complete. In complete injuries, the prostate and bladder shear off from the membranous urethra and are displaced superiorly, creating the classically described "pie-in-the-sky" defect on

Supplementary Information The online version of this chapter (https://doi.org/10.1007/978-3-030-50196-9_31) contains supplementary material, which is available to authorized users.

M. S. Jan
Crane Center for Transgender Surgery, Greenbae California, New York, NY, USA

L. C. Zhao (✉)
NYU Langone Health, New York, NY, USA
e-mail: Lee.zhao@nyulangone.org

© Springer Nature Switzerland AG 2022
M. D. Stifelman et al. (eds.), *Techniques of Robotic Urinary Tract Reconstruction*, https://doi.org/10.1007/978-3-030-50196-9_31

cystography. Scar eventually forms between the distracted ends of the urethra, creating a wall of scar that is located directly posterior to the pubic bone. Turner-Warwick and Waterhouse would popularize the transpubic approach to treat this entity in which a wedge of pubic bone is resected to expose the scar and posterior urethra behind it [1, 2]. While exposure was excellent, it came at the cost of complications such as bleeding, pelvic instability, incontinence, and bladder herniation [3, 4]. This approach eventually gave way to the effective and less morbid perineal approach popularized by Webster in the 1980s [5]. An abdominoperineal approach remains a commonly used technique in complex urethral injuries, especially when there is a great deal of superior dislocation of the prostate and bladder [6]. In the current age of robotic assistance, we now have a means to regain the advantages of exposure and access that the abdominal and transpubic approach provided while reducing the morbidity of pubectomy.

We believe downward mobilization is prudent in cases where the primary defect is a complete transection of the posterior urethra with upward displacement of the bladder and prostate. A purely perineal approach requires four lengthening techniques to allow for a tension-free anastomosis. These include urethral dissection (often transecting the bulbar artery), corporal splitting, inferior pubectomy, and supracrural rerouting. These maneuvers amount to creating a defect to make up for the primary defect of upward dislocation. Our philosophy is to strive to returning organs to their pre-PFUI orthotopic location. While perineal dissection may ultimately be necessary, we believe that the upward dislocation of the posterior urethra and bladder should be addressed directly through downward mobilization. If downward mobilization is inadequate to perform a tension free, watertight anastomosis, we perform a perineal dissection after minimizing the distance between the proximal and distal ends of the stenosis. Of note, since the rationale for the robotic transabdominal approach is downward mobilization of the bladder and prostate, the robotic approach is unnecessary if PFUI only involves bulbar urethral injury without any dislocation of the of the bladder or prostate.

Minimizing urethral manipulation may have significant benefits. The first pertains to bulbar urethral necrosis (BUN), a condition described by Kulkarni et al. in which there is complete necrosis of the bulbar artery and obliteration of the lumen. This occurs because urethral mobilization requires transection of the bulbar and perforator arteries, leaving the bulbar urethra reliant on retrograde blood flow from the corpus cavernosa. This puts the anastomotic segment at most risk for necrosis, scarring, and ultimately failure of the repair [7]. A recent multicenter analysis of posterior urethroplasty following PFUI showed that distraction length is significantly associated with urethroplasty failure [8]. Another situation where avoiding urethral dissection is helpful is for postoperative stress urinary incontinence (SUI) requiring an artificial urinary sphincter (AUS), since prior urethroplasty has been shown to be an independent risk factor for AUS cuff erosions [9]. Since a fully mobilized urethra must rely on retrograde blood flow, the constant constriction of the AUS cuff on the corpus spongiosum may, in theory, impair blood flow to the distal end of the anastomotic segment, increasing the risk for BUN or AUS cuff erosion.

Immediate repair is indicated for complicated bladder neck injury and PFUI in female patients. While historic reports of immediate repair is complicated by erectile dysfunction and incontinence [10, 11], the robotic approach may allow for easier immediate repair. When there is bladder neck injury, immediate repair is indicated due to the risk of incontinence. Furthermore, left untreated, life-threatening sepsis can ensue. While PFUI is generally thought of with regard to male patients, urethral injuries occur in female PFUI 5% of the time [12]. There is emerging evidence from multiple institutions that early primary repair with robotic assistance is feasible [13].

Radiation-Induced Urethral Stenosis

Radiation-induced urethral stenosis follows 4% of brachytherapy, 2% of external beam radiotherapy (EBRT), and 11% of combined EBRT and brachytherapy [14]. One institution reported a 32% 2-year stricture risk after high-dose brachytherapy [15]. The underlying defect in radiation-induced strictures is radiation-induced apoptosis, release of inflammatory mediators, endarteritis, and eventual scarring with poor vascularity [16]. Because of the underlying pathophysiology, endoscopic treatment (urethrotomy/dilation) has proven to be a poor strategy, as Brandes reports 80% recurrence after EBRT and 100% recurrence after brachytherapy at a follow-up of 48 months [17]. Alternatively, early open surgical repair with aggressive excision of all scar and primary anastomosis (not unlike the treatment for PFUI) has proven to be more successful with 2-year patency rates of up to 70% [18]. The rate of SUI post-urethroplasty has been reported to be between 26% and 43% [19]. In this case, an AUS can be offered in a staged manner.

Adjunctive surgical maneuvers may be required the longer and more proximal the RIS. The stepwise approach is similar to the approach to PFUI, including corporal splitting, inferior pubectomy, corporal rerouting, and the combined abdomino-perineal approach. In addition, for RIS, there are the additional strategies of buccal mucosa graft urethroplasty, often requiring the support of a well-vascularized bed, such as a gracilis or rectus flap. While patency rates have improved significantly, the failure rate is still 30% with a third of these patients with SUI [18]. Furthermore, urethral mobilization and radiation have both been shown to increase rates of AUS cuff erosion [9]. Much progress has been made, but there remains room for improvement.

Vesicourethral Anastomotic Stenosis

Most retrospective studies report a 5–10% incidence of vesicourethral anastomotic stenosis after radical prostatectomy [20]. Robotically assisted radical prostatectomy has improved upon this rate, with one study reporting a 1.4% VUAS rate [21]. While this rate seems low, a 2012 study estimates that 90,000 radical prostatectomies are performed in the US annually [22]. Clearly the statistics show that VUAS will be an ongoing problem for many patients and reconstructive urologists. Endoscopic management has been shown to be successful 58% of the time after a single treatment, but 27% are refractory to 3 or more interventions [23]. Some have turned to combining endoscopic treatment with mitomycin C injection into the scar, but a recent analysis shows limited benefit with a 7% serious adverse event rate [24].

For the endoscopic treatment refractory VUAS, definitive open reconstruction is the standard of care. The approach is similar to that outlined in the previous section. Because the prostate has been removed, one must take great care during this dissection as important structures, such as the rectum and ureters, will be in close proximity and at higher risk of injury. Furthermore, repair is likely to worsen or cause de novo SUI. A recent analysis of open reconstruction (abdominal, perineal, and combined approach) of VUAS showed a patency rate of 92% but at the cost of 75% incontinence. As AUS is likely to be needed, a urethral dissection-sparing approach should be preferred. Partial pubectomy was required in 75% of patients to improve visualization [25].

Bladder Neck Contracture

Post-TURP bladder neck contracture has a reported incidence of up to 12% [26]. Endoscopic treatment may be successful with durable patency rate of 58% after a single treatment [24]. As with VUAS, a BNC refractory to endoscopic treatment can be considered for open repair as outlined previously. We will consider plastic procedures for BNC (and some VUAS). Young first described a Y-V plasty in 1953 in which a longitudinal incision is made across the stricture and a V-shaped flap is advanced into the incision to create a patent lumen [27]. Patency rates have ranged from 75% to 100% in three studies investigating robot-assisted Y-V plasty. Importantly, incontinence rates were much improved over the open approach to VUAS, with 0–29% experiencing de novo SUI [28–30] versus 73% via open approach [25]. T plasty is an attractive alternative to Y-V plasty in which two bladder flaps versus one are advanced into the stenosis. Patency was 100% with at 45-month follow-up [31].

Preoperative Preparation

Preoperative urine culture is mandatory to guide antibiotic therapy. Mechanical bowel preparation is not required. A type and screen is sufficient as there is low risk for major bleeding.

Operative Equipment

In the past, we preferred the da Vinci robotic system (Intuitive Surgical, Sunnyvale, CA) Xi since it can more easily be side docked to better facilitate perineal access. More recently, we have shifted to the SP (single port) system as its narrow profile better facilitates access deep into the pelvis with less damage to the pelvic wall from instrument movement (Fig. 31.1). Furthermore, the articulating camera allows one

Fig. 31.1 This schematic highlights the narrow profile of the SP robot, facilitating deeper access with better dexterity. This also protects the pelvic side wall from instrument clashing and damage

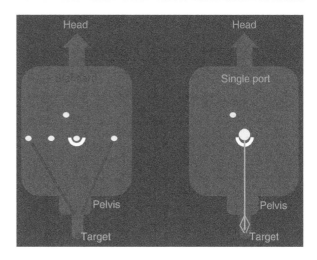

to see around corners, which is more helpful the deeper one travels into the pelvis. AirSeal (ConMed, Utica, NY) is a key component to combined abdominoperineal cases as it allows for the maintenance of pneumoperitoneum even with a large air leak. Because the open perineum is the site of escaping pressurized air, the perineal surgeon is subject to aerosolized blood. We have found an orthopedic surgical hood useful for personal protection against blood-borne pathogens, while allowing for continued visualization. A flexible cystoscope can be used to localize the distal border of the stenosis and the EUS with the aid of a near-infrared camera.

General Surgical Technique

Sequential compression devices are placed, and 5000 units of subcutaneous heparin is administered in patients with moderate to high risk for venous thromboembolism. Cephalosporin is administered 1 hour preoperatively unless preoperative urine culture dictates otherwise. Patients are placed in dorsal lithotomy with arms tucked to the sides. All pressure points are well padded, and the patient is secured to the table for safe steep Trendelenburg position.

If using the Xi system, pneumoperitoneum is established using a Veress needle or Hasson technique. Additional 8 mm robotic trocars are placed in the same configuration as a robotic prostatectomy. Instruments may be chosen at the discretion of the surgeon – our preference is monopolar scissors, bipolar Maryland forceps, and ProGrasp forceps. A 5 mm AirSeal port is used for assistance. Alternatively, a 2.7 cm vertical supraumbilical Hasson access technique is required when using the SP system. The robot is docked from the side regardless of robotic system used to allow for perineal access.

If the stenosis is 5 Fr or smaller, we prefer to approach the stenosis posteriorly to reduce the risk of rectal injury. The vas deferens are identified and used to guide dissection to the prostate where Denonvilliers' fascia is encountered. This is separated and opened using sharp dissection and judicious bipolar electrocautery. An EEA sizer may help in avoiding the rectum during this dissection. The distal limit of this dissection is the urogenital diaphragm. If the stenosis is greater than 5 Fr, we will approach anteriorly where a variety of techniques can be applied depending on the nature of the stenosis. Each technique will be discussed in the following sections. A JP drain is placed at the end of the case and the incisions closed in standard fashion.

Primary Anastomosis

Primary anastomosis is indicated in PFUI and all other obliterative or high-grade posterior urethral stenosis. As such, a circumferential dissection is required. As previously stated, the stenosis is approached posteriorly as cutting posteriorly from an anterior approach may lead to a rectal injury. Furthermore, Retzius-sparing urethroplasty may have a positive impact on continence [32].

Once the posterior urethra is exposed, cystoscopy may be performed up to the level of the stricture. The Firefly™ camera detects the near-infrared spectrum, which is coincidentally emitted from the light source for a cystoscope. This band of electromagnetic radiation penetrates through tissue more easily than the visible spectrum and essentially gives "X-ray vision" to the surgeon (Fig. 31.2). With this visual assistance, the exact location of the rhabdosphincter and the distal extent of the stricture are identified, and a urethrotomy is made. The scar tissue is then excised completely. If this cannot be fully accomplished with a posterior approach, then the bladder will be "dropped," and the space of Retzius will be developed. Another reason one might take down the bladder anteriorly is to facilitate downward mobilization to create a tension-free anastomosis. The cystoscope and Firefly will again be used to identify where the anterior urethrotomy must be made and the posterior and anterior urethrotomies will be joined. Perineal dissection is performed

Fig. 31.2 Near-infrared light emitted from the cystoscope penetrates tissue, allowing for "X-ray" vision with the Firefly camera of the Xi system

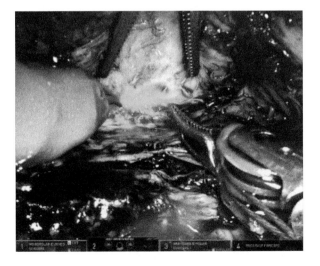

should more length be needed to create a tension-free anastomosis. The urethra will be calibrated to at least 22 French with a catheter, and the circumferential anastomosis is completed with a double-armed running 3-0 barbed suture. Upon completion, the final catheter is placed and the bladder filled to ensure a watertight anastomosis. If an anterior approach was taken, the peritoneum is closed to recreate the space of Retzius for later accommodation of an AUS pressure-regulating balloon.

If a tension-free anastomosis cannot be performed robotically, a combined perineal approach must be performed, using ancillary maneuvers previously described to reduce anastomosis tension. One can then perform a "pull-through" maneuver as first described in 1950 by Badenoch [33]. A suture is placed on the urethral stump and then passed through the perineum to the awaiting robot. The urethra is then pulled into the bladder neck where a circumferential anastomosis is performed. This approach performed in an open manner was successful in maintaining patency in 10 of 11 patients by Simonato et al.; however, one must note that all of these patients would later require AUS placement [34].

Bladder Flap Technique

When diseased segment bladder neck is short and the stenosis low grade, then the bladder neck contracture following a transurethral procedure or in some cases of vesicourethral anastomotic stenosis can be addressed with a bladder flap technique. Importantly, neither surgical fields have been subject to radiation in these cases, and the surrounding tissue is relatively supple and well vascularized. Upon identifying the stenosis with cystoscopy and Firefly, the offending segment is approached anteriorly and opened longitudinally. In the case of Y-V plasty, a V-shaped wedge of the bladder is advanced into this longitudinal incision, widening the lumen. A T plasty may be required when more scar tissue has been resected, leaving a larger defect. A longitudinal incision is extended along the anterior bladder midline, creating two bladder flaps. These are advanced into the defect and a watertight closure is made (Fig. 31.3a, b).

Buccal Mucosal Graft

If an anterior urethrotomy is made and the posterior urethral plate is noted to be adequate, we may opt for a dorsal onlay buccal mucosa graft substitution urethroplasty. Alternatively, one may take a transvesical approach and perform an anterior inlay posterior urethroplasty (Fig. 31.4). If the prostate is in situ, as is the case with RIS and BNC, we will perform a robotic retropubic or suprapubic simple prostatectomy concurrently when indicated and apply buccal mucosa over the defect. If the stenosis spans both sides of the rhabdosphincter, one should additionally approach the stenosis perineally. A continuous dorsal urethrotomy can be made spanning the membranous urethra, and the distal portion of the graft is delivered transurethrally for the perineal surgeon to complete the dorsal onlay urethroplasty.

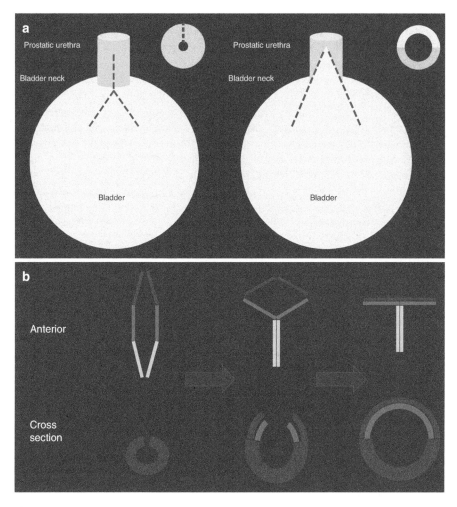

Fig. 31.3 a. Schematic of Y-V plasty of the bladder neck. **b**. Schematic of T plasty of the bladder neck

If a posterior approach is taken and the urethra is wider caliber than expected, a posterior buccal onlay urethroplasty may be performed. Irrespective of approach, due to impaired vascular supply in patients with RIS, we support buccal mucosa graft with a gracilis or rectus flap.

Postoperative Care

Patients are admitted to 23-hour observation and are usually discharged on post-operative day 1. Urethral and suprapubic (if present) catheters are kept to gravity drainage. The urethral Foley is plugged prior to discharge if a suprapubic tube is

Fig. 31.4 Anterior buccal mucosal graft transvesical inlay in a 70-year-old male with vesicourethral anastomotic stenosis after radical prostatectomy

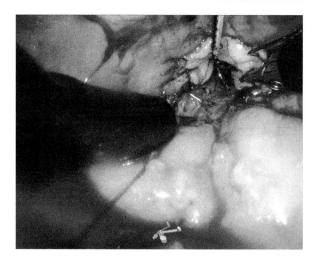

present. A JP fluid creatinine is checked prior to removal if output is high. Voiding cystourethrogram is performed in 2 weeks to ensure no leak. In cases where a suprapubic tube is present, it will be capped. The patient will record post-void residuals to ensure adequate bladder emptying prior to removal.

Conclusion

Posterior urethroplasty remains a challenging endeavor for even the most seasoned reconstructive urologists. The emergence of robotic-assisted laparoscopy has allowed for improved visualization and unprecedented exposure without the morbidity associated with open techniques such the transpubic approach with total pubectomy. Moreover, there is emerging evidence that robotic approaches can improve continence outcomes.

References

1. Turner-Warwick RT. A technique for posterior urethroplasty. J Urol. 1960;83(4):416–9.
2. Waterhouse K, Abrahams JI, Gruber H, Hackett RE, Patil UB, Peng BK. The transpubic approach to the lower urinary tract. J Urol. 1973;109(3):486–90.
3. Golimbu M, Al-Askari S, Morales P. Transpubic approach for lower urinary tract surgery: a 15-year experience. J Urol. 1990;143(1):72–6.
4. Lenzi R, Selli C, Stomaci N, Barbagli G. Bladder herniation after transpubic urethroplasty. J Urol. 1983;130(4):778–80.
5. Webster GD, Mathes GL, Selli C. Prostatomembranous urethral injuries: a review of the literature and a rational approach to their management. J Urol. 1983;130(5):898–902.
6. Seitzman DM. Repair of the severed membranous urethra by the combined approach. J Urol. 1963;89(3):433–8.
7. Kulkarni SB, Joshi PM, Hunter C, Surana S, Shahrour W, Alhajeri F. Complex posterior urethral injury. Arab J Urol. 2015;13(1):43–52.

8. Johnsen NV, Moses RA, Elliott SP, Vanni AJ, Baradaran N, Greear G, et al. Multicenter analysis of posterior urethroplasty complexity and outcomes following pelvic fracture urethral injury. World J Urol [Internet]. 2019. [cited 2019 Sep 8]; Available from: https://doi.org/10.1007/s00345-019-02824-5.
9. McKibben MJ, Shakir N, Fuchs JS, Scott JM, Morey AF. Erosion rates of 3.5-cm artificial urinary sphincter cuffs are similar to larger cuffs. BJU Int. 2019;123(2):335–41.
10. Blaschko SD, Sanford MT, Schlomer BJ, Alwaal A, Yang G, Villalta JD, et al. The incidence of erectile dysfunction after pelvic fracture urethral injury: a systematic review and meta-analysis. Arab J Urol. 2015;13(1):68–74.
11. Koraitim MM. Pelvic fracture urethral injuries: evaluation of various methods of management. J Urol. 1996;156(4):1288–91.
12. Perry MO, Husmann DA. Urethral injuries in female subjects following pelvic fractures. J Urol. 1992;147(1):139–43.
13. Vineet A, Levey HR, Robert D, Jean J. V12-08 extraperitoneal robot-assisted repair of a pelvic fracture associated urethral injury. J Urol. 2015;193(4S):e979.
14. Mohammed N, Kestin L, Ghilezan M, Krauss D, Vicini F, Brabbins D, et al. Comparison of acute and late toxicities for three modern high-dose radiation treatment techniques for localized prostate cancer. Int J Radiat Oncol. 2012;82(1):204–12.
15. Hindson BR, Millar JL, Matheson B. Urethral strictures following high-dose-rate brachytherapy for prostate cancer: analysis of risk factors. Brachytherapy. 2013;12(1):50–5.
16. Moltzahn F, Dal Pra A, Furrer M, Thalmann G, Spahn M. Urethral strictures after radiation therapy for prostate cancer. Investig Clin Urol. 2016;57(5):309–15.
17. Brandes SB, Morey AF, editors. Advanced male urethral and genital reconstructive surgery [Internet]. 2nd ed: Humana Press; 2014. [cited 2019 Sep 10]. (Current Clinical Urology). Available from: https://www.springer.com/gp/book/9781461477075
18. Hofer MD, Zhao LC, Morey AF, Scott JF, Chang AJ, Brandes SB, et al. Outcomes after urethroplasty for radiotherapy induced bulbomembranous urethral stricture disease. J Urol. 2014;191(5):1307–12.
19. Fuchs JS, Hofer MD, Sheth KR, Cordon BH, Scott JM, Morey AF. Improving outcomes of bulbomembranous urethroplasty for radiation-induced urethral strictures in post-urolume era. Urology. 2017;99:240–5.
20. Mundy AR, Andrich DE. Posterior urethral complications of the treatment of prostate cancer. BJU Int. 2012;110(3):304–25.
21. Breyer BN, Davis CB, Cowan JE, Kane CJ, Carroll PR. Incidence of bladder neck contracture after robot-assisted laparoscopic and open radical prostatectomy. BJU Int. 2010;106(11):1734–8.
22. Lowrance WT, Eastham JA, Savage C, Maschino AC, Laudone VP, Dechet CB, et al. Contemporary open and robotic radical prostatectomy practice patterns among urologists in the United States. J Urol. 2012;187(6):2087–92.
23. Borboroglu PG, Sands JP, Roberts JL, Amling CL. Risk factors for vesicourethral anastomotic stricture after radical prostatectomy11The Chief, Bureau of Medicine and Surgery, Navy Department, Washington, D.C., Clinical Investigation Program, sponsored this report S99-070 as required by NSHSBETHINST 6000.41A. The views expressed in this article are those of the authors and do not reflect the official policy or position of the Department of the Navy, Department of Defense, or the United States Government. Urology. 2000;56(1):96–100.
24. Redshaw JD, Broghammer JA, Smith TG, Voelzke BB, Erickson BA, McClung CD, et al. Intralesional injection of mitomycin C at transurethral incision of bladder neck contracture may offer limited benefit: TURNS study group. J Urol. 2015;193(2):587–92.
25. Nikolavsky D, Blakely SA, Hadley DA, Knoll P, Windsperger AP, Terlecki RP, et al. Open reconstruction of recurrent vesicourethral anastomotic stricture after radical prostatectomy. Int Urol Nephrol. 2014;46(11):2147–52.
26. Lee Y-H, Chiu AW, Huang J-K. Comprehensive study of bladder neck contracture after transurethral resection of prostate. Urology. 2005;65(3):498–503.

27. Young BW. The retropubic approach to vesical neck obstruction in children. Surg Gynecol Obstet. 1953;96(2):150–4.
28. Kirshenbaum EJ, Zhao LC, Myers JB, Elliott SP, Vanni AJ, Baradaran N, et al. Patency and incontinence rates after robotic bladder neck reconstruction for vesicourethral anastomotic stenosis and recalcitrant bladder neck contractures: the trauma and urologic reconstructive network of surgeons experience. Urology. 2018;118:227–33.
29. Musch M, Hohenhorst JL, Vogel A, Loewen H, Krege S, Kroepfl D. Robot-assisted laparoscopic Y-V plasty in 12 patients with refractory bladder neck contracture. J Robot Surg. 2018;12(1):139–45.
30. Granieri MA, Weinberg AC, Sun JY, Stifelman MD, Zhao LC. Robotic Y-V plasty for recalcitrant bladder neck contracture. Urology. 2018;117:163–5.
31. Rosenbaum CM, Dahlem R, Maurer V, Kluth LA, Vetterlein MW, Fisch M, et al. The T-plasty as therapy for recurrent bladder neck stenosis: success rate, functional outcome, and patient satisfaction. World J Urol. 2017;35(12):1907–11.
32. Sayyid RK, Simpson WG, Lu C, Terris MK, Klaassen Z, Madi R. Retzius-sparing robotic-assisted laparoscopic radical prostatectomy: a safe surgical technique with superior continence outcomes. J Endourol. 2017;31(12):1244–50.
33. Badenoch AW. A pull-through operation for impassable traumatic stricture of the urethra. Br J Urol. 1950;22(4):404–9.
34. Simonato A, Gregori A, Lissiani A, Varca V, Carmignani G. Use of Solovov–Badenoch principle in treating severe and recurrent vesico-urethral anastomosis stricture after radical retropubic prostatectomy: technique and long-term results. BJU Int. 2012;110(11b):E456–60.

Index

© Springer Nature Switzerland AG 2022

M. D. Stifelman et al. (eds.), *Techniques of Robotic Urinary Tract Reconstruction*, https://doi.org/10.1007/978-3-030-50196-9